Hospital Unit Secretary

MARGARET A. GALLOWAY, R.N.
Clinical Instructor, Health Unit Clerk Program
Albuquerque Technical-Vocational Institute
Albuquerque, New Mexico

An addition to allied health training materials published by:

Robert J. Brady Co., Bowie, MD 20715
A Prentice-Hall Publishing & Communications Company

and

The Hospital Research and Educational Trust, Chicago, IL 60611

Editor-in-Chief: David Culverwell
Acquisitions Editor: Richard A. Weimer
Production Editor: Janis K. Oppelt
Art Director: Don Sellers, AMI
Assistant Art Director: Bernard Vervin
Cover Design & Chapter Opening Art: Randy Galloway

Typesetter: Automated Graphic Systems, White Plains, Maryland
Printer: R. R. Donnelley & Sons Co., Harrisonburg, Virginia
Typefaces: Trump for display; optima for text

Hospital Unit Secretary

Library of Congress Cataloging in Publication Data

Galloway, Margaret A., date
  Hospital unit secretary.

  Includes index.
  1. Hospital ward clerks. I. Title. [DNLM: 1. Medical
secretaries. 2. Hospital units—Manpower. W 80 G174h]
RA972.55.G35   1984   651.3'74   83-21347
ISBN 0-89303-268-9

Prentice-Hall International, Inc., London
Prentice-Hall Canada, Inc., Scarborough, Ontario
Prentice-Hall of Australia, Pty., Ltd., Sydney
Prentice-Hall of India Private Limited, New Delhi
Prentice-Hall of Japan, Inc., Tokyo
Prentice-Hall of Southeast Asia Pte. Ltd., Singapore
Whitehall Books, Limited, Petone, New Zealand
Editora Prentice-Hall Do Brasil LTDA., Rio de Janeiro

Printed in the United States of America

84 85 86 87 88 89 90 91 92 93 94   10 9 8 7 6 5 4 3 2 1

Contents

Preface

The role of the unit secretary in hospitals and other health care institutions is expanding. As the role expands, so does the need for more information concerning the position of unit secretary. Information needed to perform secretarial or clerical duties on a nursing unit is presented in a correlated fashion. This is intended to promote more interest while learning and to provide a greater understanding of the various functions involved in those duties.

Routine procedures are discussed in the first section of the book with explanations that may easily be adapted to any hospital or health care institution. Pharmacology is explained so that orders written by doctors may be understood.

The second section of the book explains each body system so that structural terms used in Physician's Orders and other hospital forms become meaningful. The more common diseases, disorders, surgeries and procedures, laboratory tests, special tests, radiology and nuclear medicine examinations, and medications are correlated with each system for increased learning memory by association. Samples of Physician's Orders are included for each system.

The textbook answers students' questions regarding diseases and surgeries so that the instructor may utilize the classroom time to discuss specific procedures, to practice the use of forms, and to give individual attention to each student. The additional practice time promotes better performance during practicum or clinical experience in the hospitals.

Students need not carry other textbooks home with them for study. All necessary information is presented. The PDR, Physician's Desk Reference, will need to be used in practicum and during transcription practice in the classroom.

Hospital Unit Secretary can also be useful as a resource for hospital procedures and the functions of a unit secretary. A greater understanding of the complexity of patient care promotes improved public relations between health care providers and health care consumers.

Acknowledgments

Many people assisted in the development of this book and my sincere thanks is extended to all of them. Special thanks to:

My family for their support and encouragement

My son, Randy, for designing the cover and drawing the illustrations for the chapter headings

University of New Mexico Hospital/Bernalillo County Medical Center (UNMH/BCMC) for full cooperation in development of this book, for permission to photograph a patient room, a nursing station and hospital equipment, and for permission to use hospital forms

Cynthia Behrendt, Unit Management, UNMH/BCMC

Janet O'Grady and Robert Hlady, Public Relations, UNMH/BCMC

St. Joseph Hospital for full cooperation in development of this book, permission to photograph equipment and permission to use medication cards and hospital forms

All the unit secretaries and the entire nursing staff of St. Joseph Hospital for their courtesy and help

Robert D. Fenton, Director of Public Relations, St. Joseph Hospital

Carolyn Hinken, colleague, for her encouragement and counsel

Mary Helen Esquibel, friend and neighbor, without whose help I could never have completed this project.

Dedication

To the memory of my mother, Nina Frances Copeland, who taught me at an early age that learning can be a lifetime pleasure.

SECTION I

In Section I, you will be introduced to the duties of the unit secretary and to the environment in which you will work. The material presented includes:

- The hospital organization
- How to complete forms for each department
- A discussion on the importance of communication
- An explanation of the mechanical devices you will use
- The forms used in patients' charts
- Drug information
- Steps necessary for transcribing Physician's Orders
- An explanation of routine hospital procedures.

Appendix III is a list of commonly used abbreviations in a hospital setting. These abbreviations are used throughout the text. You should begin studying these immediately and use Appendix III when encountering them in the text. The more important abbreviations are emphasized in the chapters where appropriate.

The book is designed to be used in the classroom and to be used with forms from the actual work situation. Your instructor will provide the forms from the hospitals in your area. A procedure will first be explained in the text. You will then practice that procedure in the classroom and on your own time. In order to feel more comfortable when you go into the clinical area, you need to practice, practice, practice so you will be efficient and confident. Explanation of procedures is a combination of the hospital procedures used in several hospitals. The names of patients, nurses and doctors are purely fictional and in no way refer to any person.

Reference books you will use most frequently are:

- Physician's Desk Reference (PDR)
- Medical dictionary
- Merck Manual
- Procedure manuals from hospitals in your area.

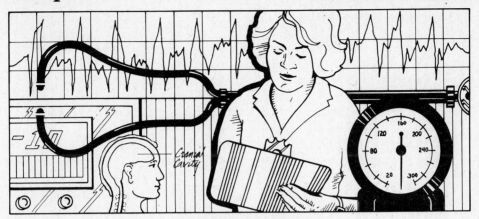

OBJECTIVES

Study of this chapter will enable you to:

1. Discuss the general responsibility of a unit secretary.
2. List the specific duties of a unit secretary.
3. List the job qualifications for a unit secretary.
4. List characteristics that help obtain and keep a job as a unit secretary.

Ward secretary, ward clerk, unit secretary, health unit clerk are all titles for the same job. Each hospital utilizes a job description that suits the philosophy and needs of that particular hospital. Although job descriptions may vary as do the titles, the basic functions are the same. The professional association for this occupation, the National Association of Health Unit Clerk/Coordinator, hopes to see the title health unit clerk/coordinator adopted by all health care institutions.

Hospital secretaries on a nursing unit work in an area of intense, varied activity which can create a high level of stress. Unit secretaries must be able to keep calm and maintain a level of efficiency regardless of surrounding distractions. The duties cover a wide range. Typing skills are needed to work in some areas such as the Emergency Room (ER) and the scheduling desk in the Operating Room (OR). Basic typing may be needed to use some computers. How computers are used in your area will be explained by your instructor.

SAMPLE JOB DESCRIPTION

General Duties

The unit secretary is responsible for all clerical duties of the unit and communications to and from the unit. The head nurse is responsible for supervising the secretary. The unit secretary supervises only the students assigned to work with her.

Specific Duties:

1. **Acts as receptionist for the unit.** Greets new admissions with friendly professionalism. Greets and directs visitors. Dispenses correct information to the patients and their families. Directs personnel from other departments.

2. **Answers the telephone.** This duty takes up a great deal of time. Many different people will be calling for and giving information (e.g., families and friends of the patients, other departments within the hospital, and doctors giving instructions).

3. **Initiates telephone calls from the unit.** The secretary places the majority of calls necessary for the functioning of the unit. These include calls to doctors' offices, pages for doctors in the hospital, calls to other departments for test results, appointments, and equipment, calls to the nursing administration office, and other calls as needed.

4. **Acts as communication liaison.** Uses the intercommunication system to answer patient's calls and relays requests to proper personnel. Relays messages from one unit member to another to save time for those involved in direct patient care. Relays information to the doctors. Records messages from other departments and from outside the hospital and relays to proper person.

5. **Transcribes Physician's Orders.** Each time a doctor writes an order on a patient's chart, the secretary has to take some action. This may mean completing a departmental requisition, filling out a medication card, or making a telephone call. Whatever the action, the secretary **must be accurate** so the patient will receive the care needed. Transcription also includes transferring the doctor's order to a patient care card which is usually called a kardex.

6. **Assists physicians by locating charts and obtaining examination equipment.** Charts are located and handed to each doctor as he/she arrives on the unit. Equipment that is commonly requested by a doctor includes a **sphygmomanometer** (blood pressure cuff) to measure blood pressure, a **stethoscope** to listen to sounds from within the body, an **otoscope** for examining the ears, an **ophthalmoscope** for examination of the interior of the eye, and a flashlight to test the reaction of the eyes to light. (See Figure 1-1.)

7. **Completes clerical duties for admissions, discharges, transfers, deaths, and passes.** There are routine functions for each of the above. Omission of any function may cause a delay in the care of the patient or inconvenience for the family or the hospital staff.

8. **Keeps accurate census records.** Each nursing unit records admissions, discharges, transfers, and deaths on a **census sheet.** The totals on the census sheet must correspond with the actual number of patients on the unit at the end of each eight hour shift.

9. **Charts vital signs on the graphic sheet.** Patient's temperature, pulse, respiration, and blood pressure are taken at routine times as well as times specified by the doctor. The secretary transfers these from a unit list to individual graphic sheets on patients' charts.

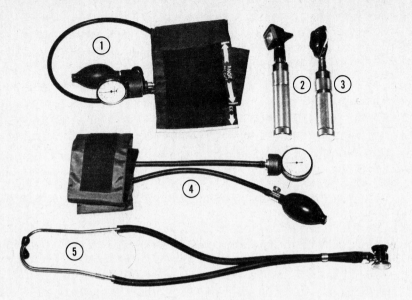

1. Adult blood pressure cuff
2. Otoscope
3. Ophthalmoscope
4. Pediatric blood pressure cuff
5. Stethoscope

Figure 1-1. Equipment a doctor may request for examinations.

10. **Files forms in individual charts.** Results from tests and examinations may be sent to the unit. The secretary then places them in the patient chart in the correct section and in correct sequence.

11. **Checks patient charts for proper identification and forms.** Every sheet in a chart must be addressographed (imprinted with the identification card). Each patient is given a medical record number, a hospital number, or both. A birth date is also an identifying number. The secretary checks all charts each morning and adds Physician's Order sheets, Progress Notes, and other forms as needed. Charts are also checked to make sure all orders have been transcribed.

12. **Maintains a current dietary list.** Each time a patient's diet is changed, the secretary enters that information on a **dietary sheet.** This sheet goes to the dietary department before each meal. If changes occur after the sheet leaves the unit, a call is made to dietary and the secretary there records the change. A list is kept of the patients having tests that require delayed meals or no meals. When the test is completed, dietary is notified so the meal may be delivered.

13. **Orders secretarial supplies at designated times.** Each unit has a budget that requires strict adherence. The secretary is responsible for proper use of supplies with as little waste as possible. Order only what is needed until the next ordering date.

14. **Transports specimens to the laboratory.** The nurse or doctor collects specimens of blood, urine, tissue, etc. from the patient in order to

perform different kinds of tests. Secretaries complete patient identification labels for the specimen containers when the requisition for the test is completed. When you transport specimens, be sure the container is labeled correctly, that the specimen is taken to the correct lab, and that someone in the lab is informed of the specimen.

15. **Transports patients.** Many hospitals teach the secretaries body mechanics so they may assist in the transport of patients when necessary. Other hospitals' philosophy dictates that the secretary should be at the desk.

16. **Runs errands as designated.** Nursing personnel may need blood from the blood bank and cannot leave the patient, so the secretary is sent for the blood. An item may be needed from the pharmacy immediately or part of a patient chart may need to be photocopied which necessitates the secretary leaving the unit.

17. **Helps maintain safety rules.** The secretary is always on the alert for dangerous situations. Spilled material is cleaned up quickly to prevent accidents. Policies for emergency situations such as fire, electrical failures, and disaster drills are reviewed periodically so that performance is organized if an emergency arises.

18. **Assists in locating lost and found items.** The items found in a patient's room after discharge are kept for a certain period of time by housekeeping or whichever department the hospital designates. Patients usually call the unit to inquire about missing items. The secretary will direct them to the proper department. If an item is lost while the patient is still in the hospital, the secretary notifies security and completes the proper forms.

19. **Maintains unit equipment.** The engineering department is notified of faulty equipment. The secretary is responsible for keeping the equipment in the nursing station in functioning order. The nurses will notify the secretary of faulty equipment in patients' rooms.

20. **Assists in completing forms for nursing administration.** The supervisors who work out of the nursing office need to know about the condition of the patients on each unit. The secretary may either write a list of patients with their diagnosis or this information may be in the form of a computerized list. The admissions, discharges, and transfers are kept up to date. The nurses enter comments regarding the condition of the patient.

21. **Completes other tasks as requested by the head nurse.** It is impossible to list every task a secretary may be called upon to perform. Many unexpected happenings occur and each person on the unit is expected to work at whatever task the head nurse assigns them in accordance with each person's job responsibilities.

You can see by the job description that the unit secretary is the hub of the unit activity. Although there is a certain amount of time spent at the desk, there is also activity on the unit as well as travel to other departments.

JOB QUALIFICATIONS:

1. Must have a high school diploma or a general education diploma (GED) in most states
2. Writing must be legible
3. Spelling skills must be average or above
4. Must have good communication skills
5. An anatomy or biology course in high school is beneficial
6. Must be able to concentrate in a noisy setting
7. Must be able to function under stressful conditions
8. Must be able to move about quickly and efficiently
9. Must be adaptable so changes in routine may be made easily
10. Must present a neat, clean appearance
11. Must be dependable; previous work records must show good attendance
12. Must have a genuine liking for people and be able to relate well with various personalities.

Helpful Characteristics:

There are several traits that are helpful in obtaining a job as a unit secretary and in achieving good job evaluations.

1. Pleasant personality. A quick smile and cheerful manner make the work easier for everyone.
2. Ability to be tactful.
3. Willingness to learn. Careful attention to instructions and asking questions when necessary show interest.
4. Willingness to help others.
5. Ability to accept constructive criticism. It is often necessary to be shown how to do something in a particular fashion to promote efficiency. It is always necessary that mistakes be corrected.
6. Ability to establish priorities. When work accumulates, it is necessary to decide what to do first and proceed in an orderly fashion.
7. Personal cleanliness. The appearance of one's hair, teeth, fingernails, and dress are important. The majority of hospitals have a dress code that limits jewelry and certain types of footwear. Uniforms are sometimes furnished. Strong perfumes should not be used as they are offensive to many people.

Working as a unit secretary can be rewarding. There are a variety of ingredients to maintain your interest:

- It is stimulating to work with so many different professions.
- Much of the knowledge learned is useful in everyday living.
- Many are inspired to further their education in the health field.
- Advancement to other jobs in the hospital is possible.
- Some hospitals have different grades of unit secretaries; advancement is dependent on performance and knowledge of procedures.

REVIEW QUESTIONS

1. The general duties of a unit secretary include _____
   _____
   _____

2. The specific duty that requires the most time and communication with all different departments is _____

3. List some of the ways in which you will be using the telephone.
   _____
   _____
   _____

4. Explain how you might assist a doctor who has just arrived on the unit.
   _____

5. Explain what transcription of Physician's Orders includes.
   _____
   _____

6. Census records include _____, _____
   , _____, _____.

7. List 3 duties relating directly to patient's charts.
   _____, _____
   _____, _____.

8. What specific duty would you not perform daily? _____
   _____.

9. List the specific duties that would require that you leave the unit. ____
   _____

10. List 7 qualifications for a job as a unit secretary.
    _____   _____
    _____   _____
    _____   _____
    _____

11. List 5 characteristics that would help in obtaining a job as a unit secretary.
    _____   _____
    _____   _____
    _____

Situational Application

Apply the knowledge you have gained from this chapter to the following situations. Circle the letter in front of the correct action.

12. A volunteer brings a new patient to your desk and gives you the admitting papers. You would:
    a. Take the papers and go on with your work
    b. Ignore the patient and talk only with the volunteer
    c. Greet the new patient and ask the volunteer to escort the patient to the assigned room.

13. A new admission arrives just as the lunch trays arrive. Physician's Orders accompany the patient and read "regular diet." You:
    a. Send a family member to the snack bar for food for the patient
    b. Call dietary and order a lunch tray for the patient
    c. Tell the patient it is too late to obtain lunch.

14. Two months in a row the supplies have run out a few days before the reorder date. This necessitates a special requisition and involves more work for you and for the purchasing department. You would:
    a. Borrow from another floor
    b. Continue making a special requisition to obtain supplies
    c. Ask permission from the head nurse to increase the order quantity for each order date.

15. It has been a very tiring day. You get into your car to go home and remember that you forgot to enter the last admission on the Census Report. You would:
    a. Return to the unit and correct the omission
    b. Go on home, call the unit and ask the secretary to correct the omission
    c. Assume that the mistake will be found and corrected when the 24 hour total is determined.

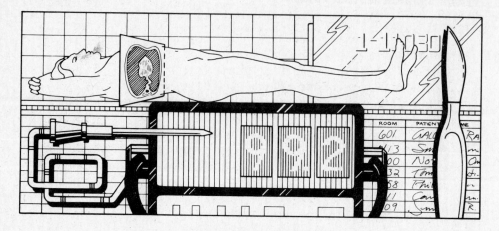

OBJECTIVES

When you complete study of this chapter, you will be able to:

1. Explain the responsibilities of the Board of Trustees.
2. Explain the responsibility of the Administrator.
3. Explain the duties of the Assistant Administrators.
4. Explain the duties of a Department Director.
5. Understand the role each department plays in the care of patients.
6. List the chain of command under which Unit Secretaries work.
7. Understand completion of departmental requisitions.

A hospital is one type of health care institution. The majority of hospitals provide care for people of all ages with a variety of health problems. Other hospitals provide care for special age groups or special diseases. This book deals with the general hospital providing care for all ages and all diseases except mental illnesses.

A hospital's primary function is to provide care for the health problems of the patient. Other functions are:

- Education of the hospital employees
- Education of the public to promote individual and community health
- Participation in community health services
- Research to promote better quality care.

The structural organization of responsibility depends on whether the hospital is privately owned or tax-supported and whether it is teaching or non-teaching. The explanation of organization may differ slightly from the plan shown since the plan shown in this chapter is from a teaching institution.

ADMINISTRATION

Board of Trustees or Governing Board

The Board is composed of interested community members who donate their time. The Board is responsible for the philosophy of the hospital, the personnel policies, and the standard of care.

Administrator

The Administrator is appointed by the Board. He/she is responsible for the overall operation of the hospital to see that the policies and standards set forth by the Board are maintained.

Assistant Administrator

The size of the hospital determines how many assistants are needed. Each is responsible for the operation of designated areas and reports to the Administrator.

Medical Director

The medical staff is approved by the Board after careful consideration of each application. The Medical Director supervises all the staff members who are responsible for student doctors and residents. Residents have completed their schooling and are working in a special area under the supervision of the doctors in that area.

Department Directors

Each department director is responsible for the particular function of that department. Duties of the Department Director include hiring and firing personnel, supervising department personnel, and maintaining policies and standards. This individual reports to the Assistant Administrator.

Public Information Officer (PI) or Public Relations Officer (PR)

As liaison officer between the hospital and the public, the P.I. Officer is responsible for news releases to the media for advances in patient care, new technological tools the hospital acquires, and statements concerning patients who are in the public eye.

Director of Volunteer Services

Training and supervising the people who donate services to the hospital is the responsibility of the volunteer director. Volunteers usually manage a gift shop within the hospital; provide a coffee cart for patients and visitors; provide

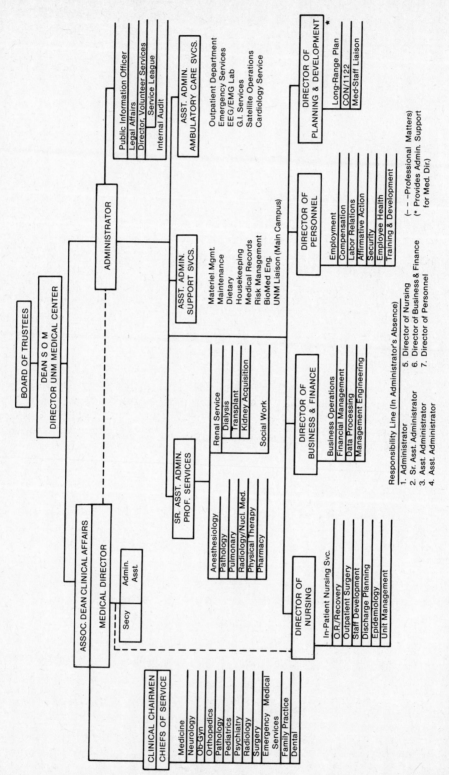

Figure 2-1. Hospital Organizational Chart.

a library cart; assist with distribution and collection of menus; staff the information desk; and act as receptionist in the surgical waiting room to keep relatives posted on patient's condition. Volunteers also perform a variety of other tasks which benefit the patient. The Director may also be responsible for a Service League or Auxiliary which sponsors fund-raising functions to purchase hospital equipment.

PROFESSIONAL SERVICES

Anesthesiology Department

An **anesthetic** is a drug or gas that produces a state of unconsciousness with loss of sensation or a relaxed state with loss of sensation. The main types of anesthesia are **general, local** and **spinal.**

An **anesthesiologist** is a doctor who specializes in the administration of an anesthetic. He/she may also be referred to as an **anesthetist.** Nurses who specialize in this field are **nurse anesthetists.** The anesthesiology department works with the patient's doctor to provide care during surgery and in the recovery room. Each evening, the anesthetists visit the patients on the schedule for surgery the next day and question them about allergies and past experiences with anesthesia. At this time, the patient receives an explanation of what to expect before surgery. The patient is taken to the RR (recovery room) following surgery and remains there until fully reacted from the anesthetic. The anesthetist checks the patient and writes orders for the patient's return to the unit. Someone from the anesthesiology department visits the patient the following day to make sure there are no problems related to anesthesia.

Laboratory

The laboratory (lab) performs examinations on specimens as ordered by the doctor. There are many divisions of the lab, each having a specific function. Be sure to find out the hours the lab is open in the hospital where you will be working.

Requisitions

Computers are used in many hospitals instead of requisitions. However, the use of requisitions is explained since requisitions are the back-up system when a computer is not functioning.

Laboratory requisitions are completed in the same manner even though each section has individualized requisitions. The information you need to place on the requisitions is as follows:

1. Addressograph the requisition with the patient's identification card. Be sure the ID (identification) is in the space provided.
2. The patient's room number must be on the requisition.
3. Designate the test the doctor ordered by placing an X in the proper space.

4. Write in the requesting doctor's name. This may not be the doctor who admitted the patient; therefore, the name on the identification card would not be the name of the doctor who wrote the order.
5. Fill in specified blanks according to your hospital's forms. This information usually includes:
   - The date ordered
   - The date and time the test is to be performed
   - The name or initials of the person completing the requisition
   - The name of the person who collected the specimen if the collecting was done by unit personnel.
6. Specify if STAT or ASAP. **STAT** means immediately and is used whenever the patient's condition is serious and the test results are needed to determine treatment. **ASAP** means as soon as possible and is used when the patient's condition is not quite as serious but when time is still an element of concern. Your instructor will show you the routine for STAT and ASAP orders in your area.
7. Labels for the containers of specimens collected by unit personnel are completed when the requisition is completed.

Keep in mind that all the forms shown may differ in physical form from the one you will work with in class; but, the information you will be placing on the forms is the same. Most of you will not spend your entire working years in one place and will benefit from exposure to various methods of ordering tests.

General Lab

This section of the lab performs routine urinalysis (UA) and complete blood count (CBC) examinations. The receptionist can answer questions you may have regarding tests or examinations that may not be listed in the hospital laboratory manual.

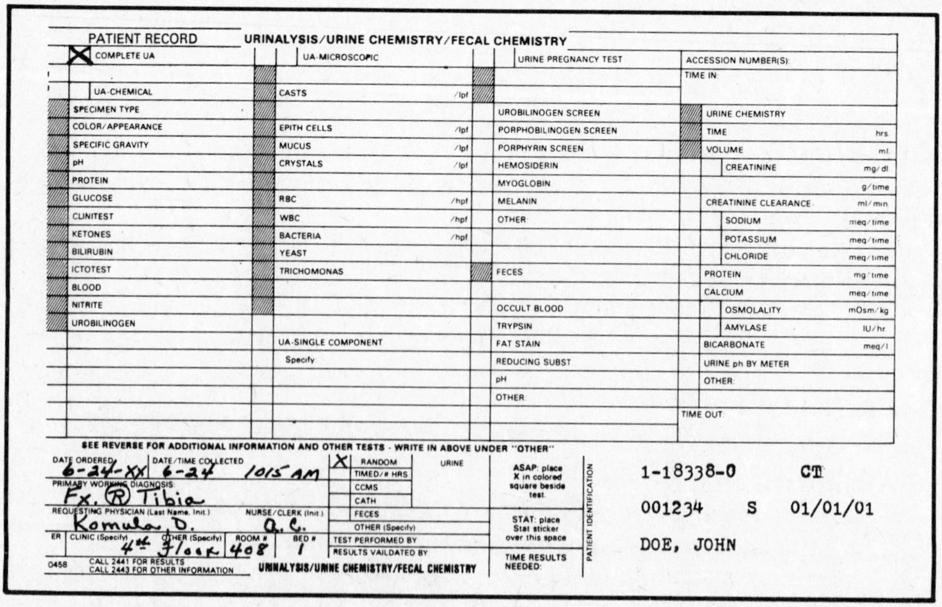
PATIENT RECORD
URINALYSIS/URINE CHEMISTRY/FECAL CHEMISTRY
X COMPLETE UA
UA-MICROSCOPIC
URINE PREGNANCY TEST
ACCESSION NUMBER(S):
TIME IN:
UA-CHEMICAL
SPECIMEN TYPE
COLOR/APPEARANCE
SPECIFIC GRAVITY
pH
PROTEIN
GLUCOSE
CLINITEST
KETONES
BILIRUBIN
ICTOTEST
BLOOD
NITRITE
UROBILINOGEN
CASTS /lpf
EPITH CELLS /lpf
MUCUS /lpf
CRYSTALS /lpf
RBC /hpf
WBC /hpf
BACTERIA /hpf
YEAST
TRICHOMONAS
UA-SINGLE COMPONENT
Specify:
UROBILINOGEN SCREEN
PORPHOBILINOGEN SCREEN
PORPHYRIN SCREEN
HEMOSIDERIN
MYOGLOBIN
MELANIN
OTHER:
FECES
OCCULT BLOOD
TRYPSIN
FAT STAIN
REDUCING SUBST
pH
OTHER:
URINE CHEMISTRY
TIME hrs.
VOLUME ml.
CREATININE mg/dl
g/time
CREATININE CLEARANCE ml/min
SODIUM meq/time
POTASSIUM meq/time
CHLORIDE meq/time
PROTEIN mg/time
CALCIUM meq/time
OSMOLALITY mOsm/kg
AMYLASE IU/hr
BICARBONATE meq/l
URINE ph BY METER
OTHER:
TIME OUT:
SEE REVERSE FOR ADDITIONAL INFORMATION AND OTHER TESTS - WRITE IN ABOVE UNDER "OTHER"
DATE ORDERED: 6-24-XX
DATE/TIME COLLECTED: 6-24 1015 AM
PRIMARY WORKING DIAGNOSIS: Fx. Ⓡ Tibia
REQUESTING PHYSICIAN (Last Name, Init.): Komula, D.
NURSE/CLERK (Init.): A. C.
ER | CLINIC (Specify) | OTHER (Specify): 4th Floor | ROOM #: 408 | BED #: 1
URINE: X RANDOM | TIMED/# HRS | CCMS | CATH | FECES | OTHER (Specify)
TEST PERFORMED BY
RESULTS VAILDATED BY
ASAP: place X in colored square beside test.
STAT: place Stat sticker over this space
TIME RESULTS NEEDED:
PATIENT IDENTIFICATION
1-18338-0 CT
001234 S 01/01/01
DOE, JOHN
0458 CALL 2441 FOR RESULTS
CALL 2443 FOR OTHER INFORMATION
URINALYSIS/URINE CHEMISTRY/FECAL CHEMISTRY

Figure 2-2a. Urinalysis Requisition.

Hematology/Coagulation Section

Hematology is the study of the components of blood and the blood-forming tissues. Coagulation is the clotting process of blood. Certain coagulation tests are changed by medications (you will learn these medications later in Chapter 11). If the patient is receiving one of these particular medications, the requisition should contain that fact.

2-2b. Hematology Requisition for CBC and Differential (ASAP order).

Chemistry Section

The chemistry lab performs tests on blood, urine, and other body fluids to determine the amount of chemicals present in relation to normal amounts. Some of these tests require that a specimen be collected, then a medication be administered, and another specimen collected at a specified time. The requisitions for such tests must be absolutely correct as to specimen collection time. Be sure you understand the order before preparing the requisitions. Examples of such tests are given in Chapter 15 so you will be able to practice the procedure.

Toxicology Section

Toxicology is the study of poisons. The toxicology section studies specimens of blood, urine, and body fluids or tissues to determine if a poison is present, to identify the poison, and to ascertain the amount of poison in the specimen. The doctor ordering such tests usually specifies which toxic substance he suspects is present.

Immunology Section

To be immune to a disease is to be safe from the disease. Our bodies have an immune system that aids in fighting and resisting disease. The immunology lab conducts tests to determine if the body's own defenses are in proper order. It studies substances (antibodies), found in persons with an infectious disease, which are formed by the tissues and possess the ability to destroy or injure the agent that caused the disease.

Radioimmunoassay Section

Radioimmunoassay determines the concentration of substances in the blood, especially the proteins in hormones. Hormones are substances produced by certain glands of the body and travel through the bloodstream to influence or stimulate other areas of the body. Radioactive material is used to complete the test.

Microbiology Section

Microbiology is the study of an organism that is too small to be seen without the aid of the microscope. An example are **bacteria,** disease-causing organisms found in three different forms: spherical shaped bacteria called *cocci,* rod-shaped called *bacilli,* and spiral shapes called *spirilla, spirochetes,* or *vibrios.*

Gram's method for staining bacteria is important in identification. Gram-positive bacteria retain the color of the stain; gram-negative bacteria do not retain the original stain but take the color of a counter stain.

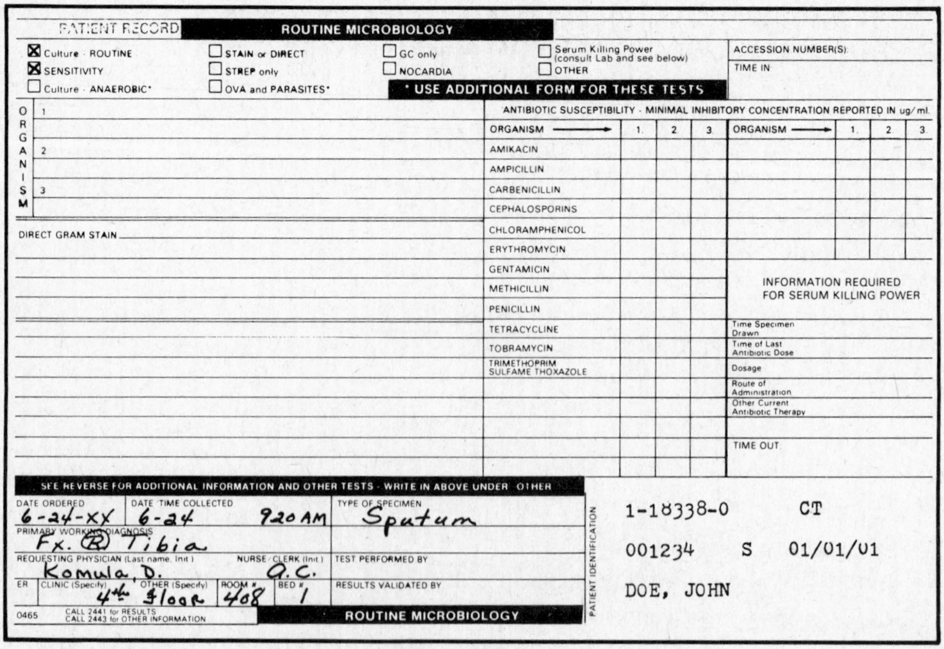
PATIENT RECORD
ROUTINE MICROBIOLOGY
☒ Culture - ROUTINE
☒ SENSITIVITY
☐ Culture - ANAEROBIC*
☐ STAIN or DIRECT
☐ STREP only
☐ OVA and PARASITES*
☐ GC only
☐ NOCARDIA
☐ Serum Killing Power (consult Lab and see below)
☐ OTHER
* USE ADDITIONAL FORM FOR THESE TESTS
ACCESSION NUMBER(S):
TIME IN
ORGANISM 1 2 3
ANTIBIOTIC SUSCEPTIBILITY - MINIMAL INHIBITORY CONCENTRATION REPORTED IN ug/ml.
ORGANISM → 1. 2. 3.
AMIKACIN
AMPICILLIN
CARBENICILLIN
CEPHALOSPORINS
CHLORAMPHENICOL
ERYTHROMYCIN
GENTAMICIN
METHICILLIN
PENICILLIN
TETRACYCLINE
TOBRAMYCIN
TRIMETHOPRIM SULFAME THOXAZOLE
DIRECT GRAM STAIN
INFORMATION REQUIRED FOR SERUM KILLING POWER
Time Specimen Drawn
Time of Last Antibiotic Dose
Dosage
Route of Administration
Other Current Antibiotic Therapy
TIME OUT
SEE REVERSE FOR ADDITIONAL INFORMATION AND OTHER TESTS - WRITE IN ABOVE UNDER OTHER
DATE ORDERED 6-24-XX
DATE TIME COLLECTED 6-24 9:20 AM
TYPE OF SPECIMEN Sputum
PRIMARY WORKING DIAGNOSIS Fx. Ⓡ Tibia
REQUESTING PHYSICIAN (Last name, Init.) Komula, D.
NURSE-CLERK (Init.) A.C.
TEST PERFORMED BY
ER CLINIC (Specify) OTHER (Specify) 4th floor ROOM # 408 BED # 1
RESULTS VALIDATED BY
0465 CALL 2441 for RESULTS CALL 2443 for OTHER INFORMATION
ROUTINE MICROBIOLOGY
PATIENT IDENTIFICATION
1-18338-0 CT
001234 S 01/01/01
DOE, JOHN

Figure 2-3a. Requisition for Culture and Sensitivity Test.

A **culture** determines the type of bacteria, and **sensitivity testing** determines which medication will destroy the bacteria. Specimens for cultures must be taken to the lab immediately. Culture requisitions must contain the source of the specimen; that is, you must specify if the specimen is blood, urine, drainage from a wound, a swab from a certain area of the body, or fluid taken from the body. Anaerobic cultures (without air) are usually collected in surgery.

The microbiology section also conducts tests for fungi, parasites, protozoa, rickettsia, and viruses. Some hospitals have a virology section for virus studies because there are over 200 varieties.

2-3b. Requisition for AFB Culture and AF Stain.

Blood Bank Section

The blood bank studies blood to determine blood type, crossmatches blood for transfusions, and dispenses blood and blood products to the units. Blood products are discussed in Chapter 6. The requisitions for blood and blood products have a space for the quantity needed. The majority of hospitals will also have a requisition to be completed and taken to the blood bank when a product is obtained. Your instructor will demonstrate the method used in your area.

If a patient has a reaction to a blood transfusion, the container is returned to the blood bank with a report so further testing can be done to determine the reason for the reaction.

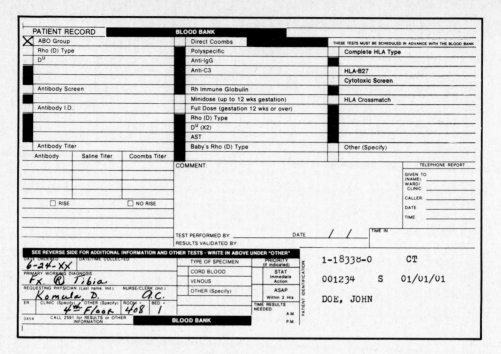

Figure 2-4a. Requisition for Blood Typing.

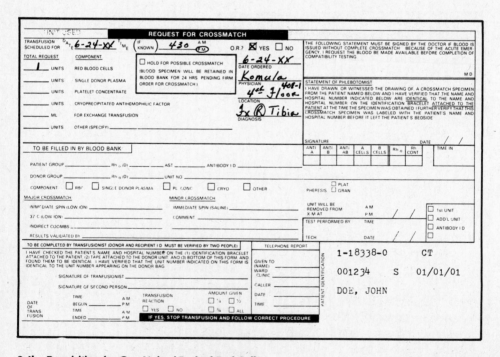

2-4b. Requisition for One Unit of Packed Red Cells.

Pathology/Cytology Section

This section studies cells and tissues for abnormal growth and development, aids in diagnosis and treatment of disease, and performs autopsies.

All tissue removed from a person during surgery is sent to the pathology section for study by a **pathologist,** a medical doctor who specializes in the study of cells and tissues and the changes caused by disease. The pathologist performs autopsies.

UNIVERSITY OF NEW MEXICO HOSPITAL
BERNALILLO COUNTY
MEDICAL CENTER
CYTOLOGY LABORATORY

Ward _5 West_

CLINICAL INFORMATION: Age _56_ Race _C_ If Indian, Tribe or Group _____ Accession Number _1-18338-0_

Significant History _Chest X-ray reveals spot in middle right lobe. Patient is heavy smoker. Emphysema diagnosed 5 years ago._

GYNECOLOGY:

A. History: LMP_____ PMP_____ Previous Smear_____ with date Recent Therapy: Radiation_____

Pregnant_____ (EDC_____) Endocrine_____ Surgical_____

Grav._____ Para_____ Other (Trich., Cervicitis, etc.)_____

B. Material Submitted: Fast Smear ☐ (Combined) Cervical Scraping ☐ Vaginal Pool ☐

Endocervical ☐ Endometrial Aspiration ☐ Nipple Secretion ☐

C. Report
Unsatisfactory Smears ☐ Reason_____
Maturation Index (Basal/Intermediate/Superficial) _/ /_
Inflammatory Reaction: Mild ☐ Moderate ☐ Severe ☐
Flora: Bacteria ☐ Trichomonas ☐ Fungi ☐ Other_____

Evaluation for Neoplasia: NEGATIVE ☐   SUSPECTED ☐ POSITIVE ☐

Slight Dysplasia ☐   Squamous Lesion - In Situ ☐ Invasive ☐
Moderate Dysplasia ☐   Glandular Lesion - Endometrial ☐ Endocervical ☐
Severe Dysplasia ☐
Recommend: Repeat Smear In ___Months ☐
Tissue Confirmation ☐

RESPIRATORY SYSTEM:
A. Material Submitted: Sputum ☐ Bronchial Washing ☒ Other_____
B. Report
Unsatisfactory ☐ Reason_____
Evaluation for Neoplasia: NEGATIVE ☐ SUSPECTED ☐ POSITIVE ☐
Lesion Suspected_____
MISCELLANEOUS: (Urine, G.I., Fluids, etc.)
A. Material Submitted_____
B. Report: Unsatisfactory ☐ Reason_____
Evaluation for Neoplasia: NEGATIVE ☐ SUSPECTED ☐ POSITIVE ☐

Lesion Suspected_____
Screener_____
COMMENT:

Sex _M_
Date _5-19-XX_
Doctor _Samson, J._
Hospital _UNMH/BCMC_

1-18338-0   CT
001234   S   01/01/01
DOE, JOHN

PATIENT INDENTIFICATION
ADDRESSOGRAPH

PATIENT RECORD

_____, M.D.
PATHOLOGIST
P00040 Rev. 8/77

Figure 2-5. Cytology Laboratory Requisition.

SURGICAL PATHOLOGY REQUISITION

CLINICAL HISTORY, DIAGNOSIS & CRITICAL LAB DATA

Hx: Food intolerance - pork, fat, spices past six months. Occasional pain RUQ. Severe pain two days ago. Radiating to back.

Dx: Cholecystitis c cholelithiasis X-Rays show multiple stones in gallbladder with inflammation.

OB-GYN:

Gr. _____ P _____

LMP _____

PMP _____

If abnormal describe:

_____

_____

Hormonal Therapy including Contraceptives _____

_____

Tissue passed spontaneously

_____

_____

Cytology _____

_____

Print Age **48**

1-18338-0   CT

001234   S   01/01/01

DOE, JOHN

Physician: Wilcott, M.

Operation: Cholecystectomy

Specimen Required: Gallbladder

Service/Ward/Clinic: Surgical service Rm504

Special Requests:

ADDRESSOGRAPH   PL1005 (8/80)

Figure 2-6. Surgical Pathology Requisition.

EEG (Electroencephalogram) Department

An EEG is a recording of the electrical activity of the brain (see Chapter 16 for a discussion of the types of tests). Complete the requisition by addressograph-ing in the proper space and filling out the appropriate blanks according to your hospital's policy. The EEG department usually requires an appointment. Be sure you know why the test is ordered and the condition of the patient before calling for the appointment; the department secretary may also ask you the condition of the patient—alert, comatose, or semi-comatose.

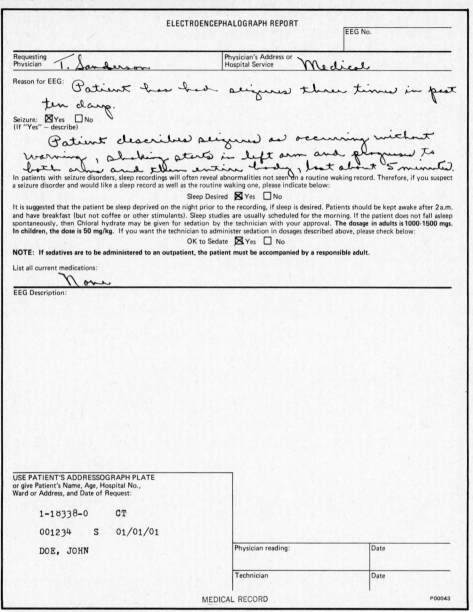

ELECTROENCEPHALOGRAPH REPORT

EEG No.

Requesting Physician *T. Sanderson*

Physician's Address or Hospital Service *Medical*

Reason for EEG: *Patient has had seizures three times in past ten days.*

Seizure: ☒ Yes ☐ No
(If "Yes" — describe)

Patient describes seizures as occurring without warning, shaking starts in left arm and progresses to both arms and then entire body, last about 5 minutes.

In patients with seizure disorders, sleep recordings will often reveal abnormalities not seen on a routine waking record. Therefore, if you suspect a seizure disorder and would like a sleep record as well as the routine waking one, please indicate below:

Sleep Desired ☒ Yes ☐ No

It is suggested that the patient be sleep deprived on the night prior to the recording, if sleep is desired. Patients should be kept awake after 2 a.m. and have breakfast (but not coffee or other stimulants). Sleep studies are usually scheduled for the morning. If the patient does not fall asleep spontaneously, then Chloral hydrate may be given for sedation by the technician with your approval. **The dosage in adults is 1000-1500 mgs. In children, the dose is 50 mg/kg.** If you want the technician to administer sedation in dosages described above, please check below:

OK to Sedate ☒ Yes ☐ No

NOTE: If sedatives are to be administered to an outpatient, the patient must be accompanied by a responsible adult.

List all current medications: *None*

EEG Description:

USE PATIENT'S ADDRESSOGRAPH PLATE
or give Patient's Name, Age, Hospital No.,
Ward or Address, and Date of Request:

1-18338-0   CT

001234   S   01/01/01

DOE, JOHN

Physician reading:	Date
Technician	Date

MEDICAL RECORD

P00043

Figure 2-7. EEG Requisition.

Cardiology Testing Department

Cardiology is the study of the heart. The EKG or ECG (electrocardiogram) is a recording of the electrical activity of the heart and is a common examination. Other tests are usually listed on a separate requisition. The requisition is addressographed and the blanks are completed according to your hospital's policy. Many tests require an appointment. Chapter 11 explains the various tests and the medications that may affect the tests.

```
DEPARTMENT OF DIAGNOSTIC CARDIOLOGY    **
NON-INVASIVE MEDICINE, 2ND FLOOR - WEST
PHONE:  843-2403 ECG AND 843-2672 ECHO

TEST DESIRED:
ECG/EKG  12 LEAD  ____✓____        VCG _____
*TREADMILL _____        PHONO _____
*TREADMILL WITH THALLIUM _____   *HOLTER MONITOR 24 HR ____
*ECHO M-MODE _____      *HOLTER MONITOR 12 HR ____
*ECHO 2-D _____         RHYTHM STRIP _____
*ECHO MM/2-D (AS INDICATED) ____

INPATIENT _____    OUTPATIENT _____    E.R. _____    ROOM _____
HOME PHONE _____    HEIGHT ____    AGE ____    DATE OF BIRTH _____
                        WEIGHT ____
PERTINENT CLINICAL DATA:
1. _Cholecystitis c̄ Cholelithiasis_____
2. _____
3. _____
4. _____

CARDIAC MEDICATIONS AND DOSAGE:
1.  DIGOXIN:                      2.  QUINIDINE:
3.  INDERAL:                      4.  DIURETICS:
5.  NITRATES:                     6.  ANTI-HYPERTENSIVES:
7.  K+ :                          8.  OTHER:

REASON FOR EXAM: _Pre-op Surgery scheduled for_
_1100 Am 6-26-XX_____
REQUESTED BY: ____R. Ahamuha____ M.D.
RESULTS TO ___4 West_____

*ALL INFORMATION MUST BE FILLED OUT OR THE PROCEDURE WILL NOT BE SCHEDULED OR DONE.
**LAB IS LOCATED ACROSS THE HALL FROM THE PATHOLOGY (BLOOD) LAB.

NAME: _Doe, John_____
UNMH/BCMC # __001234__
DATE TEST SCHEDULED: __6-25-XX  330 p___
```

ADDRESSOGRAPH		
1-18338-0	CT	
001234	S	01/01/01
DOE, JOHN		

```
1026 (1/81)
```

Figure 2-8. Diagnostic Cardiology Requisition.

Radiology Department

Radiology is the study of x-rays in the diagnosis and treatment of disease. An **x-ray** produces a picture of internal structures. Barium is sometimes given before an x-ray to give contrast. If a dye is injected or a catheter is inserted into an artery or vein, the procedure is termed an **invasive study.**

You complete the requisition by filling in the spaces as designated by your instructor. State the type of x-ray that the doctor ordered, the diagnosis of the patient, why the x-ray is needed, the mode of transportation and the name of the doctor who wrote the order. Be sure the addressograph is in the proper space.

If the doctor did not supply complete information as to why the test is needed, consult the nurse working with you. The information can usually be found in the Progress Notes. Example: A patient has been treated for a fractured tibia and the doctor writes an order for a **GI Series** (an examination of the esophagus, stomach and small intestines). The diagnosis of a fractured tibia means nothing to the x-ray department in connection with a GI Series. The Progress Notes will

---

RADIOLOGY CONSULTATION REQUEST   DATE _3-18-XX_

EXAMINATION REQUESTED: _Chest and Lumbar spine_

PERTINENT CLINICAL DATA: _Low back pain_

PATIENT: AMBULATORY ( )   INFANT IN ARMS ( )   IN WHEELCHAIR (X)   STRETCHER ( )   ISOLATION ( )

HOSPITAL NUMBER	AGE	SEX	RACE	CLINIC OR SERVICE	ROOM	HEIGHT	WEIGHT
_001234_	_56_	_M_	_C_	_Ortho_	_403_	_5'11"_	_160_

REQUESTED BY: DR _Komula_   ATTENDING PHYSICIAN: DR _Komula_   PREVIOUS X-RAYS HERE ☐ YES ☒ NO ☒ NEW ☐ OLD

RADIOLOGIST'S REPORT

DIAGNOSTIC ULTRASOUND CONSULTATION REQUEST   DATE _5-8-XX_ (11-15)

EXAMINATION REQUESTED: _Ultrasound abd and pelvis_

PERTINENT CLINICAL DATA: _Possible ovarian tumor_

PATIENT: AMBULATORY ( )   INFANT IN ARMS ( )   IN WHEELCHAIR (X)   STRETCHER ( )   ISOLATION ( )

HOSPITAL NUMBER	AGE	SEX	RACE	CLINIC OR SERVICE	ROOM	HEIGHT	WEIGHT
_004342_	_31_ (16-18)	_F_ (9)	_C_ (10)	_Gyn_ (28-31)	_332_	_5'6½"_	_130_

REQUESTED BY: DR _A. Johnson_   ATTENDING PHYSICIAN: DR _G. Antre_   PREVIOUS STUDIES HERE ☒ YES ☐ NO (35) PATIENT ☐ NEW ☒ OLD

DATE OF REPORT: ULTRASONOGRAPHER'S REPORT

NUCLEAR MEDICINE CONSULTATION REQUEST   DATE _4-29-XX_

EXAMINATION REQUESTED: _Brain Scan_

PERTINENT CLINICAL DATA: _Ca Lung   R/o metastasis_

PATIENT: AMBULATORY ( )   INFANT IN ARMS ( )   IN WHEELCHAIR (X)   STRETCHER ( )   ISOLATION ( )

HOSPITAL NUMBER	AGE	SEX	RACE	CLINIC OR SERVICE	ROOM	HEIGHT	WEIGHT
_001234_	_62_	_F_	_S_	_Medical_	_521_	_5'4"_	_115_

REQUESTED BY: DR _L. Marsten_   ATTENDING PHYSICIAN: DR _L. Marsten_   PREVIOUS X-RAYS HERE ☒ YES ☐ NO ☐ NEW ☒ OLD

RADIOISOTOPE DIAGNOSTIC REPORT

Figure 2-9. Headings of Radiology, Ultrasound, and Nuclear Medicine Consultation Requisitions to Show Completion Procedure.

probably reveal something like this: patient has periods of pain, heartburn, and gastric distress. Write this information on the requisition in quotation marks to show it was taken from the chart.

Computerized Tomography (CT scan) is more sensitive than regular x-ray and allows detailed examination of the body's softer tissues. A rapidly rotating, pencil-thin beam of x-ray is passed through the body or head taking pictures which a computer compiles into horizontal cross-sectional pictures. Tumors or infections can be quickly determined. A dye may be injected into a vein to obtain a better outline of an abnormality; this procedure is ordered as a CT scan with contrast.

Nuclear Magnetic Resonance (NMR) produces pictures of anatomical slices as does the CT scan but no x-rays or contrast material is used. The patient is placed in a static magnetic field and a second alternating magnetic field is applied at right angles to the first field. Cells react to the vibration of the field. When the second field is turned off, cells release detectable signals which a computer can process and record as an image or as chemical data. NMR gives information about the contents and surroundings of cells, helps identify cancers of the breast, kidney, lung and liver, and produces pictures of blood vessels without the use of contrast material.

Xeroradiography is a type of x-ray that uses Xerox® paper in place of the usual x-ray film to give a more realistic picture of the soft tissues of the body. This is usually used for locating the position of a foreign object such as a piece of metal in a foot.

Ultrasound is a division of radiology. Inaudible sounds of a very high frequency are passed through the body and their echoes are recorded as they strike tissues of different densities. The echoes produce an image of organs, tumors, or fetus. Ultrasonic studies are also called echograms and sonograms.

Nuclear medicine is another division of radiology. Different tissues have an attraction for certain radioactive elements. Nuclear medicine utilizes this fact to study diseases and to treat diseases. Radioactive material is given to the patient and then the area to be studied is scanned.

Rehabilitation Department

Physical therapy and occupational therapy are the divisions of this department. **Physical therapy** helps improve circulation, strengthen muscles, restores motion, corrects deformities, relieves pain, and speeds recovery from illness or injury. **Occupational therapy** trains the patient in self-care skills, helps build morale and physical fitness through hobbies, and assists the patient and family to return to community life.

The types of treatments used by physical therapy are:

1. **Hydrotherapy**—the use of water to make motion easier and less painful. This includes the whirlpool, Hubbard Tank (a tank large enough to immerse the entire body in moving water), ice packs, hot packs, hot and cold baths, and a swimming pool.

2. **Heat and light**—to relieve pain and improve circulation. This includes heating pads, paraffin wax applications, infrared heat, diathermy, ultrasound, and ultraviolet light treatments.

3. **Exercises**—to strengthen muscles, correct limitation of motion, and promote independence.

ORIGINAL

UNIVERSITY OF NEW MEXICO HOSPITAL
BERNALILLO COUNTY MEDICAL CENTER
DEPARTMENT OF PHYSICAL THERAPY

PHYSICAL THERAPY REQUISITION

NAME _Doe, John_   RM.NO./ER/OPD _408-1_   DATE _7-12-XX_

ADDRESS _2702 West Arboles_   TEL NO _893-2071_ AGE _42_ SEX _M_

HOSPITAL NO _001234_   CLASS NO _S_   DPW OR CASE NO _____

Physician's Information, Plan and Order Section

Diagnosis: _Low back pain_

Area(s) To Be Treated _Lumbar spine_

Physical Therapy Modality Ordered:

__ Electrical Stimulation (Faradic 'Galvanic)	__ Test and Measurements (R.O.M.)
__ Ultrasound	__ Manual Muscle Test
__ Medcosonlator	__ Passive, Active-Assistive Range of Motion
__ Short Wave Diathermy	__ Active Range of Motion
__ Microwave Diathermy	__ Active Resistive Exercise
__ Ultraviolet	__ Crutches and Crutch Walking
__ Infrared (Radiant Heat)	__ Cane and Cane Instructions
__ Paraffin Bath	__ Ambulation and/or Gait Training
__ Hydrocolator Packs (Hot Packs)	__ Jobst Intermittent Compression
__ Cold Packs or Ice Massage	__ Splinting (Construction)
__ Whirlpool	__ Home Care Instructions (Exercise Program)
__ Moistaire Cabinet	__ Others
__ Massage	
__ Traction (Cervical)	
X Traction (Lumbar)	

Space below for narrative treatment plan if preferred:

Teach muscle strengthening exercises for back.

Treatment Frequency:

X Daily
__ Tri-weekly
__ Bi-weekly
__ Weekly
__ Other_____

Estimated Duration of Treatment Course:

__ Single Treatment
X Weeks (Enter No.)
__ Other (Explain)

Treatment Goal:

To strengthen muscles, reduce pain and increase mobility.

Precautions and Additional Remarks:

D. [signature]
Physician's Signature

--- Patient Imprint Information ---

1- 18338-0   CT

001234   S   01/01/01

DOE, JOHN

P00065

PHYSICAL THERAPY REQUISITION   MR-20
PREPARE IN DUPLICATE: ORIGINAL TO PT CLINIC, COPY TO MEDICAL RECORDS

Figure 2-10. Physical Therapy Requisition.

The types of treatments used by occupational therapy are:

1. **Evaluating** the **ability** of the patient and the extent of any disability.
2. Selected **activities** to build strength in order to reduce the patient's limitations due to injury or disease. Light handicrafts, manual skills, and group activities such as sports or music are beneficial and enjoyable.
3. **Training** to overcome disabilities and to perform tasks necessary for daily living.
4. Assist patients in **developing job skills,** help them in finding new jobs, and help them in adjusting to those jobs.

To complete requisitions, addressograph the sheet in the proper space, state the name of the doctor who wrote the order, designate the treatment ordered, state the patient's diagnosis and information concerning disability.

Respiratory Therapy Department (RT)

This department may be called the Inhalation Therapy Department in some hospitals. This department conducts tests to aid in the diagnosis and treatment of breathing disorders and lung diseases. Various treatments are performed (the treatments and the tests are discussed in Chapter 12). Oxygen therapy is the most common treatment. Requisitions for the RT Department are completed in the same manner as those previously discussed. The sheet is addressographed, you designate the treatment ordered, the name of the doctor ordering the treatment, the diagnosis of the patient. Some tests require an appointment.

Pharmacy Department

Pharmacy supplies patient medications to the hospital units. This may be done by sending unit doses (single doses) at certain times or by sending several days' supply at one time.

The carbon of the Physician's Order Sheet is sent to pharmacy, and orders are filled in the same way prescriptions are filled in a local drugstore.

You may be required to send an additional requisition for intravenous medication orders. A special form is required to order stock drugs. You should keep a supply of this form in your cabinet so the nurses will have them to order drugs when necessary. Drugs that remain when a patient is discharged will be returned to the pharmacy with a credit slip. Your only responsibility is to addressograph the credit slip; the nurses take care of the rest.

Home Health Care Department (HHC)

A staff of registered nurses assist the unit nurses by teaching patients self-care procedures such as how to give themselves insulin and teach the patient and family how to care for wounds. These nurses also visit patients in their homes after discharge from the hospital and work with Social Services to place patients in nursing homes. Requisitions for HHC must specify what type of service the patient needs. The staff wil review the patient's chart before seeing the patient.

UNIVERSITY OF NEW MEXICO HOSPITAL
RESPIRATORY THERAPY ORDER FORM

DIAGNOSIS *Pneumonia, right lower lobe*

THERAPEUTIC OBJECTIVES
- ☐ Atelectasis Treatment/Prevention
- ☒ Mobilize secretions/improve bronchial hygiene
- ☐ Treat Bronchospasm
- ☐ Treat Hypoxemia
- ☐ _____
- Treat Respiratory Failure due to
- ☐ Alveolar Hypoventilation
- ☐ Hypoxemia

☐ **RESPIRATORY THERAPY CONSULTATION**   Sig. *D. Komula*   MD

***NOTE**   1. IF RESPIRATORY THERAPY CONSULTATION IS CHECKED, RESPIRATORY THERAPY WILL DETERMINE THE BEST MODALITY TO ACHIEVE THE THERAPEUTIC OBJECTIVES.

ALL THERAPY ORDERS ARE DISCONTINUED AFTER THREE (3) DAYS UNLESS REORDERED

THERAPY ORDERS

THERAPY:	FREQUENCY:	MEDICATION:
☒ Postural Drainage and Percussion	☒ QID CIRCLE ONE	☐ _____ cc Isuprel 1:200
☐ Percussion, No Trendelenburg	☐ TID Q1	☐ _____ cc Bronkosol
☐ Ultrasonic Nebulization (USN)	☐ BID 2	☐ _____ cc Racemic Epinephrine
☐ Incentive Spirometry	☐ PRN 3	☐ _____ cc Mycomyst
☐ Nebulizer	4	☐ _____ cc Other _____
☐ IPPB	5	With
☐ Sputum induction	6	☐ _____ cc Normal Saline
☐ Other _____	7	☐ _____ cc Water
	8	
	☐ During Night Hours Hours	
	(9 PM - 6 AM)	

OXYGEN THERAPY ORDERS
- ☒ _2_ L/Min by Nasal Cannula
- ☐ _____ L/Min by Oxygen Mask
- ☐ Venti Mask
  Approximate O_2 concentration desired:
- ☐ 24%   ☐ 28%   ☐ 31%   ☐ 35%   ☐ 40%
- ☐ _____%

- ☐ Aerosol Mask _____ % Oxygen
- ☐ T-Tube _____ % Oxygen
- ☐ Hood _____ % Oxygen
- ☐ Mist Tent _____ % Oxygen
- ☐ Face Tent _____ % Oxygen
- ☐ CPAP _____ CM H_2O _____ % Oxygen

- ☐ Heated
- ☐ Cool

INITIAL VENTILATOR ORDERS   (Additional orders or changes please use physician order sheet in Patient Chart)

Place Patient on _____   ☐ Assist/control   ☐ IMV

Tidal Volume _____ Rate _____ FIO_2 _____ Peep _____

(For correct ventilator settings please see respiratory therapy physician manual)

DIAGNOSTIC PROCEDURES
- ☐ Bedside Spirometry
- ☐ Pre and Post Bronchodilator Spirometry (FEV_1)
- ☐ Arterial Blood Gases
- ☐ Therapeutic Bronchoscopy - Set-Up & Assistance
- ☐ Diagnostic Bronchoscopy - Set-Up & Assistance
- ☐ Laryngoscopy
- ☐ Other _____

Comments: *Patient has rheumatoid arthritis which causes difficulty in moving.*

DATE *8-14-XX*   ROOM NO. *519*

PATIENT INFORMATION

```
1-18338-0        CT
001234      S    01/01/01
DOE, JOHN
```

1014

MEDICAL RECORDS

Figure 2-11. Respiratory Therapy Requisition.

Pastoral Care Department

The personnel in Pastoral Care have completed special training in helping people with the problems of serious and terminal illnesses. Patients or nursing personnel may request the service or a doctor may order the service. The cancer unit (oncology) usually notifies Pastoral Care of each admission. The emotional support given to patients and their families by this department is extremely valuable.

Your hospital may have requisitions or the policy may be that you notify the department by telephone only.

Outpatient Clinic

The clinic serves patients who do not need to be hospitalized. Patients may be sent from a doctor's office for lab or x-ray exams; patients being discharged may need follow-up testing. The doctor writes the order for follow-up testing, and the secretary makes the appointment and gives the patient an appointment card.

Social Services Department

Personnel help place patients in nursing homes, assist in the acquisition of financial aid, and assist with Medicaid and Medicare benefits. The department is usually notified of requests by telephone.

| SUPPORT SERVICES

Communications Department

The switchboard handles incoming calls and provides information about departments. Volunteers staff an information desk to give information concerning patients' room numbers. The switchboard uses the address system to page doctors or other personnel as requested, makes announcements, and announces emergency situations according to hospital policies.

The mailroom receives and distributes mail to patients, departments, and doctor's individual mailboxes; it also forwards mail to patients who have been discharged.

Central Supply Department (CS)

Items needed for patient comfort, administration of IV fluids and blood, care of wounds, catheters, and trays for special examinations are dispensed by this department. Each unit may have a cart filled with the most commonly used items. Each item will have a charge form attached and when an item is used the form must be addressographed with the patient ID. The RN may do this or may write in a room number and leave for the secretary to addressograph. CS collects the forms daily. When trays for special exams are needed, request the tray by calling the department. If a doctor needs the tray in a hurry, you may have to go to CS to obtain the tray.

Dietary Department

The director of the department is an **administrative dietitian** who oversees the operation of the department, purchases food, and handles all administrative duties. The **therapeutic dietitian** prepares the menus for patients' meals, visits patients at request of nurse or doctor, provides teaching of diets for patients

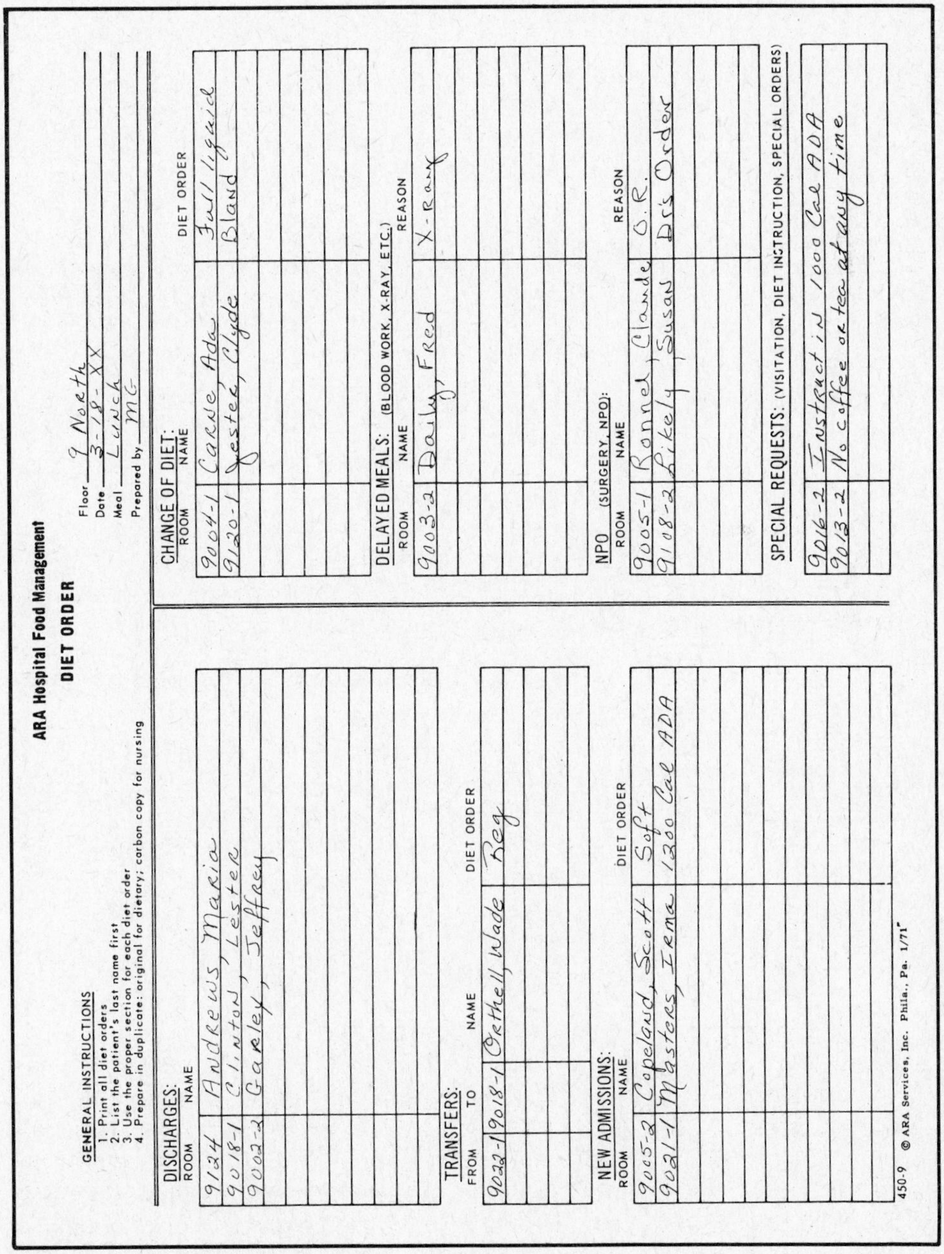

ARA Hospital Food Management
DIET ORDER

Floor 9 North
Date 3-18-XX
Meal Lunch
Prepared by MG

GENERAL INSTRUCTIONS
1. Print all diet orders
2. List the patient's last name first
3. Use the proper section for each diet order
4. Prepare in duplicate: original for dietary; carbon copy for nursing

DISCHARGES:

ROOM	NAME
9124	Andrews, Maria
9018-1	Clinton, Lester
9002-2	Garley, Jeffrey

TRANSFERS:

FROM	TO	NAME	DIET ORDER
9022-1	9018-1	Orthell, Wade	Reg

NEW ADMISSIONS:

ROOM	NAME	DIET ORDER
9005-2	Copeland, Scott	Soft
9021-1	Masters, Irma	1300 Cal ADA

CHANGE OF DIET:

ROOM	NAME	DIET ORDER
9004-1	Carne, Ada	Full liquid
9120-1	Jester, Clyde	Bland

DELAYED MEALS: (BLOOD WORK, X-RAY, ETC.)

ROOM	NAME	REASON
9003-2	Daily, Fred	X-Ray

NPO (SURGERY, NPO):

ROOM	NAME	REASON
9005-1	Ronnel, Claude	O.R.
9108-2	Likely, Susan	Dr's Order

SPECIAL REQUESTS: (VISITATION, DIET INSTRUCTION, SPECIAL ORDERS)

ROOM	
9016-2	Instruct in 1000 Cal ADA
9013-2	No coffee or tea at any time

450-9 © ARA Services, Inc. Phila., Pa. 1/71

Figure 2-12. Dietary Order Form.

and their families, and counsels hospital personnel who have dietary problems. Each unit should have a manual explaining the various diets provided and the foods each diet includes. Each unit sends a diet list to the department before each meal for notification of admissions, discharges, changes, and patients who may not eat (NPO) due to tests or by order of the doctor.

Escort Service Department

Personnel are instructed in body mechanics so they can assist patients into and out of wheelchairs, manuever stretchers to take patients to other departments, and assist patients getting onto and off of a stretcher. This service transports patients to departments for testing, to the operating room from the unit, to the unit from recovery room, from emergency room to designated area, and from unit to car when discharged. Personnel coming to a unit for a patient will have a verification slip with patient's name, room number, time, and where patient is to be transported.

Housekeeping Department

Hospitals must be kept clean and free from germs that might be carried from one patient to the next. The housekeeping department is responsible for this cleanliness. A maid will be assigned to each nursing unit to clean the rooms each day and prepare rooms for new patients when one is discharged. Special procedures are followed if the patient is in isolation. A janitor is also assigned to each unit to keep the corridors, nursing station, utility rooms, and bathrooms clean.

Housekeeping supplies the units with linen for the patients' needs. A one day supply, or pack, for each patient is distributed to the rooms early each morning. A cart in the clean utility room contains extra linen and patient gowns or pajamas. Sterile linen may be needed for some cases. Notify housekeeping and these packs will be made, sent to Central Supply, and sterilized before delivery to the unit. Rooms used for isolation cases will be supplied a cart containing gowns, masks, gloves, etc., according to the type of isolation (some hospitals may have CS dispense isolation carts). Some hospitals have a Linen Department for dispensing linen.

Maintenance and Engineering Department

Personnel in this department include plumbers, electricians, gardeners, painters, and air-conditioning and heating repair persons. The department is responsible for maintenance of equipment and inspections for safety, upkeep of the hospital grounds, periodic painting of patient rooms and physical appearance of the entire hospital. Notify this department by telephone for emergencies involving patient safety or major utility problems and send a requisition for all other types of service.

Medical Records Department (MR)

Patient charts are kept on file indefinitely. When a patient is discharged, the chart is kept in the MR department and incorporated into any previous chart. This provides a reference if the patient is admitted at some future date. Charts may be microfilmed to reduce storage space. Charts are checked to make sure that the rules established by the Joint Commission for Accreditation of Hospitals (JCAH) are met. The staff doctors who have not signed all necessary forms on the charts are notified by the department so they may correct the omission.

Medical transcriptionists type the history, physicals, and consultations recorded on the dictaphones in each nursing unit. The typed pages are then placed in the patients' charts.

Materials Management or Purchasing Department

This department handles the ordering of all equipment and makes sure each department in the hospital adheres to the budget for that department. Purchasing keeps routine supplies on hand and dispenses them to the departments upon receipt of a written request.

BUSINESS AND FINANCE

Admitting Office

The admitting office receives information from doctors' offices for admission of patients, keeps up-to-the-minute census records to show available beds,

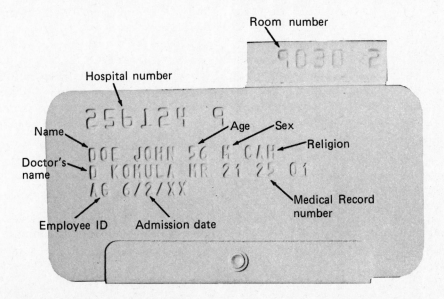

Figure 2-13a. Sample Addressograph Card.

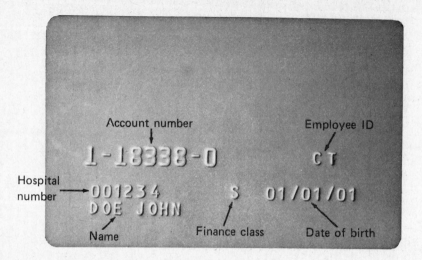

Figure 2-13b. Sample Addressograph Card.

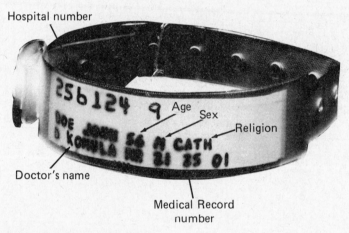

Figure 2-13c. Sample Identification Bracelet.

gathers information from patients or relatives regarding hospitalization insurance, and completes a Patient Identification Sheet for the chart, the ID bracelet for the patient, and the addressograph card. The office works with the units on intra- and interunit transfers. Admitting helps patients with financial arrangements for their hospital bills.

Business Office

The business office receives charges from all the departments to compute each patient's bill and calculates the amount of the bill covered by insurance, Medicaid, or Medicare. It sends monthly statements to those with outstanding bills.

This office also pays the monthly bills of the hospital and handles the payroll for all personnel.

Data Processing

The data processing section collects data pertaining to patients' financial charges, charges incurred by the hospital, and puts it all into accessible form for the business office.

PERSONNEL SERVICES

Personnel Office

The personnel office receives applications for employment, advertises for employment vacancies, and interviews and screens applicants before referring them to a department director. The office maintains benefit records of employees, explains benefits to the applicants and new employees, and, possibly assists in counseling and termination of employees.

Employee Health

The hospital has a responsibility for maintaining good health of their employees. Many hospitals hire a nurse practitioner to do physical examinations of new employees, to perform yearly physicals of all employees, and to care for ill employees. The secretary for this department sends notices to employees for physical exams and sets up appointments.

Security Department

Security guards provide for protection of property and for protection of patients, employees, and visitors. Any disturbance in the hospital should be reported to security. Missing items, whether those of a patient, visitor, or employee, are reported and investigated by the security department.

Training and Development

Employees have an orientation period, when hired, to acquaint them with the hospital's philosophy, background, and procedures. The training and development department assumes the responsibility for this orientation. The department also conducts continuing education classes to keep employees up-to-date on new developments.

NURSING SERVICES

The nursing department conducts the care of the patient and implements the doctors' orders. There are many points of care that are basic to the comfort of the patient that the nursing staff does without specific orders. A registered nurse (RN) has completed a course of study in a three-year hospital-based diploma program or a two-year college associate degree program or a four-year college Bachelor of Science in Nursing program and has passed a state examination for licensure. A licensed practical nurse (LPN) or a vocational nurse (VN) is a graduate of an approved program and has passed a state examination. Programs for practical or vocational nurses are usually one year. Nursing assistants (NAs) may have completed a training program or may have on-the-job training at a hospital. Most states issue a certificate to graduates of a Nursing Assistant program. Technicians (Techs) may be trained in many different areas and may be graduates of a program or be trained on-the-job. Techs do specialized work in the operating room, the emergency room, day surgery unit, orthopedic unit, and cardiology testing department.

Director of Nurses

The director of nursing services is an RN with an advanced degree. He/she is responsible for all nursing administrative duties and reports to the Administrator.

Assistant Directors

The number of assistants depends on the size of the hospital and the budget. Assistant directors may be called supervisors. Each assistant will have specified areas to supervise and will assist the head nurses of those areas, see seriously ill patients, and help with work schedules. All assistants assist the director with administrative duties and report to him/her.

Staff Development

A group of RNs conduct classes to make sure that RNs, LPNs, NAs, Techs, and Unit Secretaries are aware of new developments in their field. Many states require that RNs and LPNs acquire a specified number of hours in continuing education credit for licensure renewal. A hospital may assume some responsibility for this education. The classes which are conducted are approved for credit and are considered as duty time.

Unit Management

There are many clerical tasks connected with patient care. Each hospital has their own philosophy on the duties of the Unit Management Department. Basically, this department assumes the clerical tasks of each unit in order to free the nursing personnel for actual nursing duties. This usually includes

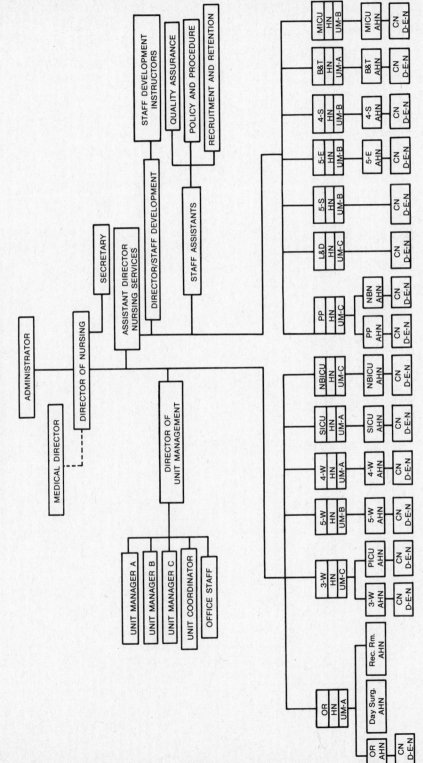

Figure 2-14. Nursing Organizational Chart.

supervising the unit secretaries, helping with budget planning, helping security with reports of missing items, and orienting new employees to the clerical duties of a unit.

Nurse Specialists

Each patient care category may employ an RN with special training. This individual acts as a consultant for the unit personnel and aids in the care of patients. The hospital may have a medical specialist who works on the medical unit, in the CCU (Coronary Care Unit), and with the medical patients in the ICU (Intensive Care Unit), a pediatric specialist who works on the Pediatric Unit, and a surgical specialist who works with all the surgical patients.

The epidemiology RN checks all infections that exist in the hospital, conducts studies to determine if the environment of the hospital contributes to disease, assists doctors in setting standards for prevention of infections, and assists the nursing staff in isolation techniques. Infections are reported to the state health agencies when necessary.

Head Nurse

The head nurse assumes responsibility for the overall function of a nursing unit. He/she supervises the unit staff, sees each patient daily, discusses patient care with doctors and staff, conducts staff meetings, assists with orientation of new unit employees, hires, counsels, and terminates employees, compiles the unit budget, and completes a work schedule for unit employees.

Staff Nurse

A staff nurse may be an RN or an LPN. The duties of each depend on the type of nursing care system the hospital is using. **Team nursing** is a system which divides the patients into groups or teams with an RN or an LPN as the team leader. The team leader is responsible for everything that happens to each patient during a shift. All members of the team are responsible to the team leader. LPNs may be assigned patients, or they may be assigned the task of giving all medications except intravenous ones to all the patients on the team. NAs and Techs do bedside patient care.

Total patient care is a system in which an RN or LPN is assigned only a few patients and performs all the care for those patients. NAs and Techs are not utilized in this type of a system. The RN performs all the bedside care and distributes medications. In addition, she/he supervises all the activities of the patient so that tests and other treatments are correlated, consults with the doctors concerning problems and reactions to treatment, assists the other departments in their treatments of the patient, and explains the treatment to the family.

Primary nursing care is a system in which an RN is assigned to a patient when the patient is admitted; the RN is responsible for the care of that patient for the full 24 hours each day until that patient is discharged. The primary nurse supervises the other RNs who care for the patient, sees the patient each day, acts as a patient advocate, consults with the doctors concerning the care, and correlates all the treatment the patient receives. Patients consider a primary nurse "their" nurse just as a doctor is "their" doctor.

Nursing Assistant

NAs help with the physical aspect of patient care. They give baths, help patients walk, and do simple treatments. Since they are in closer contact with the patient for longer periods of time, they are helpful in reporting any change in the patient's condition or behaviour.

Unit Secretaries

The job description for unit secretaries was discussed in Chapter 1. The head nurse is the immediate supervisor, unit management is an indirect supervisor, and all RNs on the unit act as supervisors when necessary.

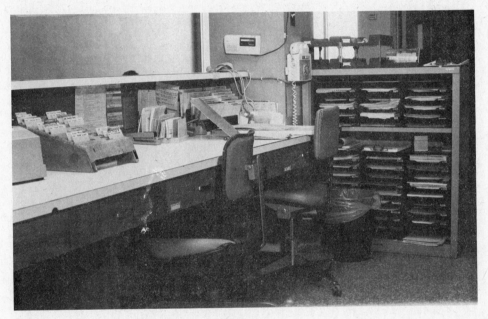

Figure 2-15. Secretary Section of a Nursing Station.

Nursing Units

A nursing unit consists of a number of patient rooms, a nursing station, a medication room, a place for doctors to use the dictaphone and review charts, a conference room, tub and shower rooms for patients, a clean utility room for supplies, a dirty utility room for used supplies, bathrooms for employees and visitors, and a waiting room for visitors.

The nursing station contains a desk for all the supplies and equipment needed by the unit secretary. The telephone, addressograph machine, chart rack, intercommunication device, and all paper supplies are easily accessible. The medication room and the area for the dictaphone are a part of the nursing station.

Nursing units are designated by numbers and location such as 4-West, 4-South, and each unit cares for a specific type of patient.

Day surgery unit (DSU), ambulatory surgery unit (ASU), out-patient surgery (OPS) are units caring for patients having minor surgery or examinations which require careful monitoring. RNs and LPNs in this area prepare the patient for surgery, assist with the surgery or examination, and monitor recovery from anesthesia. The patient arrives in the morning and goes home that afternoon. If the surgery proves to be more complicated than expected, the patient will be admitted to the hospital as an in-house patient.

Emergency room (ER) is equipped to care for all types of emergency cases. There will be an admitting desk, a conference room, and a number of examining rooms. A doctor will be on duty and do urgent care before calling the patient's private physician. A patient may be treated and released or may have to be admitted to the hospital.

Eye, ear, nose and throat unit (EENT) takes care of medical and surgical patients with problems involving either the eye, ear, nose, or throat or a combination of any of those structures. Doctors using this area have various titles:

- *Laryngologist* specializes in diseases of the throat, particularly the voice-box (larynx).
- *Opthalmologist* specializes in care of the eye.
- *Otologist* specializes in care of the ears.
- *Otorhinolaryngologist* specializes in care of the ear, nose and throat.
- *Rhinologist* specializes in care of the nose.

Genito-urinary (GU) unit cares for patients with problems of the urinary system and reproductive-urinary system combined in the male patients. Doctors specializing in this field are *urologists*.

Gynecology (GYN) unit treats females with reproductive system problems. Gynecologists are doctors who specialize in this field.

Intensive care unit (ICU) cares for either medical or surgical cases that need constant, intense care. The RNs and LPNs in this area have additional training. Any doctor may use this unit.

Medical unit contains all types of illnesses, acute and chronic. Medical doctors specialize in many areas with titles such as:

- *Allergists* treat illnesses due to sensitivity to a substance.
- *Cardiologists* diagnose and treat diseases of the heart and the blood vessels.
- *Dermatologists* deal with problems of the skin.
- *Endocrinologists* diagnose and treat diseases of glands that produce an internal secretion (endocrine glands).
- *Family practice* includes all types of illnesses and all ages.
- *Gastroenterologists* specialize in diseases of the esophagus, stomach, intestines, liver, gallbladder, and pancreas.
- *Hematologists* diagnose and treat diseases of the blood.
- *Internal medicine* includes problems of the circulatory, respiratory, endocrine, and gastrointestinal systems.

- *Pulmonary specialists* diagnose and treat diseases of the respiratory system.

Coronary Care Unit (CCU) is a special medical unit that cares for patients who need constant monitoring of their heart activity. RNs and LPNs in this unit have additional training. The unit may have *Monitor Techs* who watch the heart monitors and report abnormal activity to the nursing staff.

Neurological Unit cares for patients with problems of the brain, spinal cord, and nerves (the nervous system).
- *Neurologists* treat medical problems of the nervous system.
- *Neurosurgeons* perform surgery on the nervous system.

Obstetrics (OB) and **newborn nursery (NBN)** are combined units to care for the mother during labor, during delivery, following delivery including care for the infant. Gynecology and obstetrics are usually combined. *Obstetricians* care for the mother; *pediatricians* care for the infant.

Oncology cares for patients who have cancer. Patients may be medical or surgical. *Oncologists* specialize in diagnosis and treatment of cancer.

Orthopedics cares for patients with musculoskeletal problems. The patient may have broken bones or may have a medical problem that interferes with movement of muscles and bones. An *orthopedic surgeon* performs surgery on the musculoskeletal system.

Pediatrics cares for infants and children up to age 16. Patients may be medical or surgical. *Pediatricians* care for infants and children.

Rehabilitation unit cares for patients needing long-term physical and occupational therapy. These patients may have orthopedic or neurological problems. A *physiatrist* is a doctor who treats disease by physical means.

Surgical units may have a variety of cases including surgery of blood vessels, respiratory system, gastrointestinal system, endocrine system, and breast surgery.

- A *cardiovascular surgeon* performs surgery on the heart and blood vessels.
- A *general surgeon* operates on the organs of the digestive system, hernias (ruptured muscles), the breasts, and may do surgery on the female reproductive system.
- The *thoracic surgeon* does surgery on structures in the chest, except the heart and blood vessels.
- A *vascular surgeon* deals with surgeries of blood vessels.
- A *plastic surgeon* does reconstructive work to correct deformities, repair injuries, correct congenital defects and for cosmetic purposes.

Surgery section consists of a holding area, the operating room, and a recovery room.

- The *holding area* receives the patient from the unit, checks to make sure all the pre-operative orders have been followed, may do the surgical prep (shaving and cleansing an area), checks for proper patient identification, and observes the patient until the operating room is ready for the patient.

- The *operating room* is where the actual surgery takes place. RNs, LPNs and Techs have additional training for this area. When the surgery is completed, the patient is taken to the recovery room.

- The *recovery room* monitors the patient until he/she is fully reacted from the anesthetic. The anesthetist then checks the patient and okays the return to the unit room. An RN or LPN will telephone a report to the unit regarding the patient's condition. Some hospitals allow secretaries to receive this report, others have RNs or LPNs receive the report. There is a special sheet on which to record the report so the information may be relayed to the unit personnel responsible for that patient. When the patient arrives on the unit, one of the nursing staff accompanies the patient to the room and checks their condition after transferring them to the bed in the room.

PATIENT ROOMS

Figure 2-16 shows a photograph of a private room. Private rooms are designated by a number, usually the first number is the floor level such as 315, 420, 743, etc. Semi-private rooms and wards containing several beds designate the beds according to hospital policy. One method is to use the numbers 1, 2, 3, 4 after the room number so the full number reads 315-1, 315-2 according to the location of the bed in the room.

Most rooms have a bathroom, at least a commode and a lavatory. There is a clothes closet for the patient's belongings. In nonprivate rooms, the closets will be marked as to which one corresponds to which bed. The beds are electrically controlled so the entire bed may be positioned differently—the head and the knees are adjustable. The controls for the bed are attached to the bed frame by a holder or clamp. The overbed table is for food trays and whatever use the patient may want while sitting in bed. The water pitcher and cup are kept within reach of the patient. Television controls and systems for calling a nurse are different in each hospital. The overhead light may be any of various types. There may be a small lamp attached to a movable arm for use during examinations. Cabinets for supplies used routinely are under the lavatory or in a convenient portion of the room.

Telephones are usually supplied for the patient's convenience. The bedside stand serves as a holder for the telephone. Items such as a wash basin, bedpan, urinal, and emesis basin are kept inside the stand. There will be a drawer for cosmetics or shaving supplies.

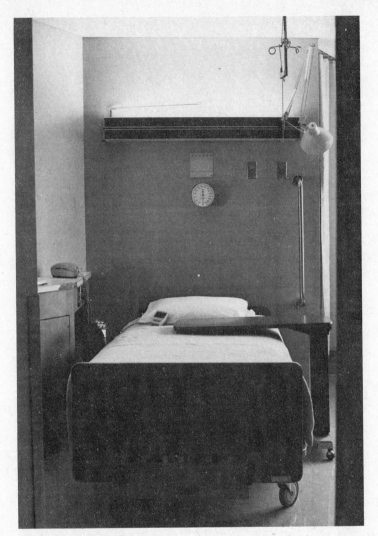

Figure 2-16. Patient Room.

REVIEW QUESTIONS

1. The _____department uses radioactive material before scanning procedures.
2. You are directly supervised by the _____.
3. Patients are taught procedures for their care after discharge by the _____department.
4. Medications are supplied by the _____.
5. Patients' bills are handled by the _____.
6. The first department the patient usually comes in contact with is the _____.

7. Blood examinations are conducted by the _____.
8. Routine x-rays are taken in the _____department.
9. Examinations of the heart are done in the _____.
10. Newspapers and other news media obtain information from the _____.
11. Applications for jobs are submitted to the _____.
12. Equipment for the hospital is ordered by the _____.
13. Meals are served by the _____.
14. When you need an isolation cart, you call the _____ department.
15. A doctor is needed immediately. How do you find one? _____.
16. Treating patients by physical means is done by the _____.
17. You need a special tray for a spinal puncture examination. You obtain it from the _____.
18. The _____sets the policies for the hospital.
19. A head nurse needs help with counseling for disciplinary problems involving one of her staff. She asks the _____to assist her.
20. The _____determines the treatment for patients.
21. A patient becomes very unruly and the nurses cannot control the patient. What do you do? _____.
22. You have a terrific idea for an educational class for all unit secretaries. Who would you ask to conduct the class? _____.
23. The _____is responsible for the overall operation of the hospital and maintains the policies and standards.
24. Departments are supervised by _____who report to the _____.
25. Requisitions are different for each department; however, all requisitions must be _____by you.

Situational Application

Apply the knowledge gained from this chapter to the following situations Circle the letter in front of the appropriate action.

26. A newspaper reporter calls and asks for information concerning a patient who holds a prominent political office. You would
   a. Refer the reporter to the head nurse
   b. Give the information requested
   c. Refer the reporter to the public relations officer.

27. A person stops at your desk and states that he is supposed to have some breathing tests and has forgotten where the Out Patient Clinic told him to report for the tests. You direct the person to the
    a. Respiratory therapy department
    b. Cardiology lab
    c. Rehabilitation department.

28. A visitor inquires about a patient who is not on your patient roster. You would
    a. Tell the visitor to go to the next floor
    b. Tell the visitor that you don't have that patient and go on with your work
    c. Call the Information Desk, locate the patient, and direct the visitor to the correct unit.

29. A patient's neighbor comes to the desk and tells you that the patient has no family and wonders what can be done to obtain help for the patient when she goes home.
    a. Advise the neighbor that you will relay the information to the Head Nurse who will probably contact the Home Health Care Department
    b. Say you will leave a note on the chart for the doctor with that information
    c. Tell the neighbor she will have to find someone or the patient will have to find someone herself

30. A patient's family tells you that the patient will need financial help to take care of the hospital bill. You would
    a. Tell them you can do nothing about their problem
    b. Ask them to wait while you find the Head Nurse so she may discuss the situation and contact the Social Services Department
    c. Call the Social Services Department yourself

Chapter 3 | Communication

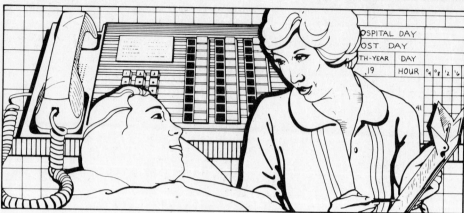

OBJECTIVES

After careful study of this chapter, you will be able to:

1. Discuss the meaning of communication.
2. List the steps in giving and receiving a message.
3. Use a telephone effectively.
4. Use an addressograph machine.
5. Use an intercommunication device.
6. Use a tube system.
7. Use a dumbwaiter.
8. Explain the function of the kardex.
9. Explain the uses of the unit blackboard.
10. Explain the use of assignment sheets.
11. Explain the use of the communication notebook.
12. Discuss points to keep in mind when communicating with patients.
13. Discuss how communication builds good interpersonal relationships.
14. Discuss the importance of body language.

Communication is defined by Webster as "the art of delivering, conferring or imparting knowledge, opinion or fact." This tells us that someone is **giving the message,** and that someone is **receiving the message.** What it does not tell us is the difficulty involved in **clarifying the message**—making sure the message is understood. If you do not listen attentively, you will not understand a message. If you do not speak distinctly and concisely when giving a message, the receiver will not understand the message.

In a hospital setting, the person giving the message must:

- Identify herself/himself
- Identify the hospital if necessary
- Identify the unit
- Identify the person to whom the message is to be delivered
- Give the message in simple language and make sure the message is understood.

The receiver of the message must:

1. *Write* down:
   - The name of the person or department calling
   - The name of the person for whom the message is intended
   - The message itself
2. Repeat the message to check accuracy
3. Give the message to the correct person.

Messages must be written, there is too much activity to try to remember everything. In summary, three different devices help with communication: giving a message, receiving a message, and clarifying a message.

Giving a message:

"I would like to speak to a member of Ida Stuart's family, please. This is the secretary on 7 East at _____Hospital."

"I am Ida's mother."

"The doctor caring for Ida, Dr. Mason, would like for you to call him at his office before 11 A.M. today. I have the number if you want to write it down. The number is 216-7803. That is Dr. Mason at number 216-7803."

Wait for the person to reply before hanging up.

Relaying a message after writing it:

"Joan, x-ray called and would like to have Ruth Atkins returned to x-ray at 1:30 P.M. for some follow-up work. I told them she would be through with her treatments by then. Is that alright with you?"

"Yes, I will have her there."

"Good. I won't have to call them back."

Receiving a message:

Special forms or blank sheets can be used to record a message. Do so in the following manner:

Nursing office called—Mary Lemar, LPN on 3–11 is ill, 3-North will send a replacement. (11:45)

For—Head nurse.

Be sure the head nurse receives the message. If it needs to be recorded on the work schedule, do so immediately. Write messages as you hear them over the phone and fill in the name of the person for whom the message is intended and the time you received the message. Repeat the message to the caller to check accuracy.

TELEPHONE

The telephone is the most frequently used communication device. Figure 3-1 shows a telephone system that contains several outside lines, a hold button, a button for transferring calls to other phones on the unit and to other departments or to a patient's room, and direct lines to all the hospital departments. The direct line button is depressed instead of dialing to connect you to a department. The system shown in the photograph would be located at the unit secretary's desk. Other phones on the unit would contain only the outside lines and a hold button. Some telephones have a computer-like entry feature to enter bed availability and to automatically transfer calls when a patient is moved from one room to another. Your instructor will demonstrate the use of the system you will be using.

The "Dial a Doc" index (Figure 3-1) is a quick telephone directory for the doctors on the staff. Individual cards arranged alphabetically contain the name of the doctor, the specialty of practice, the office phone number, and the answering service phone number.

Using the Hold Button

To place a person on hold—ask their permission, depress the hold button, and hang up. Be sure to remember who is on which line. The light designating a line on hold flashes at a faster frequency than the light designating an incoming call. All available lines may be on hold at the same time. Even if you think you remember who is on which line, when you return to a line, identify the caller again.

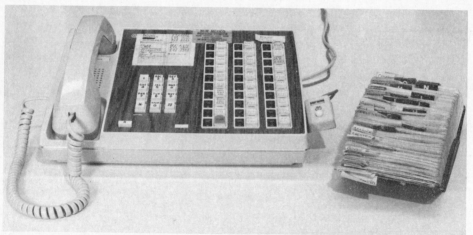

Figure 3-1. Telephone System with "Dial a Doc" File (Courtesy of Mountain Bell).

The following examples of how to handle calls will help you practice in the classroom.

Answering Calls

Greeting the caller:
"4 West, Unit Secretary Ann, may I help you?"
"_____ Hospital, 4 West, Secretary Ann speaking."
"4 West, student secretary, may I help you?" Some hospitals prefer that you answer in this manner while still a student. It identifies you more than your name and saves time.
Clarifying the message:
"Would you repeat that, please?"

"I'm sorry, I did not understand the name. Would you repeat it, please?"

"Would you spell that for me, please?"

If called person is busy:

"Ms. Allen is busy and cannot come to the phone. May I take a message, or may someone else help you?"

"Ms. Allen is unable to talk with you just now. May I have her call you, or would you like to call back?"

When called person is not on unit:

"Ms. Allen is in a meeting and is expected back at (state time)."

"Ms. Allen is in a workshop and cannot be reached. May someone else help you?"

"Ms. Allen is not on duty today. May someone else help you?" Do not give home phone numbers of employees to anyone. If it is an emergency, the secretary in the nursing office will help the caller.

"Ms. Allen is at lunch. Shall I page her or may I give her a message when she returns?"

When leaving line to obtain information:

"Would you mind waiting while I check?"

"I'm sorry, I do not have that information. Will you hold, please, while I find someone who can help you?" Always give the caller some satisfaction. Do not say "I do not know," and dismiss them.

"It will take a few minutes to find that information. Would you like to hold, or may I call you back?"

Acknowledging a request:

"I will be glad to give Ms. Allen the message."

"Yes, Mr. Cole, I will be happy to do that for you."

"You are welcome. I'm glad I could help."

Completing the conversation:

"Thank you for calling, Mr. Cole."

"You are welcome. Good-bye." Avoid "Bye-bye," "That's ok," or "So long."

Calling outside the hospital:

Have all the information you will need to complete the call in front of you before you dial. Suppose you need to call for a back brace for a patient. Have the chart in front of you and then dial the shop. The shop answers, "Orthopedic Appliance Shop, Mr. Thomas."

You reply, "This is _____Hospital, 4 South, Unit Secretary Anne. Dr. Brown has ordered a back brace for Antonio Marcel in Room 422."

The shop may ask for the patient's home address, home phone number, place of employment, and name of hospitalization insurance company. Since you have the chart in front of you, it is easy to give the information quickly.

Mr. Thomas then says, "Someone will be there this afternoon."

You respond, "Thank you. I will tell Mr. Marcel that you will be here." Hang up. Record the time called on the Physician's Order sheet and tell Mr. Marcel's nurse so she may explain to the patient.

Calling inside the hospital:

A doctor arrives on the unit and asks for a lab report that has not been filed on the patient's chart. You call the lab:

"Laboratory, this is Mary, may I help you?"

"Mary, this is Pat on 5 West. Dr. Lew is on the unit and needs the CBC report on Madeline North in Room 561." Mary finds the report and reads it to you. You record the report on the proper form, read it back to Mary for accuracy check.

"Thank you, Mary." Hang up, find Dr. Lew, and hand him the report.

Telephone Manners

Use the phone in the classroom enough so that you feel comfortable in all types of situations. There will be times when you answer the phone at work and the caller reprimands you for something about which you know absolutely nothing. But just because someone else has forgotten their manners, don't forget yours. Remain cool and ask the person to start from the beginning so that you may help him/her. If you remain calm and keep your voice pleasant at such stressful times, the other person usually calms down and responds in kind. Do not let personal feelings interfere with your professional performance.

PAGING SYSTEMS

The **loudspeaker** is a commonly used type of paging system. To page someone over the loudspeaker, dial the switchboard operator and ask that (name of person) be paged. Give the operator the extension number where you are or the name of the unit where you are. *Example: "Please page Dr. Moore for Intensive Care."* When you request a page, do not leave the desk. If you must leave, tell someone that you are expecting an answer to a page and give them the message to be delivered. Do not keep a person answering a page waiting while someone hunts for the person requesting the page.

Silent page systems may be used. These systems utilize a vertical light panel which is placed in hallways on each unit. Key personnel will have assigned numbers which correspond to numbers built into the light panel. When the switchboard operator lights a number, the person assigned that number calls the operator for messages.

Individual pagers are small enough to fit into a pocket or hook onto a belt. Each pager has a number. The operator will dial the number causing the pager to buzz. The person carrying the pager turns it on and receives the message.

A **nurse pager** may be on each unit. This pager is a box-like machine with a row of metal-lined, hollow tubes into which a solid metal rod fits. Each tube has a number above it, and each person on the unit has a number to correspond with a tube number. A soft-toned beeper is activated when the rod is placed inside a tube and turned. The number of beeps is the same as the number above the tube. The beeps are audible in every area of the unit. Unit personnel may be called to the desk without disturbing the patients.

COMPUTERS

Because computers are great time savers, many hospital departments utilize them. The unit secretary will also use a computer—primarily to transcribe physician's orders (see Chapter 6, Transcribing Physician's Orders, for the computer's function); the secretary may also assist, or be promoted to, other departments utilizing them. The specific role the computer plays in other departments is discussed below.

Admitting enters identifying information into the computer when they are notified that a patient will be admitted. Additions to this data base are an ongoing process. Patient information may be retrieved at any time. For example, if a patient returns to a clinic after discharge, personal and/or medical information is easy to obtain instead of looking through a complete chart.

The **laboratory** can easily retrieve all tests on a specific patient so a consultant may review the case. Also, a cumulative lab summary provides a list of all the tests ordered for a specific day and helps to schedule the work.

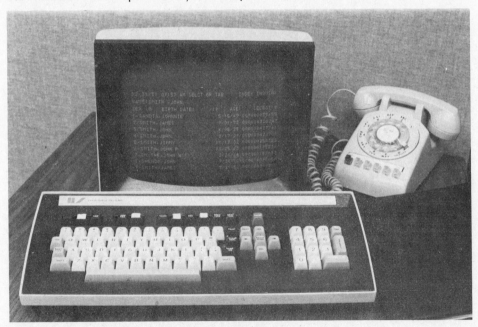

Figure 3-2. Computer Terminal *(Courtesy of Four-Phase Systems, Inc.).*

Pharmacy uses the computer to dispense patient medication records to the nurse, send charges to the business office for each patient, compile reports on drugs controlled by the Harrison Narcotic Act (see Chapter 5, Pharmacology), and schedule the work for pharmacy personnel.

Dietary can receive orders from the various units and make diet labels for trays. Printouts show diet census and other information which helps to order supplies.

Medical Records are easier to index by using a computer. Summary data such as number of deaths in a given period of time, categories of diseases including numbers for each, discharge statistics by service, total discharge statistics, operation indexing, and procedure indexing can be quickly retrieved.

ADDRESSOGRAPH MACHINE

The addressograph machine imprints the information on the addressograph card (Figure 2-13) onto hospital forms. The cards are placed in a file rack, each slot of the rack is labeled with a room number, and the rack is located near the addressograph machine.

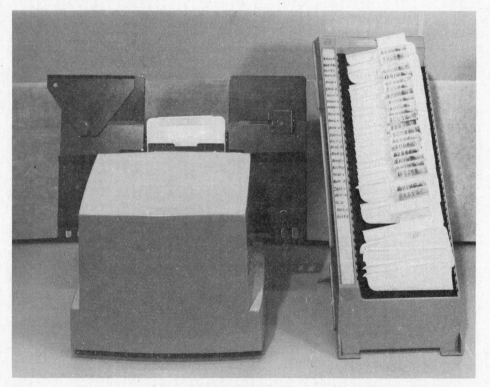

Figure 3-3. Addressograph Machine and Card Rack *(Courtesy Addressograph Farrington, Inc.).*

Your instructor will demonstrate the use of the type of machine you will be using. To use any addressograph machine, you should:

1. Be sure you have the correct addressograph card.
2. Insert the card into the machine in the receptacle provided.
3. Insert the form to be imprinted into the machine so that the addressograph space on the form is aligned with the card. The side to be imprinted

is toward the ink supply of the machine.

4. Be sure your fingers are away from the imprinting area before you activate the machine.

5. Remove the card and place it in the proper slot of the card rack when you have completed that patient's forms.

6. If you must leave the machine during the process of imprinting a number of forms, make sure the correct card is still in the machine when you return. Everyone on the unit uses the machine and someone may remove the card you were using, use another card, and leave it in the machine. Checking prevents an imprinting error which would necessitate discarding the form.

INTERCOMMUNICATION DEVICE: THE INTERCOM

The intercom allows you to:

1. Talk to patients without going into their room.

2. Locate and talk to nursing personnel. In addition to being able to locate a nurse with an intercom, you can talk with nurses when they are in conference. This causes less disturbance than going into the room.

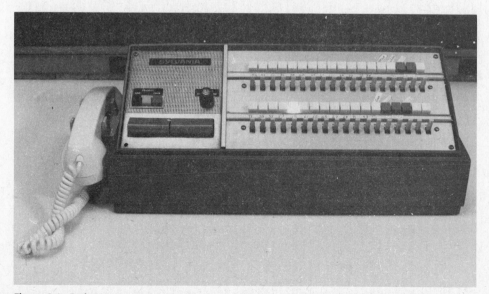

Figure 3-4. Patient Intercommunication System *(Courtesy Philips Communication and Television Systems).*

The intercom contains a receiver space for the person using it to talk into, a control switch for two-way conversation, and individual buttons for each room on the unit which you depress for connection to the room. It may have a button which opens all rooms at once for announcements in case of emergency. When a patient presses the "nurse call" control in the room, a light goes on over the door of the room and the individual button for that room on the intercom lights up as a buzzer sounds.

Answering a patient's call:

1. The buzzer tells you a patient needs assistance. The light on the intercom shows you which room is calling. Depress the lighted button.
2. Switch the control button to the **on** position and ask the patient if you may help him/her.
3. If the patient needs something you cannot provide, be sure to relay that message to someone who can. *Be careful not to discuss any confidential information on the intercom.*

Initiating a call:

1. Depress the button for the room you wish to call.
2. Switch the control to **on** and proceed as you would for a phone call. Identify the person to whom you wish to speak and identify yourself.
3. Always return the control for two-way conversation to the **off** position when you have completed a conversation. An intercom saves time and steps.

| PNEUMATIC TUBE SYSTEM

The tube system is located in the nursing station and is used to transport papers throughout the entire hospital. The system operates in the following manner:

1. Papers are placed in a tube; the tube is securely fastened.
2. Letters and/or numbers on the tube are aligned as per instructions on the system to code the tube for its destination.
3. The tube is placed in the sending compartment and the compartment is closed. The tube automatically goes to the department for which it is coded.
4. When a tube arrives on the unit, a light above the receiving unit goes on and/or a bell rings. The light goes off when the receiving unit is opened.

Some systems have a metal tube that allows small containers of medicine to be sent to the nursing units from pharmacy.

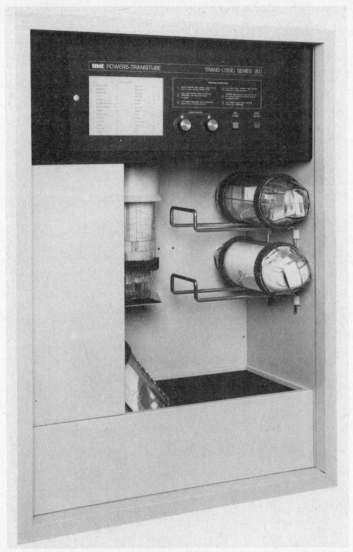

Figure 3-5. Powers-Transitube System, a Pneumatic Tube System *(Courtesy MCC Powers-Transitube, a Unit of Mark Controls Corporation).*

| DUMBWAITER

The dumbwaiter is a transport system for items other than papers, such as food or central supply items. This box-like structure travels up and down like an elevator and is usually located in a central location in a hallway convenient to all nursing stations. The dumbwaiter may transport supplies and patient trays to/from the dietary department, to/from the nursing units; it may also transport supplies to/from central supply and pharmacy. The operation of this system is simple when you follow these basic steps:

1. Place the item to be transported on the dumbwaiter. If there are des-

ignated shelves for certain departments, be sure you place the item on the correct shelf.

2. There are two doors—one opens into the hallway, the other opens the dumbwaiter. Be sure both doors are closed. BOTH MUST BE CLOSED FOR THE SYSTEM TO OPERATE.

3. The control buttons are on the wall beside the unit and are numbered according to the floors in the building. Push the appropriate floor number.

4. When something arrives on the receiving floor, a light above the dumbwaiter goes on. A corresponding light, used only for the dumbwaiter, goes on in the nursing station or the department so someone knows to remove items from the transport system. Some systems may require a telephone call from the sending department to the receiving department in place of the light signal.

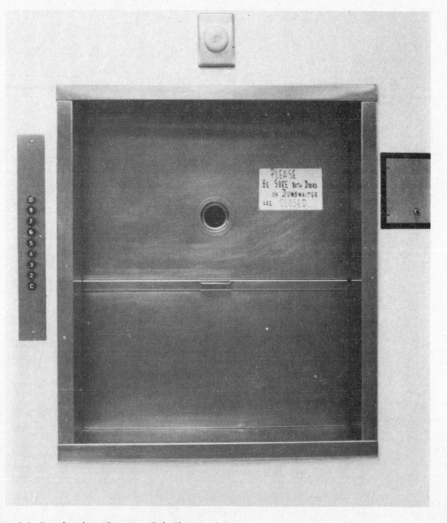

Figure 3-6. Dumbwaiter *(Courtesy Otis Elevator Co.).*

PATIENT CARE CARDS AND HOLDER

Kardex is the name commonly used for the holder and the cards that contain a record of treatment for each patient. All the unit personnel use the kardex for information about patients. It is also used to report available beds to the admitting office. Chapter 6 explains how you transfer the orders written by doctors onto the kardex cards.

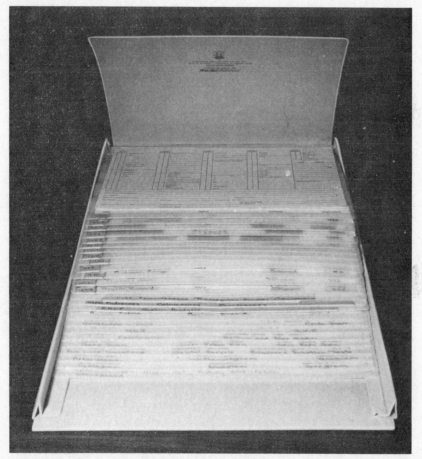

Figure 3-7. Medic-Visitray® for Patient Care Cards (Courtesy Carstens Health Industries, Inc.).

UNIT BLACKBOARD

The blackboard is used according to the preference of the Head Nurse on the unit. It is often used as a record of patient examinations for the day. Names of those patients going to surgery or to other departments for examinations are listed, including the exam and the time scheduled. When each patient returns to his/her room, the name is erased. This system provides a quick reference for all unit personnel.

Some units use the blackboard for personnel assignments. The name of each employee and his/her duty for that shift are listed. This helps the unit secretary locate personnel and gives information on who is taking care of which patient.

ASSIGNMENT SHEET

Some units do not use the blackboard for assignments. Instead, a special sheet called an assignment sheet is completed for each shift and left at the desk. There is also an assignment sheet for each nursing assistant (NA) which includes all the care each patient is to receive for that day. The NA assignment sheet is not kept at the desk, each NA keeps his/her own.

COMMUNICATION NOTEBOOK

Many secretaries keep a notebook to record messages and to remind them of a task. Telephone calls that could not be completed immediately are noted. If you called a doctor's office for some medication for a patient and the doctor was not in, keep that information in the notebook. When the doctor calls back with the information and the patient's needs are met, the notation is lined through. This serves two functions:
1. A reference for the secretary on the next shift
2. A reference which may need to be checked the next day.

PERSON TO PERSON COMMUNICATIONS

First Impressions

You may be the first person on the unit to greet new patients. First impressions are important. A friendly greeting with a cheerful smile will put the patient at ease. Each person coming into the hospital will be worried—worried about his/her illness, about the family, about the cost of the illness. Each will also have fears—fear of the unknown that they are facing, fear of how the family will cope with the situation, fear of not being in control of what is happening, fear of being considered ignorant if he/she does not understand procedures. Patients are subjected to an almost intolerable invasion of privacy. This is not the fault of the personnel, it is just the nature of the setting. You can help alleviate the worries and fears by being kind and considerate. Dispense accurate information to patients and families regarding tests and procedures. Answer all questions—if you do not know how to answer, find someone who can.

Cultural Differences

You also need to know about the different cultures in your area. You need to know how many interpreters for what languages are available. Cultural beliefs and rituals must be respected. For example:

1. You may have an elderly patient who has always eaten the food of his/her native country and will not eat any of the hospital food. You will work with the nurse, the dietitian, and the family to make sure that the patient's nutritional needs are met. The family may have to bring the food to the hospital.
2. Perhaps you have a patient whose religious belief dictates that any portion of the body that is removed surgically or for purposes of surgical preparation must be buried instead of being disposed of by the hospital. If a person with those beliefs were to have the head shaved before surgery, the hair must be saved and given to the patient's family.

Some rituals may be necessary for the welfare of the patient even though they seem out of place in the hospital. As long as the welfare of the other patients is not compromised, these rituals should be allowed. Keep these points in mind when communicating with patients.

Communicating with Unit Personnel

Good communication skills build good interpersonal relationships that are essential for the efficient functioning of a unit. Some characteristics of good interpersonal relationships are:

1. **Emotional maturity**—being able to express oneself with restraint and courtesy
2. **Dependability**—being accurate and doing your share
3. **Tact**—always consider the feelings of others
4. **Respect**—listen to others' beliefs and opinions
5. **Trustworthiness**—all information concerning patients is strictly confidential. Discussion of the information is for purposes of care and only with those involved in that care. Never carry any information regarding a patient outside the hospital. All employee information is also confidential.
6. **Acceptance of authority**—respond willingly to instructions from those supervising you
7. **Tolerance**—do not be critical of others just because they do not have your values. Everyone is entitled to their own.
8. **Sincerity**—speak honestly. If there is a problem on the unit, talk it over honestly and openly. Let others know how you feel.
9. **Professionalism**—treat others in a dignified manner. Do not ask doctors for professional advice while you are on duty. Keep your personal life and professional life separate.

BODY LANGUAGE

The way you sit at your desk, how you look at a person, and how you move tells others a great deal about you. If you slump in your chair and rest your elbow on the desk with head in hand, it tells people that you are not interested in your job. If you are talking with someone but looking off in the distance, it appears that you are not listening. If someone corrects you and you respond affirmatively verbally but toss your head in a defiant way, you are speaking louder with your body than with words.

If you are proud of your job and proud to be a part of the institution that employs you, you can show it by presenting an alert appearance. Sit up straight at your desk. Look people straight in the eye. Be careful about abrupt body movements. In conferences, try to sit in a relaxed position. Sitting with feet tightly tucked under the chair and arms folded tightly across the chest might give others the impression that you are not willing to engage in honest discussion. Watch other people and practice reading their body language so that you are more aware of your own.

To sum it all up: in every communication, be polite, prompt, helpful, courteous—and human. Ralph Waldo Emerson wrote, "Common sense is genius dressed in its working clothes." Let common sense be your guide.

REVIEW QUESTIONS

1. Define communication. _____ .
2. The steps in receiving a message are _____
   _____
   _____.
3. The steps in giving a message are _____
   _____
   _____.
4. _____ is as important as speaking.
5. You cannot answer a question so you tell the caller _____
   _____.
6. Addressograph machines are for _____purposes.
7. You can talk with a patient by using the _____.
8. To send papers to another department, you would use the _____
   _____.
9. Dietary might use the _____to send a food tray at a time other than meal time.

10. The _____ contains all the treatment information of a patient.

11. Several ethnic groups are represented by the patients on your unit. Does this fact have anything to do with their care? _____.

12. The _____ tells you what person is responsible for which patients.

13. A unit blackboard may be used for _____ or _____.

14. A _____ helps keep track of the messages in and out for the day and completion of those messages.

15. How can you communicate with a patient to put them at ease?

_____

_____.

16. List five communication skills which build good personal relationships.

_____

_____

_____

_____

_____.

17. List some ways in which body language tells others about your feelings.

_____

_____

_____.

Situational Application

Use the knowledge gained in this chapter to answer the following questions. Circle the letter in front of the correct action.

18. An employee from another unit asks to see the kardex for a patient, explaining that the patient is a friend. You would:
    a. Locate the kardex and let the employee read it
    b. Refuse to show the kardex to the employee and suggest that the employee speak with the Head Nurse for information
    c. Tell the employee you can't give the kardex to her but she can find it and look at it.

19. You have three phone lines on hold. Line one is a doctor who wants to give orders to a nurse, line two is a relative asking for information on a patient, line three is a supervisor asking to speak to the head nurse. You would complete the calls in the following sequence:
    a. Locate a nurse to take the doctor's orders, locate the head nurse (she may be in her office), and locate the nurse who is taking care

of the patient in question to talk to the relative
b. Locate the head nurse, locate a nurse to take the call from the relative, and then have the head nurse talk to the doctor when she finishes talking to the supervisor
c. Tell the head nurse you have three calls for her without explaining the type of calls.

20. One nurse on the floor is constantly asking you to do things that you feel she/he should do. You would:
    a. Have a frank talk with the nurse and tell her/him how you feel so an understanding can be reached
    b. Gripe about the situation to everyone on the floor
    c. Talk to the head nurse and ask her/him to settle the problem.

21. You answer the telephone and someone in the chemistry lab starts reprimanding you because a specimen was not handled correctly. You would:
    a. Angrily tell him/her that you know nothing about it
    b. Tell the person to relay the message to a nurse and find a nurse
    c. Very calmly tell the person that if you can have all the information (patient's name, type of specimen, when specimen was sent) you will check on it and return the call or have a nurse return the call.

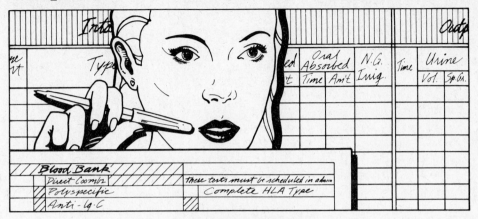

OBJECTIVES

Upon completion of study of this chapter, you will be able to:

1. Explain the purpose of a chart.
2. List some legal points regarding charts.
3. Know where to locate information in the chart.
4. List the standard forms for a chart.
5. List some of the supplementary forms for a chart.

A patient's chart is a record of everything that happens to the patient during the time of hospitalization. The chart protects the patient, the doctor, and the nursing personnel by the factual report of all activities of the patient and all the treatments received by the patient.

The chart is the property of the hospital. It is a legal document and can be entered as evidence in the courtroom. The chart should never be taken from the hospital except in cases where it is evidence in a trial.

An increasing number of states have statutes that allow the patient to see the chart. If no statute exists, the medical staff and the medical records department may establish guidelines in regard to permission to see the chart.

Since the chart is a legal document, no erasures are allowed at any time on any form. Mistakes are corrected by drawing a line in ink through the mistake, signing and dating the correction, and then making the correct statement. Black ink is used so that the forms may be photocopied. Some hospitals may use two colors to denote different times, the colors are usually black and red. Blue will not photocopy.

Many states have a privileged communication statute which protects the privacy of information in a chart. Even if no statute exists, the patient has a right to confidentiality. It is universally accepted that confidential material is furnished only on the written authority of the patient, the patient's guardian if the patient is a minor, the patient's committee if the patient has been judged insane, or the representative of the patient's estate if the patient is deceased. If a patient is unable to give consent and information in the chart is vital to the welfare of that patient, the proper officer of the hospital may assume responsibility for the release of information. Information is usually given in the form of photo-copies. Consent is not needed where information is to be reported by law (i.e., venereal and contagious diseases are reported to health agencies, wounds caused by criminal acts are reported to the police, and child abuse cases are reported to the police).

A patient may request that his/her record be amended. This is accomplished by a notation being made at the end of the chart which states the change and that the patient requested the change. The patient must explain the request if the chart is used in court.

Incident and accident reports during hospitalization are not a part of the record. These are not allowed to be used as evidence in a trial as they constitute hearsay evidence.

Local laws dictate how long the records must be kept.

The Joint Commission on Accreditation of Hospitals have the following rules for charts but do not dictate the types of forms a hospital must use:

1. There must be an accurate and complete medical record on all patients.
2. Charts must be filed in an accessible place in the hospital.
3. Complete records should include:
   - Patient identification
   - Sociological data
   - Physical examination
   - Special exams such as laboratory and x-ray
   - Provisional diagnosis
   - Medical or surgical treatment
   - Pathological findings
   - Progress notes
   - Final diagnosis
   - Condition on discharge
   - Follow-up plan
   - Autopsy findings when applicable

CHART BACKS

Charts are kept in holders ordinarily referred to as chart backs. These may be plastic or metal and may open like a tablet or like a loose-leaf notebook. The patient's name and the name of the doctor will be written on strips of paper and inserted into the slot at the top of the chart back. Some charts have slots at both ends. A unit may designate different colors for different doctors; if so, there will be a list at the desk as to which color is for which doctor. The colored strips are easily seen and doctors can more readily identify the charts of their patients.

The charts are filed in a chart rack when not in use. The chart rack may be stationary or mobile.

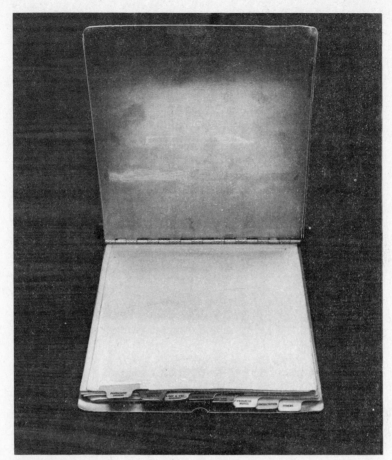

Figure 4-1. Patient Chart Back.

CHART FORMS

Chart forms are referred to as **standard** and **supplementary**. The standard forms are used for all patients. Supplementary forms are used for specific reasons in specific cases. Standard forms include:

1. Identification Sheet or Face Sheet
2. Physician's Order Sheet
3. Progress Notes
4. History and Physical
5. Graphic Sheet
6. Admission Summary
7. Nurse's Notes
8. Laboratory Sheets

Standard forms for surgery include:

1. Surgical Consent

2. Pre-op Checklist
3. Pre and Post Anesthesia Record

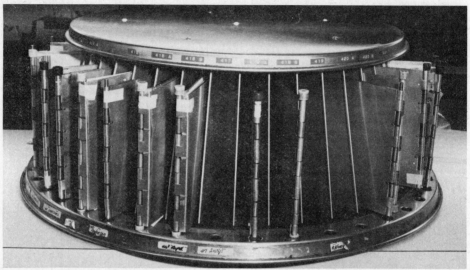

Figure 4-2. Roto Chart Caddy *(Courtesy Carstens Health Industries, Inc.).*

Standard Forms

Identification Sheet

This may be called the Face Sheet and is placed at the beginning of the chart. Admitting completes the information when the patient is admitted. The sheet contains the patient's name, address, telephone number, nearest of kin with their address and telephone number, type of insurance, place of employment, birthdate, diagnosis, the name of the admitting physician, date and time of admission. This sheet is a reference whenever you need to call an outside agency to arrange for services. Discharge information is entered by the doctor at the time of discharge.

Physician's Order Sheet

The physician writes the tests, treatment, and medications the patient is to receive on an order sheet. You will transfer the orders to requisitions, medication and treatment cards, and to a kardex card.

By law, the doctor is required to sign all orders. Telephone orders (TO) and verbal orders (VO) should be signed the next time the doctor visits the patient. Medical Records requires that the chart be completed in every detail within so many hours after the patient is discharged. Doctors are reminded of omissions by the MR department.

The sheets have self-carbons so that a copy may be sent to the pharmacy for their use in filling medication orders. It is your responsibility to see that each chart has sufficient space on the sheet for orders to be written. An extra blank sheet may be inserted and folded up to reveal the partially used one beneath it. This assures adequate writing space in case several doctors see the patient and each writes orders.

Progress Notes

It is the responsibility of the doctor to record the condition of the patient daily. If the patient is seen more than once a day, the doctor should record it more often. One of the methods used for writing progress notes is called SOAPing:

- **S** stands for symptoms and records what the patient tells the doctor about how he/she feels
- **O** is for observation—what the doctor sees and finds on physical examination
- **A** is assessment and consists of the conclusions regarding the patient's condition after tests and observation since the last visit
- **P** is for plan—what the doctor intends to do for the patient's problems.

This shows that the doctor is aware of everything happening to the patient and is doing everything possible to restore that patient to the best possible condition.

Other health workers may use the progress notes to notify the doctor of what they are doing for the patient. The dietitian may make notes on how the patient is responding to diet and instructions, the Social Services personnel may write what the department is doing to help the financial situation of the patient, and Home Health Care may write about their efforts to place the patient in a nursing home or other facility.

History and Physical Form

The doctor may either write on these forms or dictate the information and MR department will type it and place it on the chart.

A medical history of the patient and the patient's family is obtained. If the patient is unable to give a history, the doctor may talk to a family member.

The physical consists of the actual findings during a physical examination. Each part of the body is examined.

The Short Form is a very brief history and the physical exam may be only a heart and lung check plus examination of whatever body part caused the hospitalization.

Graphic Sheet

Temperature, pulse, respirations, and blood pressure are called **vital signs.** They are recorded when the patient is admitted and at routine times unless the doctor specifies differently. The vital signs are recorded as a graph so variations may be seen quickly.

Whether the unit secretary or the nursing assistants chart the vital signs depends on the rules of the hospital. Your instructor will show you how to graph if that is one of your responsibilities. The vital signs may be either written on a patient list sheet, or each of the nursing personnel may have a list of only assigned patients.

The sheet may contain other information such as weight and a space for recording the number of bowel movements the patient has.

Admission Summary

This is a record of the patient's admission. An NA or a RN (according to the rules of the hospital) records information regarding the patient:

- Why the patient is being hospitalized
- How the patient feels
- What medications the patient is taking routinely
- The mental status of the patient
- If patient has eye glasses or dentures
- What allergies to medication and food the patient has
- By what means the patient arrived on the unit

The NA may complete the routine summary, and the RN may do a complete physical assessment which would be recorded on another form.

This is omitted if the patient arrives on the unit from the RR. The nursing notes constitute the admission in that case.

Nurse's Notes

The hospital's medical staff and nursing staff develop policies concerning the type and extent of nursing notes to be kept. The Joint Commission on Accreditation of Hospitals has no list of standards. Items that need inclusion for legal evidence are:

1. Doctor's visits should be recorded
2. Method of admission—ambulatory, wheelchair, stretcher, ambulance
3. Complete description of patient's condition on arrival and on discharge
4. Vital signs on admission
5. Record of routine and special procedures
6. Medications, dosage and mode, times given, and by whom
7. Objective signs and subjective symptoms
8. Changes in appearance and mental condition
9. Complaints of the patient
10. Signature of nurse or person charting.

Who may chart on the Nurse's Notes is a matter of individual hospital policy. If the hospital where you will work allows unit secretaries to chart, some of the things you would record are:

1. Time, destination, and mode of transportation when a patient leaves the unit
2. Time of patient's return to the unit
3. Notification of a telephone call to a family member for which the doctor had written an order.

Medication Record

The medication record is quite often on the back of the graphic sheet. Medications are written as ordered and the person giving the medication records the time and signs his/her initials beside the time. The sheet has a space for the full name of the person giving the medications on each shift.

You will record the orders if the hospital is using the Medication Administration Record (MAR) method instead of medication cards.

Laboratory Sheets

The majority of hospitals have two or more blank sheets on which laboratory requisitions are attached after completion of the tests. There is usually one for hematology tests and one for other tests. The filing is started at the bottom of the page and new ones are placed on top so that the most recent one is visible.

Surgical Forms

Operative Permit

The patient must sign a permit before the surgery can be performed. The permit must be without error—no mistakes are allowed to be corrected and abbreviations may not be used. The doctor writes the order for the permit with the name of the procedure. Do not depend on the order to have correct spelling. If there is any doubt, use the dictionary. Doctors may use abbreviations on the order sheet but you *must* use the complete word on the permit. A hospital may use one form for all surgical and diagnostic procedures, or there may be a special permit for several types of surgeries and a special one for each diagnostic procedure.

The age of majority or consent is 18 by law in many states; if no statute exists, common law sets the age of consent at 21.

Unit secretaries are not allowed to witness the signing of a surgical permit since they are not qualified to answer any and all questions the patient may wish to ask regarding the procedure.

Preoperative Checklist

The checklist insures that the chart is in proper order and that the patient is properly prepared for surgery. You are responsible for the section regarding the chart. The RN who is in charge of the patient for that day is responsible for the completion of the rest of the checklist.

Pre and Post Anesthesia Record

Your responsibility is to addressograph the sheet. The anesthesiologist visits the patient the evening before surgery to talk about allergies and past experience with anesthesia. An explanation of what will take place in the operating room and in the recovery room is given to the patient. Someone from anesthesia visits the patient the day after surgery to make sure there are no problems related to the anesthesia.

Anesthesia Record

This form is placed in the chart in the holding area. The anesthesiologist charts all drugs given to the patient and graphs the vital signs before and during the surgery. The condition of the patient following surgery is noted. Become familiar with this form so you can see what drugs the patient had if you are requested to relay that information.

Recovery Room Record

The holding area also places this form on the chart. The nurses in the recovery room chart the arrival of the patient, the type of IV if one is running, and the patient's condition; they also check the VS as ordered. When the patient is reacted from the anesthesia, an anesthesiologist will check and release the patient. You will use this form to transcribe the VS order on the chart when the patient is received on the unit. If the order reads *VS every 15 minutes for 1 hr then every 30 minutes for 2 hrs, then every hour till stable,* you can see how much of that order has already been completed.

O.R. Record Slip

An RN in the operating room keeps a record of the exact surgery performed, the names of the doctors and nurses doing the surgery, positioning of the patient, sponge count, and type of drains inserted. You will use this form to copy the exact surgical procedure onto the kardex card.

Supplementary Forms

Anticoagulant Flow Sheet

Blood coagulation studies are performed daily when a patient is first given anticoagulants. The tests' results are recorded and the anticoagulant dose is recorded so the doctor may see the changes and correlate the test results with the drug dosage.

Consents

The usual approach is to have the patient sign a consent for treatment when admitted. This constitutes an informal consent for each laboratory test, each drug administration, and each treatment considered routine.

Admitting also has the patient sign a permit for release of information to the patient's insurance company for payment.

Other consents are for examinations or procedures with a risk involved, for taking before and after photographs for reference, use of investigational drugs, and experimental procedures.

Consents for emergency situations may be signed by two doctors when the patient is unable to sign and there are no relatives available to assume the responsibility of signing. A telephoned consent from a family member may be obtained if a physician and a nurse or two nurses witness the call and both sign the consent form verifying that the emergency exists and the family member has stated that the doctors may have permission to perform the necessary procedure or surgery.

Consultations

A doctor who is called in by another doctor as a consultant will probably dictate his/her findings and the transcriptionists in MR type the report and place it in the chart. The consultant may make a brief note on the Progress Notes to relay information to the admitting doctor immediately.

Forms are filed according to date when more than one consultant is called on the case.

Departmental Therapy Reports

Each department that gives treatments has a special form on which to record the treatment and the patient's reaction to the treatment. Departments using forms for charts would be Physical Therapy, Occupational Therapy, Respiratory Therapy, and Radiation Therapy.

Diabetic Record

Patients who have diabetes will have urine or blood tests at certain times. The tests help the doctor to decide how much insulin the patient needs. The test results, time of test, insulin dosage, type of insulin, time insulin is given, and site of injection are recorded so all pertinent information is in one place.

Fluid Balance Sheet

Knowing exactly how much fluid is taken into the body and by what route it is taken and knowing exactly the amount lost by the body and by what route the fluid is lost are extremely important in a variety of illnesses. The nurses and nursing assistants keep a running record of fluid balance at the bedside and transfer the information to the chart form at the end of each eight hour shift.

Laboratory Flow Sheet

Special units such as ICU, CCU, and SAC use a laboratory flow sheet to chart lab results. With this form, the doctor may see all the tests which have been performed instead of looking at several different sheets. Patients who are very ill may have lab work performed several times a day. It is easier to compare the results when everything is on one sheet.

Neurological Signs

Patients who have brain and spinal cord injuries need special monitoring. Neurological signs record how the eyes react to light, the level of consciousness, strength and motion of extremities, and VS.

Pathology Report

All tissue taken from a patient in surgery is examined by a pathologist. All surgical cases will have this form placed on the chart when MR completes the typing. Other charts may have this form if a biopsy is done in the room.

Refusal Forms

Patients may refuse some form of treatment; if the doctor feels that this treatment is necessary, the patient must sign a refusal statement. Some patients refuse blood transfusions, others refuse certain medications, or refuse to have tests that are considered necessary for recovery from their illness. Each hospital devises their own format for this.

Test Reports

Each department that performs tests has a form where the test results are recorded. These are either placed on the chart by the department personnel or are sent to the unit and filed by the unit secretary.

MAINTENANCE OF THE CHART

Chart dividers keep the chart in order while in use. It is your job as unit secretary to see that forms are in the proper section. The chart may be rearranged when the patient goes to surgery for the convenience of the anesthesiologist but must be arranged in working order when the patient returns to the unit.

Thinning a Chart

Thinning or splitting a chart is done when the chart becomes so thick that the chart back cannot hold all of it. Remove the parts that the doctors and the nursing staff will not need for reference. Nurse's Notes, Progress Notes, and Physician's Orders that are over a week from the present date may be removed as well as Departmental Therapy Records. The thinned portion is secured by placing a rubber band around it or by placing it in an envelope addressographed with the patient's ID. The thinned part is placed in a drawer marked for that purpose and reincorporated into the chart when the patient is discharged. A sticker is placed on the inside of the chart back to show the chart has been thinned.

Transporting Charts

The escort service will ask for the chart when escorting a patient to a department for tests or treatment. The addressograph card should be attached to the chart. Chart backs may have a pocket or a clip for this purpose. Many hospitals have a rule that a note must be made on the Nurse's Notes when a patient leaves the unit. You are usually allowed to make the entry on the chart. Escort personnel are instructed to keep the chart where the patient does not have the opportunity to read it. An entry is also made when the patient returns to the unit, and the addressograph card is placed in the rack.

SAMPLE CHART

The following forms represent a surgical patient's chart in the sequence ordinarily used. The forms are completed to show you the information each form includes. Your instructor will give you the forms for your area and explain any changes you need to know. The addressograph corresponds to the institution supplying the form so you will notice two types of addressographs.

- Patient Identification Sheet or Face Sheet (Figure 4-3)
- Physician's Order Sheet (Figure 4-4)
- Intake and Output, Fluid Balance Sheet (Figure 4-5)
- Laboratory Report File Sheet (Figure 4-6)
- Radiology Report (Figure 4-7)
- Consent for Surgery (Figure 4-8)
- Emergency Situation Verification (Figure 4-9)
- Preoperative Checklist (Figure 4-10)

- Pre and Post Anesthesia Record (Figure 4-11)
- Anesthesia Record (Figure 4-12)
- Recovery Room Record (Figure 4-13)
- O.R. Record Slip (Figure 4-14)
- Pathology Report (Figure 4-15)
- History Form Headings; Physical Examination, in part (Figure 4-16)
- Doctor's Progress Notes (Figure 4-17)
- Graphic Sheet (Figure 4-18)
- Medication Administration Record (Figure 4-19)
- Nurse's Admission Summary (Figure 4-20)
- Laboratory Flow Sheet (Figure 4-21)

Nurse's Notes are not shown because of the tremendous differences in format. Your instructor will supply a copy of the type you will see.

MEDICAL RECORDS

UNIVERSITY OF NEW MEXICO HOSPITAL
BERNALILLO COUNTY MEDICAL CENTER
2211 LOMAS BOULEVARD, N.E. • ALBUQUERQUE, NEW MEXICO 87106 • (505) 843-2111

FORM	INTERVIEWER
Sally Munfro	

MEDICAL RECORD NO.	DATE & TIME OF ADMISSION	DATE & TIME OF DISCHARGE	LOS	PSR	ACCOUNT NO.	FC
21 25 01	3/18/xx 0810				1-18338-0	

PATIENT'S NAME, ADDRESS, TELEPHONE	(PREVIOUS NAME)	BIRTHDATE	AGE	BIRTHPLACE	SEX	EO	MARIT. STATUS
Doe, John		5/8/XX	56	Ohio	M		M
2708 Canyon Drive, Albuquerque, NM		NEXT OF KIN			RELATIONSHIP		
Phone--893-2071		Clara Doe			Wife		

PERSON TO NOTIFY IN CASE OF EMERGENCY	RELATIONSHIP	ADDRESS	TELEPHONE
Clara Doe	wife	2708 Canyon Drive, Albuquerque	893-2071

PATIENT'S OCCUPATION	PATIENT'S EMPLOYER	ADDRESS	TELEPHONE
Salesman	Sandia Appliances	4726 Madrid Ave SW	364-2195

GUARANTOR'S NAME, ADDRESS, TELEPHONE	RELATIONSHIP/GUARANTOR NO.	GUARANTOR'S EMPLOYER, ADDRESS, TELEPHONE	OCCUPATION/HOW LONG
Self			

PRIMARY SOURCE OF PAYMENT	INS. PLAN	COV. TYPE	SUBSCRIBER	IDENT. NO.(S)	VERIF.
Blue Cross, Blue Shield		A	Sandia Appliances	7530837	
SECONDARY SOURCE OF PAYMENT	INS. PLAN	COV. TYPE	SUBSCRIBER	IDENT. NO.(S)	VERIF.
TERTIARY SOURCE OF PAYMENT	INS. PLAN	COV. TYPE	SUBSCRIBER	IDENT. NO.(S)	VERIF.

ACC.	DATE & TIME OF ACCIDENT	W/C	ATTENDING PHYSICIAN
			D. Komula / K. Statler

Dx: Possible Cholelithiasis

Final Diagnosis/Concomitant Conditions/Complications

Nosocomial infection? Yes / / No / / If yes, define:

D/C Summary Dictated by :   Date:

Operations/Procedures (Include date performed):

Discharged: HOME / / AMA / /   EXPIRED: Under 48 hrs / / Over 48 hrs / /

Transferred to: HOSP / / OTHER / / NAME OF FACILITY:

Recommendations upon discharge:

Copy of Discharge Summary to :

Address:

DISCHARGING PHYSICIAN: SR RESIDENT/ATTENDING PHYSICIAN

Figure 4-3. Patient Identification Sheet.

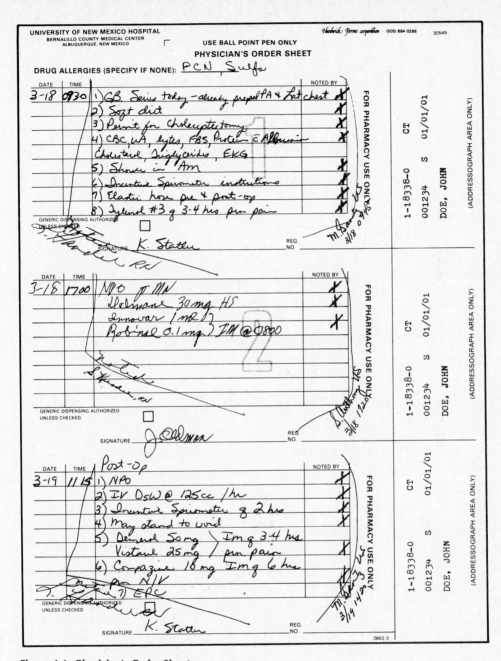

Figure 4-4. Physician's Order Sheet.

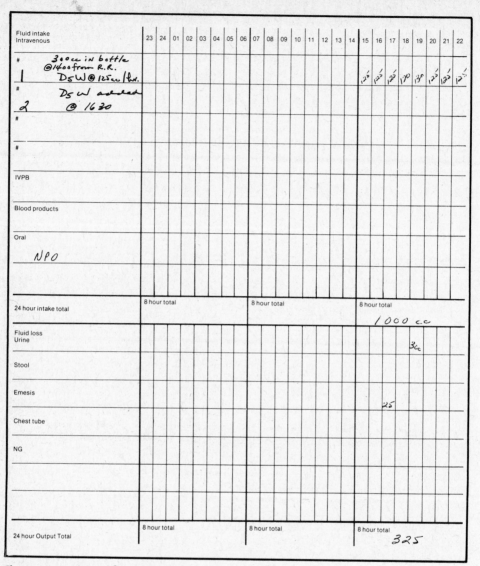

Figure 4-5. Intake and Output Record.

LABORATORY REPORTS

UNIVERSITY OF NEW MEXICO HOSPITAL / B.C.M.C.

PATIENT RECORD		CHEMISTRY		UNMH BCMC 2211 LOMAS BLVD. NE ALBUQUERQUE, N.M. 87106	
		AMMONIA µmol l	ALK PHOS IU l	BLOOD GASES	ACCESSION NUMBER(S)
		ALCOHOL mg dl	ALK PHOS ISOENZYMES	ARTERIAL	
X	SODIUM 137 meq l	SALICYLATE mg dl		VENOUS	TIME IN
X	POTASSIUM 4.5 meq l	AMYLASE IU l		pH	
X	CHLORIDE 102 meq l	SGOT IU l		pCO mmHg	GLUCOSE TOL 3 HRS
X	CO 27 meq l	SGPT IU l	CIP	pO mmHg	GLUCOSE TOL 5 HRS
	UREA NITROGEN mg dl	GGT IU l	LDH TOTAL IU l	DELTA BASE	FAST mg dl
	GLUCOSE RANDOM mg dl	ACID PHOS IU l	LDH ISOENZYMES	BICARB	HR mg dl
X	GLUCOSE FASTING 110 mg dl	X TOTAL PROTEIN 6.7 g dl	LDH 1	TOTAL CO	1 HR mg dl
	GLUCOSE 2 HR PP mg dl	X ALBUMIN 4.5 g dl	LDH 2	PT TEMP	2 HR mg dl
	CREATININE mg dl	URIC ACID mg dl	LDH 3	FIO	3 HR mg dl
	CALCIUM meq l	LACTATE meq l	LDH 4	Hgb	4 HR mg dl
	MAGNESIUM meq l	PYRUVATE mg dl	LDH 5	MEAS O SAT	5 HR mg dl
	PHOSPHORUS mg dl	X CHOLESTEROL 174 mg dl	CK TOTAL IU l	CARBON MONOXIDE	KETONES
	OSMOLALITY mOsm kg	HDL CHOLESTEROL mg dl	CK MB		OTHER
	BILIRUBIN MICRO mg dl	X TRIGLYCERIDES 72 mg dl	SWEAT CHLORIDE TEST		TIME OUT
	BILIRUBIN TOTAL mg dl	SERUM IRON µg dl			
	BILIRUBIN DIRECT mg dl	SERUM TIBC µg dl			

SEE REVERSE SIDE FOR ADDITIONAL INFORMATION AND OTHER TESTS-WRITE IN ABOVE UNDER 'OTHER'

DATE ORDERED 3-18-XX	DATE TIME COLLECTED 3-18 10:40 AM	X FASTING	ASAP place X in colored square beside test
PRIMARY WORKING DIAGNOSIS Cholelithiasis		ARTERIAL BLOOD	
		X VENOUS	
REQUESTING PHYSICIAN (Last Name, Initial) Komula D.	NURSE CLERK (init) a.c.	CAPILLARY	STAT place Stat sticker over this space
		SERUM	
		PLASMA	
ER	CLINIC (Specify) 9th floor	OTHER (Specify) ROOM # 9030 BED # 2	TEST PERFORMED BY TL	TIME RESULTS NEEDED
0457	CALL 2441 FOR RESULTS CALL 2443 FOR OTHER INFORMATION	TEST VALIDATED BY OG CHEMISTRY	

1 -18338-0   CT

001234   S   01/01/01

DOE, JOHN

LABORATORY REPORTS

P00124

Figure 4-6. Laboratory Report File Sheet.

UNIVERSITY OF NEW MEXICO HOSPITAL
BERNALILLO COUNTY MEDICAL CENTER
ALBUQUERQUE, NEW MEXICO

RADIOLOGY CONSULTATION REQUEST   DATE *3-18-XX*

EXAMINATION REQUESTED: *G. B. Series, PA & Lat chest this AM*
PERTINENT CLINICAL DATA: *Dx: Cholelithiasis.*

PATIENT:	AMBULATORY ( )	INFANT IN ARMS ( )		IN WHEELCHAIR (X)		STRETCHER ( )	ISOLATION ( )	
HOSPITAL NUMBER	AGE	SEX	RACE	CLINIC OR SERVICE	ROOM	HEIGHT	WEIGHT	
001234	*56*	*M*	*C*	*Surgical*	*9030-2*	*5'11"*	*160*	
REQUESTED BY			ATTENDING PHYSICIAN			PREVIOUS X-RAYS HERE		
DR *S. Turbin* MS III		DR *D. Komala / K. Stattew*				☒ YES ☐ NO		
						☐ NEW ☒ OLD		

RADIOLOGIST'S REPORT

Cholecystogram shows good vizualization of the gallbladder.
There are numerous stones visible.   No obstruction seen.
IMPRESSION: Cholelithiasis.

PA and Lat. chest -- two views of the chest are negative for
cardiac or pulmonary abnormalities.
IMPRESSION: No active pulmonary process.

L. Vanderman
RADIOLOGIST _____ M D

NOTES

ADDRESSOGRAPH PLATE

1-18338-0   CT
001234   S   01/01/01
DOE, JOHN

1008

Figure 4-7. Radiology Report.

UNIVERSITY OF NEW MEXICO HOSPITAL/BCMC

AUTHORIZATION FOR A CONSENT
TO OPERATION(S) AND PROCEDURE(S)

MY SIGNATURE CONSTITUTES MY ACKNOWLEDGEMENT THAT:

(1) I, _John Doe_ , CONSENT TO AND AUTHORIZE THE
          Print Patient's Name
UNIVERSITY OF NEW MEXICO HOSPITAL/BCMC AND DR. _Statler_
                                              Print Doctor's Name
OR HIS DESIGNEE TO PERFORM THE FOLLOWING OPERATION(S) AND PROCEDURE(S) AND ANY OTHER
OPERATION(S) OR PROCEDURE(S) THAT IN THE JUDGEMENT OF THE PHYSICIAN MAY BE ADVISABLE
ON THE BASIS OF THE FINDINGS DURING THE COURSE OF THE OPERATION(S) OR PROCEDURE(S).

Cholecystectomy

(2) THE NATURE AND PURPOSE OF THE OPERATION(S) OR PROCEDURE(S) HAVE BEEN ADE-
QUATELY EXPLAINED TO ME BY MY ATTENDING PHYSICIAN(S) OR SURGEON(S) AND I HAVE ALL
THE INFORMATION THAT I DESIRE.

(3) I UNDERSTAND THAT THESE SURGICAL OPERATION(S) AND/OR PROCEDURE(S) MAY IN-
VOLVE CALCULATED RISK OF COMPLICATION, INJURY AND IN RARE CASES EVEN DEATH FROM BOTH
KNOWN AND UNKNOWN CAUSES.

(4) ALTERNATIVE MEANS OF TREATMENT AND THERAPY HAVE BEEN EXPLAINED TO ME AND I
UNDERSTAND I HAVE THE RIGHT TO REFUSE THE OPERATION(S) OR PROCEDURE(S).

(5) I AUTHORIZE AND CONSENT TO THE ADMINISTRATION OF SUCH ANESTHETICS AS ARE
DEEMED ADVISABLE BY THE ATTENDING ANESTHESIOLOGIST AND THE POSSIBLE RISKS AND COMPLI-
CATIONS OF ANESTHESIA HAVE BEEN EXPLAINED.

(6) NO GUARANTEE OR ASSURANCE HAS BEEN MADE TO ME AS TO THE RESULTS THAT MAY BE
OBTAINED.

(7) I REQUEST THAT ANY TISSUE, ORGAN OR MEMBER SEVERED IN ANY OPERATION BE DIS-
POSED OF BY THE PATHOLOGIST IN A MEDICALLY ACCEPTABLE MANNER.

(8) I CERTIFY THAT I HAVE READ OR HAD READ TO ME THIS AUTHORIZATION AND CONSENT,
THAT ALL BLANKS REQUIRING COMPLETION WERE FILLED IN BEFORE I SIGNED AND THAT I UNDER-
STAND AND AGREE TO THE FOREGOING.

John Doe
Patient/Person Authorized to Consent

DATE: _3-18-XX_ a.m.
TIME: _1245_ (p.m.)

A. Roppe ,R.N.   _____
     Witness   Interpreter (if utilized)

THE UNDERSIGNED PHYSICIAN HEREBY CERTIFIES THAT HE/SHE HAS EXPLAINED TO THE ABOVE-NAMED
PATIENT OR OTHERWISE AUTHROIZED CONSENTING PERSON ALL OF THE MATTERS ABOVE REFERRED TO;
AND THAT THE EXPLANATION IN HIS/HER PROFESSIONAL JUDGEMENT WAS ADEQUATE AND REASONABLE.

K. Statler
      Physician

UNMH Consent Form #1   PL0304
   March, 1980

Figure 4-8. Consent for Surgery.

UNIVERSITY OF NEW MEXICO HOSPITAL/BCMC

EMERGENCY SITUATION VERIFICATION
AND/OR TELEPHONE CONSENT
(When a patient is a minor (under 18) or unable to sign)

NAME OF PATIENT _Jonathan Jones_   AGE: _15_
ATTENDING DOCTOR _J. R. Edmond_
DATE OF SIGNING _____ _7-8_ , 19_XX_ TIME _8:40_ (a.m., (p.m.))

EMERGENCY SITUATION VERIFICATION

1. The following medical treatment or surgical procedure _thoracotomy,_
   possible removal of injured lung segment.
   should be performed upon the patient and the situation at hand is an emergency
   requiring immediate action because: _of respiratory distress_
   and loss of blood.   .
   The undersign physician/hereby certifies that he/she has explained to the above-
   named patient or otherwise authorized consenting person all of the above referred
   to; and that his/her explanation in his/her professional judgement was adequate
   and reasonable.

   JR Edmond   _T. Grayson_
   _____   _____
   Physician   Consulting Physician

TELEPHONE CONSENT

2. (indicate applicable paragraphs)

   a. I have been unable to ascertain the name and address of the legally respon-
      sible representative of the patient who could consent to the emergency treat-
      ment for the patient.

   b. I have been unable to contact _____ the
      legally responsible representative of the patient to obtain a consent to the
      emergency treatment for the patient.

   (c.) I have spoken by telephone with (Name of Legally Responsible Representative
      of Patient) _Mother — Barbara C. Jones_ and have received
      consent to proceed with the above-stated emergency treatment.

   d. The emergency did not permit any attempt to obtain a consent.

   Betty Wise R.N.   _JR Edmond_
   _____   _____
   Signature, Witness Monitoring   Physician
   Telephone Call

UNMH Consent Form #3

Figure 4-9. Emergency Situation Verification.

ST. JOSEPH HOSPITAL
Albuquerque, New Mexico
PRE-OP CHECK LIST

9030-2

256124 9
DOE, JOHN   56 M CAH
D. Komula   MR 21 25 01
AG 3/18/XX

DATE: 3-19-XX

	(Initial)	
	YES	NO
1.) Operative Permit signed and on chart (Correct Surgeon's Name)	MG	
2.) History and Physical	MG	
3.) Consultation (when applicable)		ө
4.) New Progress and Doctor's Order Sheet on Chart	MG	
5.) Routine Lab: Hct: ⌐ Hgb. ✓ Urinalysis ✓ K+ ✓		
Chest x-ray ✓ Type & Cross Match ө	MG	
6.) Miscellaneous Pre-Op Lab Studies: HSMAC, Other Lyte, FBS, Pro, all, ck, E5	MG	
7.) Chart Marked for Allergies if any	MG	
Signature(s): Mary Gantz, U.S.		
8.) Skin Prep (Wash, Scrub, (Shower)	MB	
9.) Wearing Hospital Gown (no other clothing)	MB	
10.) Dentures or Removable Bridgework Removed, Capped Teeth Present		ө
11.) Hairpins and/or Wig Removed		ө
12.) Contact Lenses or Glasses Removed		ө
13.) Prosthesis (False Limb or Eyes, etc.)		ө
14.) Make-up, False Eyelashes and Nail Polish Removed		ө
15) Jewelry Removed (Rings Taped)		ө
16.) Valuables - Business Office, (Family)(Money, Medals, Credit cards)	MB	
17.) Voided (Catheterized, or Indwelling Catheter) Amount 250 cc		
Time: 0745	MB	
18.) Vital Signs (Current) B.P. 130/70 P 80 R 16 T 98⁶	MB	
Signature(s): Nina Blackburn, RN		
19.) Pre-Operative Medication Given, Time: 0860 Int. GF	GF	
20.) Side Rails Applied:	GF	
21.) Identaband Checked with Chart and O.R. Slip	GF	
22.) Chart Signed Off	GF	
23.) Addressograph on Chart:	GF	
24.) Old Chart to O.R. with Patient (If Requested)		ө
25.) Miscellaneous: _____ to O.R. with Pt. _____		ө

SJH: 6010-33
Rev. 2/82

Signature: Gladys Frost, LPN

Figure 4-10. Preoperative Checklist.

ST. JOSEPH HOSPITAL
ALBUQUERQUE, NEW MEXICO

9030-2

256124 9
DOE, JOHN 56 M CAH
D. Komula MR 21 25 01
AG   3/18/XX

PREOPERATIVE ANESTHESIA EVALUATION   DATE: 3-18-XX

PROPOSED SURGERY: Cholecystectomy

PREVIOUS SURGERY AND ANESTHESIA HX: Appendectomy 12 years ago
General - no problems

MEDICAL HX: _____ [O=NON PERTINENT HX]

CARDIAC Normal EKG

PULMONARY (INCL. ASTHMA) O

HEPATIC (INCL. JAUNDICE) O

RENAL O

OTHER

MEDICATIONS: None

ALLERGIES: Sulfas, PCN

PHYSICAL EXAM: [✓=NORMAL LIMITS]

HEENT ✓   TEETH (R) ✓ ✓ ✓ ✓ (L)

CHEST ✓

HEART ✓

ABDOMEN ✓ some tenderness over liver

EXTREMITIES ✓

ASA CLASS: _____ ANESTHESIA EXPLAINED TO PATIENT: ✓

_____ AND AGREEABLE TO: ✓

ORDERED: ECG ✓ LYTES ✓ CAP _____ OTHER: _____ J. Oldman M.D.
                                              (SIGNATURE)
COMMENT: _____

POSTOPERATIVE ANESTHESIA EVALUATION DATE: 3-20 TIME: 1300

COMPLICATIONS: None

POSTOP STATUS: Good

COMMENTS: _____ J. Oldman M.D.
                                      (SIGNATURE)

PRE AND POST OPERATIVE ANESTHESIA
EVALUATION

Figure 4-11. Pre- and Postoperative Anesthesia Record.

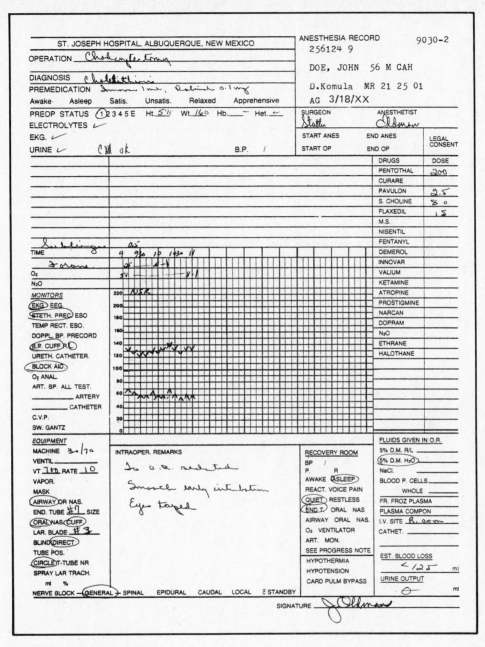

Figure 4-12. Anesthesia Record.

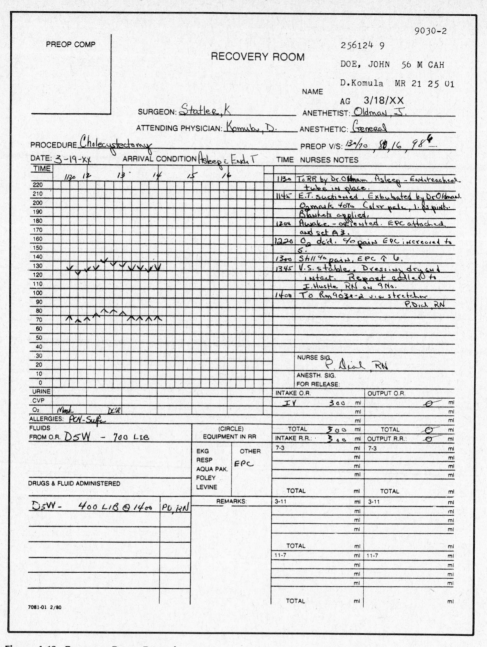

Figure 4-13. Recovery Room Record.

ST. JOSEPH HOSPITAL
Albuquerque, New Mexico

9030-2

256124 9
DOE, JOHN   56 M CAH
D. Komula   MR 21 25 01
AG   3/18/XX

Name   Rm. No.   Age   Doctor   MR. No.

Operating Room # _2_ Date _3-19-XX_

Surgeon (s): _Statler, K._

Assistant(s): _Komula, D._

Preoperative Diagnosis: _Cholelithiasis_

Postoperative Diagnosis: _Cholelithiasis č Cholangitis_

Operative Procedure (s) Performed _Cholecystectomy_

Tissue Removed: _Gallbladder_

Patient In: _0845_   Surgery Start: _0910_

Patient Out: _113_   Surgery Finish: _1100_

Patient identified by: _BB   J.O._

Class: (Major) Minor   Clean /Infected

Anesthesia Person _J. Oldham, MD_

Anesthesia: (General) Spinal Regional None

Local: _____

(ETT)   Mask

Medication given:
_Ø_
_Ø_

Skin graft donor site: _Ø_

Bone graft donor site: _0_

Tourniquet: Box(es)# _Ø_   Checked: Yes No

Padding applied: Yes No

Applied by: _____

Location: #1 _____ #2 _____

Pressure: _____

Time Up: _____

Time Down: _____

Position: (Supine) Prone Jackknife

Lateral Lithotomy Semifowlers

Other: _GB pillow under left side_

Bovie: Unit # _1_ Checked: Yes No

Plate location: _R thigh_

Applied by: _BB_

Catheter: _Ø_

Drains: _Ø_

Packing: _Ø_

Culture: _Ø_

Counts:

(Sponges) Cottonoids (Instruments) (Needles)

Pre-Op Count: _BB_

1st Count: _Correct_   _J. Gilley, RN_

2nd Count: _Correct_   _J. Gilley, RN_

Scrub Person: _E. Statler, RN_

Relief: _____

Circulating Nurse: _J. Gilley, RN_

Relief: _____

*See back for special comments

6211-01   9/79

O. R. RECORD SLIP

Figure 4-14. OR Record Slip.

ST. JOSEPH HOSPITAL
ALBUQUERQUE, NEW MEXICO

DATE 3-19-XX   PATH. NO. 175430

NAME Doe, John   ROOM NO. 9030-2

SEX M   HOSP. NO. 256124 9
AGE 56   SURGEON Statler, K.

PRE-OP DIAGNOSIS Cholelithiasis
POST-OP DIAGNOSIS Cholelithiasis, Cholecystitis
TISSUE SUBMITTED Gallbladder and several stones

GROSS DESCRIPTION:

Specimen consists of a gallbladder measuring 5.9 cm in
maximal dimensions. The serosal surface is smooth and
glistening and bile stained. The wall is of normal thickness.
Received with the gallbladder are several dark black stones
with irregular surfaces and spherical shape measuring 0.5 to
1.3 cm. Sections of the gallbladder wall are submitted.
Microscopic: sections consist of gallbladder wall segments
in which there is a minimal amount of fibrosis associated with
focal collections of small numbers of chronic inflammatory
cells.

PAS   _David Grossman, M.D_
                                        PATHOLOGIST
                                                   CHART

PATHOLOGIST'S CONSULTATION REPORT

Figure 4-15. Pathology Report.

UNIVERSITY OF NEW MEXICO HOSPITAL
BERNALILLO COUNTY MEDICAL CENTER

HISTORY - PART 1	CHIEF COMPLAINT AND HISTORY OF PRESENT ILLNESS	DATE 3/18/XX

HISTORY - PART 2   PAST HISTORY - REVIEW OF SYSTEMS   DATE 3 - 18 - XX

INSTRUCTIONS - Include 1)OCCUPATION, 2) HABITS (Alcohol, Tabacco, Drugs), 3)FAMILY HISTORY, 4)CHILDHOOD ILLNESSES, 5)ADULT ILLNESSES, 6) OPERATIONS, 7)INJURIES, 8)DRUG SENSITIVITIES AND ALLERGIC REACTIONS and 9)IMMUNIZATION HISTORY

UNIVERSITY OF NEW MEXICO HOSPITAL
BERNALILLO COUNTY MEDICAL CENTER

PHYSICAL EXAMINATION

DATE OF EXAM.	HEIGHT	WEIGHT 160	TEMPERATURE	PULSE	BLOOD PRESSURE
3 - 18 - XX	5' 11'	HEAD SIZE	36.8	78	132/78

General: Well developed, well nourished male in middle 50's.
 Alert, intelligent and communicative. Slightly uncomfortable.

Head and Neck: Normal size and contour. Thyroid not palpably
 enlarged. No lymphadenopathy.

Eyes: Pupils are round and equal, react to L & A. Sclera and
 conjunctiva are clear.

Ears: Tympanic membrane clear with no scars.

Nose: No septal abnormalities. Normal.

Mouth: Good dental hygiene. Has permanent implant of first and
 second molar, upper right. No irritation of mucous membranes.
 Tongue pink and smooth, no abnormalities.

Throat: Tonsils have been removed. Normal.

Chest: Equal expansion bilaterally. Skin clear with no cysts or
 growths.

Lungs: Clear to percussion and auscultation.

Cardiovascular: Heart tones are clearly audible and of equal
 quality. Varicose veins of both legs, not extensive or
 troublesome.

Abdomen: Tenderness over liver. Scar from previous appendectomy.
 No distention.

Genitalia: Normal male.

Rectum: No abnormal findings.

ADDRESSOGRAPH PLATE

1-18338-0   CT
001234   S   01/01/01
DOE, JOHN

Figure 4-16. History Form Headings and Physical Examination.

UNIVERSITY OF NEW MEXICO HOSPITAL
BERNALILLO COUNTY MEDICAL CENTER

PROGRESS NOTES
(sign all copies)

DATE	
3-18	Admitted to 9 No. Some discomfort Will get
0920	G B Series to verify diagnosis K. Statler
1300	X·ray shows stones Surgery risks explained
	to patient and wife Permit signed K Statler
3-19	1115 Op · cholecystectomy K. Statler
	Tolerated procedure well
	EBL < 125 cc
	To R.R. in good condition
	K. Statler

ADDRESSOGRAPH

1-18338-0   CT

001234   S   01/01/01

DOE, JOHN

(continue on reverse side)

PL0808 (9/80)

Figure 4-17. Doctor's Progress Notes.

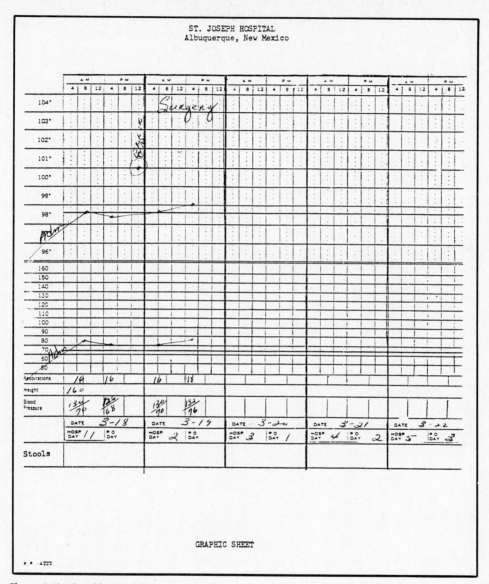

Figure 4-18. Graphic Record.

UNIVERSITY OF NEW MEXICO HOSPITAL
BERNALILLO COUNTY MEDICAL CENTER

7 DAY MEDICATION RECORD

DRUG, DOSAGE, ROUTE FREQUENCY	DATE 3-18	DATE 3-19	DATE 3-20	DATE 3-21	DATE 3-22	DATE 3-23	DATE 3-24
Tylenol #3 q 3-4 hrs prn pain	1605 m.c.						
Dalmane 30 mg HS	2100 SK						
Innovar 1 mL Im Robinal 0.1 mg		0800 m.c.					
Demerol 50 mg Im Vistaril 25 mg q 3-4 hrs prn pain		1730 SK					
Compazine 10 mg Im q 6 hrs prn N-V.		2100 S.K.					

ADDRESSOGRAPH	Personnel Initials Identification			
1-18338-0 CT	Mary Conner			
001234 S 01/01/01	Barb Kunder			
DOE, JOHN	(continue on reverse side) MR-18 (Rev. 4-71) PL0817 (REPLACES PL0038)			

Figure 4-19. Medication Administration Record.

BERNALILLO COUNTY MEDICAL CENTER   PLD041

PROGRESS NOTES
(Sign all notes)

DATE	Time: *0845*	Admission Form: Medical/Surgical

3-18

Name: *Doe, John*   Age: *56*   Sex: *M*

How Admitted: *Ambulatory*   Accompanied By: *wife*

T. P. R.: *(98⁶) 37*   B.P.: *130/70*   HT.: *5'11"* WT.: *160*

Present Complaint: *Pain right side just below ribs and travels to back.*

Observations of Mental and Physical Status: *Oriented. Some discomfort, appears healthy otherwise.*

Prostheses or Health Aids: *o*

Language/Communication Barrier: *o*

Last Meal: *supper 3-17*

Last Voiding: *this A.M.*

Last B.M.: *this A.M.*

Valuables: *given to wife.*

1. Have you been in a hospital before? *Yes*
2. Do you have any allergies to medications? *PCN - sulfa.*
3. Do you have any allergies to foods? *No*
4. Do you require special diet or foods? *Omit pork and spice*
5. Do you take medication now? *No*   Medications and disposition:

ORIENTATION TO: Call light: *Yes*   Visiting Hours: *Yes*

T.V./Bed Controls: *Yes*

Admitted By: *N. Ortega, N.A.*

1-18338-0 CT	R. N. Signature: *L. Hander, RN*
001234 S 01/01/01	Name of Doctor Notified: *Statler*
DOE, JOHN	Time: *0900* Signature: *G.C.*
ADDRESSOGRAPH:	(Med./Surg. Overprint)

MR-7 (Rev. 8/69)

Figure 4-20. Admission Summary.

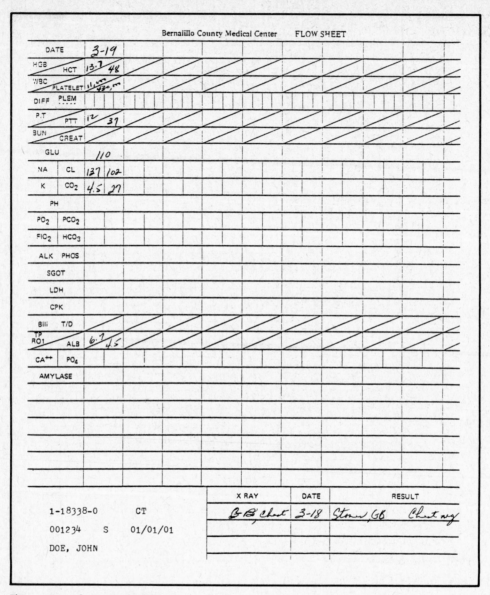

Figure 4-21. Laboratory Flow Sheet.

REVIEW QUESTIONS

1. Explain the difference in standard forms and supplementary forms.

   _____
   _____ .

2. List some legal concerns regarding a chart.

   _____
   _____ .

3. List the standard forms for a chart.

   _____
   _____
   _____ .

4. List four supplementary forms.

   _____
   _____ .

5. Maintenance of the chart is the responsibility of the _____ .

6. You need a History and Physical on a chart. You call the _____
   _____ department to request them.

7. You are calling the prosthetic appliance shop to order a brace. The
   shop needs the patient's address, telephone number, and the name of
   the hospitalization insurance company. You find this information on the
   _____ .

8. Why would you refer to the Anesthesia Record?

   _____ .

9. The Social Service worker uses the _____
   to inform the doctor of the progress in placing a patient in a nursing
   home.

10. The purpose of the patient's chart is _____
    _____ .

11. A friend knows a patient on the floor where you work. The friend asks
    you why the patient is hospitalized. How do you answer and why?

Situational Application

12. Escort personnel pick up a patient. You notice that as the patient is
    wheeled down the hall, he is reading his chart. You would:
    a. Ignore the situation

b. Politely and professionally take the chart from the patient and explain that reading the chart is not allowed and hand the chart to the escort personnel. Report this to the head nurse.

c. Report the incident to your head nurse.

13. You notice that an entry in a chart is incorrect regarding the department to which the patient was taken. You would:

    a. Ask the head nurse if you may correct the statement and do so by drawing an ink line through the statement, signing and dating it, and entering the correct statement

    b. Ignore it since you did not make the entry

    c. Black out the statement with a Magic Marker®.

14. A diabetic is admitted to the floor. You are assembling the chart. There are orders for daily blood sugar tests and insulin. You would:

    a. Add a Fluid Balance sheet to the chart

    b. Add a Laboratory Flow sheet to the chart

    c. Add a Diabetic Record sheet to the chart.

15. A new surgical returns to the unit and there are orders for an IV and to measure drainage from a stomach tube every 8 hrs. You would:

    a. Add a Vital sign sheet to the chart

    b. Add a Fluid Balance sheet to the chart

    c. Do nothing until requested to do so.

Chapter 5 | Pharmacology

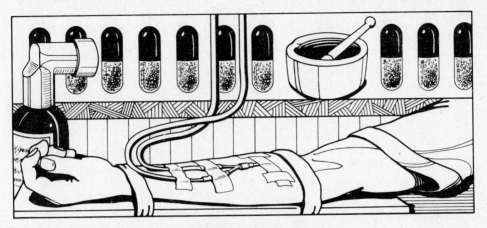

OBJECTIVES

Mastery of this chapter requires memorization of some sections. When you have completely mastered the chapter, you will be able to:

1. Define pharmacology.
2. Define controlled drugs.
3. List the types of drug preparations.
4. List modes of administering medications.
5. List the units of measure of the Apothecary System.
6. List the units of measure of the Metric System.
7. Compare units of measure of Apothecary and Metric Systems with common household measures.
8. Identify medication times and abbreviations.
9. Identify symbols and abbreviations used in administering medications.
10. Define narcotics.
11. List narcotics and give the usual adult dose/dosage range.
12. Define hypnotics.
13. List hypnotics and give the usual adult dose/dosage range.
14. Define sedative and tranquilizer.
15. List sedatives and tranquilizers and give the usual adult dose/dosage range.
16. Define analgesics.
17. List analgesics and give the usual adult dose/dosage range.
18. Define antinauseants.
19. List antinauseants and give the usual adult dose/dosage range.
20. Appreciate the importance of accuracy in orders for drugs.

The word pharmacology is derived from the Greek word *pharmakon* which means drugs and the word *logos* which means a study. Pharmacology is the study of drugs—their origin, nature, properties, and effects upon living organisms.

Pharmacy is the practice of compounding and dispensing medicinal preparations. The hospital pharmacy stores the drugs and dispenses them to the units as either stock drugs or individual patient drugs. Stock drugs are those kept on hand for emergency situations and the drugs that must be accounted for by law, such as narcotics and hypnotics. Individual patient drugs are dispensed as the physician orders them. The terms drugs and medicines are used interchangeably.

The Food and Drug Administration (FDA) enforces laws governing drugs. These laws assure that drugs:

- Comply with standards of strength and purity
- Are tested before marketing
- Have been proven effective
- Are properly labeled.

One such law is the Harrison Narcotic Act which was written in 1914 and has been amended several times. The Act regulates the importation, manufacture, sale, and use of narcotics and analgesic drugs that are habit forming or may cause a psychological dependence. **Narcotics** are drugs which produce sleep and relieve pain when given in moderate doses because they depress the central nervous system. Excessive doses produce unconsciousness and sometimes death. **Analgesics** are drugs that lessen or relieve pain. Narcotics and some analgesics are stock drugs that must be accounted for by signing for the drug whenever it is given. The accounting sheet is issued from pharmacy at the same time the drug is issued. The exact number of tablets, capsules, or vials is noted at the top of the sheet. Each time an RN or LPN gives one of the controlled drugs the sheet is signed with the patient's name, amount of drug given, time given, name of physician ordering the drug, and the name of the person giving the drug. Controlled drugs are counted at the end of each shift by two persons: one RN or LPN going off duty and one RN or LPN coming on duty. The number of each drug in the locked cabinet must match the accounting sheet. When all of a drug is used, the empty container and sheet are returned to pharmacy and a new supply is issued. These drugs are kept under lock and key; the key is in the possession of an RN or LPN at all times. If a patient is ordered a controlled drug that is not stock, pharmacy will issue a small supply in an individual prescription that is placed in the locked cabinet. If the patient goes home before all the drug is used, the remainder is hand carried to pharmacy by an RN or LPN. Hospitals usually do not allow the secretaries to handle controlled drugs.

A drug may have a variety of names. The **chemical name** is the description of the chemical constituents. The **generic name** designates the chemical family but is much simpler than the chemical name and is not capitalized. The generic name may be used in all countries and is never changed. The **trade name or brand name** is given by the manufacturer, is capitalized, and can be used only by that company. Several companies may make the same generic drug but each company will have a separate brand name.

The *Physician's Desk Reference* (PDR) is published each year with supplements all year. The PDR is the most frequently used reference for drug information—spelling, action, mode, dosage, side effects, and how supplied. Each nursing unit will have a current PDR. Make it a habit to look up drugs that are not familiar to you.

TYPES OF DRUG PREPARATIONS

Internal Administration

There are several types of preparations which are introduced *into* the body in some manner. The types are discussed below.

Ampules (amps) and vials. Both contain powdered or liquid drugs which are usually given by injection. Ampules are sealed glass containers with usually only one dose. Vials are glass containers with rubber stoppers and usually contain several doses.

Aqueous solutions (aq. sol'n). *Aqua* is the Latin word for water. These solutions have one or more substances dissolved in water. **Syrups** are aqueous solutions of sucrose (a simple sugar) in which a drug is mixed to disguise the taste or to preserve the strength of the drug. Syrups are often used for their soothing effect on irritated membranes of the throat.

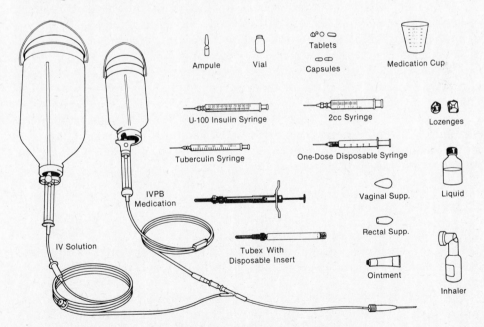

Figure 5-1. Common Ways Medications are Prepared and Administered.

Aqueous suspensions (aq. susp.). Drugs mixed with, but not dissolved in, water are called aqueous suspension drugs. **Mixtures** are aqueous preparations of two or more substances without chemical union which contain suspended particles. These must be shaken before use. **Emulsions** are a mixture of fats or oils in water added to another liquid. **Gels** are mixtures of insoluble drugs in a solid state so that particles are evenly distributed.

Capsules (caps). The Latin word capsula means little box. Capsules are gelatin containers of a single dose of a drug. The gelatin dissolves in the stomach, and the drug is released. **Enteric-coated** capsules are coated by a substance that is resistant to gastric juices and does not dissolve until the drug reaches the intestines. Time release capsules like Spansules, Timespans, and Gradumets contain small particles of a drug which dissolve at different time intervals. This allows one capsule to supply medication for a long, continuous period.

Disposable syringes contain individual doses of a drug. The syringe has an attached needle that is covered with a sealed, sterile cap.

Elixirs (elix) are drugs prepared in a sweetened, aromatic, alcoholic liquid. Some patients may have trouble swallowing caps or tablets but can swallow liquids.

Extracts (ext) are solutions of a drug using water or alcohol as the solvent and then allowing evaporation so that a solid or semi-solid preparation remains.

Fluidextracts (fl. ext) are alcoholic liquid extracts of vegetable drugs made so that 1 milliliter of the fluid extract is equal to 1 gram of the drug.

Lozenges or troches are drugs prepared in various shapes to be held in the mouth. As they dissolve, the drug is released. These give a high concentration of the drug to the mucous membranes of the mouth and throat.

Spirits (sp) are concentrated alcoholic solutions of substances that easily evaporate. The alcohol serves as a preservative as well as a solvent.

Tablets (tabs) are preparations of a powdered drug compressed into small disks. Shapes may vary. Tablets may be enteric-coated.

Tinctures (tr) are prepared by adding non-evaporative substances to a dilute alcoholic solution. The name of the drug is added after the word tincture—Tincture of Opium.

Suppositories (supp) are drugs mixed in a firm base and molded into various shapes for insertion into a body cavity or into an opening of a structure such as the rectum, vagina, or urethra. Suppositories dissolve at body temperature releasing the drug for local or systemic action.

External Preparations

The following drugs can be applied externally.

Liniments are liquid suspensions of a drug and are rubbed on the skin. These may relieve pain and swelling for a short time by improving circulation of blood to the area.

Lotions are liquid suspensions patted on the skin for either protection, cooling, cleansing, astringent action (drawing together or constricting), or anti-pruritic action (relief of itching).

Ointments (oint) are also called salves and unguents. A drug is prepared in a fatty, soft substance such as petroleum or lanolin (wool fat) and used for external application to the skin or mucous membranes. Their action is either astringent, soothing, or bacteriostatic (inhibiting or retarding bacterial growth).

Pastes are ointments with a base of nonfatty material. They soften and penetrate the skin as deeply as do ointments. They stick to the skin and absorb secretions.

Tinctures are made the same as for internal except that the drug is for external use only, such as Tincture of Iodine or Tincture of Benzoin.

MODES OF ADMINISTERING MEDICINES

Mode means the route or method by which a drug is given to the patient. The mode is determined by the doctor according to the desired effect, the site of desired action, how quickly action is needed, and the condition of the patient.

Hypodermic (H or h) means by needle under the skin.

Inhalation therapy (IT) or **respiratory therapy** (RT) refers to breathing in or inhaling a drug. This mode gives immediate absorption because of the large area of tissue with which the drug comes in contact as it is being inhaled. Most of the drugs dispensed by this mode are ordered as nebulization (a spray) and are administered by the RT department. Medihalers are small, pressurized containers that deliver the drug as a mist. Orders for Medihalers will be written as so many compressions per day. Oxygen and other gases are administered by the RT department.

Intradermal or intracutaneous injections are given by syringe and needle into the upper layer of the skin. The amount of drug is small. Used mostly in testing for allergies.

Intramuscular (IM) means into the muscle. Needles used for IM injections are from one to three inches long and gauge 19 to 22. Not more than 5cc should be given in one site. IMs are usually given in the buttocks, the side of the thigh muscle, or the muscle of the upper arm.

Intraspinal is also called intrathecal (into a sheath), subdural, subarachnoid, or lumbar injection. Drugs given by this method are always administered by a physician.

Intravenous (IV) means directly into a vein. Small amounts are given slowly by *syringe*; large amounts are given by drip method with the needle placed in a vein and tubing attached to the needle and to a bottle of solution. The *drip method* is referred to as an infusion. The doctor will write the type of solution and the rate at which it is to be infused. Sometimes medications are added to the solution.

IV Push (IVP) is given directly into the vein by syringe and needle or through a side-arm of an existing intravenous tubing. Many patients will have a continuous infusion and need medication every so many hours. To save the patient the discomfort of being stuck several times a day, tubings for infusions have projections with rubber stoppers that reseal themselves when punctured. The medication is drawn into a syringe, the needle is inserted into the side-arm, and the medication is pushed through the tubing.

IV Heparin Loc or Intermittent IV (INT) makes use of a small length of tubing connected to a needle and the other end of the tubing has a resealable stopper.

This is for patients who need medication IV every so many hours but do not need continuous infusion. The needle is kept open by flushing a heparin solution into the tubing after each medication administration. Heparin prevents clotting of blood in the needle.

IV Piggyback (IVPB) is used when a patient has a continuous infusion and needs a medication that must be mixed in solution with a volume too large to give by push. A small bottle with attached tubing is connected to a side-arm of an initial IV tubing and allowed to drip over a period of time. Most IV antibiotics must be mixed in from 50cc to 300cc to prevent irritation to the vein.

Oral (PO) per os—by mouth is the most common mode. It is the safest, most economical, and most convenient. The action of the drug is slower but lasts longer.

Parenteral refers to all the ways drugs are given by needle. Needles come in different gauges expressed in numbers. The larger the number the finer the needle. The length of the needle is expressed in inches. All parenteral drugs must be sterile.

Rectal (R) medications are in the form of a suppository that is inserted into the rectum by a gloved finger. Suppositories release drugs at a slow, steady rate. Medicines may also be given by enema or by slow drip via rectal tube.

Subcutaneous (SC, SQ, or subq) means below or beneath the skin. The drug is injected with a short needle into tissue just below the skin layers. Action is prompt.

Sublingual (subl, SL) means under the tongue. The tablet is placed under the tongue and kept there until it dissolves. The action is rapid because of the rich blood supply to this area.

Other modes used by physicians include intraarterial (into an artery), intraarticular (into a joint), intracardiac (into the heart), intraosseous (into bony tissue) and intrapericardial (into the sac that surrounds the heart).

TERMS AND ABBREVIATIONS FOR MEDICATION DOSAGES

Apothecary System

Apothecary is derived from the Greek work *apotheke* meaning a storage place and is used to designate a druggist or pharmacist. The basic unit of weight is the **grain** (gr). Other units of weight are *dram* (d or dr), *ounce* (oz) and *pound* (lb). The unit of liquid measure is **minim** (m or min). Fluid dram and fluid ounce signify a liquid but usually the fluid is omitted and just understood because of common usage. The symbol for fluid dram is ℨ, for fluid ounce is ℥. Quantities are expressed by Roman numerals or fractions after the symbol for the unit of

weight or liquid.
Examples:

Aspirin gr x, cough syrup ʒi, Mineral Oil ʒi.

Metric System

The metric system is slowly replacing the apothecary system. The **meter** (m) is the unit of linear measure. The **gram** (Gm or gm) is the unit of weight. The **liter** (L or l) is the unit of volume. A decimal system of ten and multiples of ten make the metric system an easy one to use. Prefixes for dividing a unit are deci for one-tenth (0.1), cent for one-hundreth (0.01), milli for one-thousandth (0.001), and micron (μ) for one-millioneth. Prefixes for multiplying by tens are *deca* for ten, *hecto* for hundred and *kilo* for thousand.

Medications are usually ordered in grams or milligrams with the quantity before the unit. A cubic centimeter (cc) is equal to a milliliter (ml) so liquids are ordered in either cc or ml. Kilograms are used when weighing patients since many drug dosages are calculated by amount per kilogram of body weight—i.e., 7.5 mg per kg every 12 hours.

Household Measures

Medicines used in the home need to be expressed in practical measures. The drop (gtt), tablespoon (tb or tbsp), teaspoon (tsp), cup (C), glass, pint (pt), quart (qt) and pound (lb) are commonly used and have approximate equivalents in the apothecary and the metric system as shown in Table 5-1

The apothecary system and the metric system can be converted, each to the other. Each nursing unit medication room will have a conversion table prominantly displayed. Use the table if you need to do any conversion. The most common ones that you may be using are:

- 1 gr = 0.065 gm = 60 or 65 mg
- 1½ gr = 0.1 gm = 100 mg
- 3 gr = 0.2 gm = 200 mg
- 5 gr = 0.325 gm = 325 mg

TABLE 5-1. MEASUREMENT EQUIVALENTS

Metric	Apothecary	Household
0.06 ml or cc	1 minim	1 drop
5 ml or cc	1 dram	1 teaspoon
15 ml or cc	4 drams	1 tablespoon
30 ml or cc	1 ounce	2 tablespoons
180 ml or cc	6 ounces	1 teacup
240 ml or cc	8 ounces	1 glass
500 ml or cc	1 pint	2 measuring cups
1000 ml or cc	1 quart	4 measuring cups
1 liter	1 quart	4 measuring cups
1 kilogram	35.2 ounces	2.2 pounds

MEDICATION TIMES

European time or military time is used in many hospitals because it eliminates the need to designate A.M. or P.M. European time is based on 24 numbers for the full day. Each time has four digits. Midnight would be 2400, 1 A.M. would be 0100, Noon would be 1200, 5 P.M. would be 1700. The afternoon and evening hours are determined by adding the hour to 12.

Each nursing unit will have a schedule of medication times posted at the desk. Times may vary on each unit according to the type and age of patients on that unit. Abbreviations for times and sample schedule using military time:

Abbreviation	Meaning	Military Time
d, od, qd	once daily	0900
qod	every other day	0900 plus dates
BID or bid	twice a day	0900 and 1700
TID or tid	three times a day	0900-1300-1700
QID or qid	four times a day	0900-1300-1700-2100

Some medications may be ordered as bid, tid, or qid by the doctor but should be evenly spaced throughout the 24 hours. The RN working with you will advise you until you become familiar with the routine.

Abbreviation	Meaning
qh	every hour for the full 24 hours
q 2 h	every two hours for the full 24 hours, start 0200
q 3 h	every three hours for the full 24 hours, begin 0300
q 4 h	every four hours for the full 24 hours, begin 0400
q 6 h	every six hours for the full 24 hours; begin 0600
q 8 h	every eight hours for the full 24 hours, begin 0600
q 12 h	every twelve hours—0900-2100
ac	before meals; *a* means ante or before, *c* is cibus or food. Usually one-half hour before meals—0730-1130-1630
pc	after meals; *p* means post or after, 0900-1300-1800
HS or hs	hour of sleep, bedtime. 2000 for children, 2100 or 2200 for adults
ac and hs	before meals and at bedtime, 0730-1130-1630-2200
pc and hs	after meals and at bedtime, 0900-1300-1800-2200
ac bkft and dinner	before breakfast and the evening meal, 0730-1630
ac bid	before meals twice a day, 0730-1630
pc bkft and dinner	after breakfast and evening meal, 0900-1800
pc bid	after meals twice a day, 0900-1800

Some medications need to be given with food so the order will read tid with meals. Times would then be determined by what time meals are served on that unit.

You will need to memorize the time abbreviations. Doctors use them and you will be transferring them to medication cards or other forms.

CHEMICAL SYMBOLS AND ABBREVIATIONS RELATED TO MEDICATIONS

Abbreviation/Symbol	*Meaning*
$\overline{aa}$	of each
aq	aqua, water, solution containing water
ad lib	as desired
ASAP	as soon as possible
$\bar{c}$	with
DC, dc	discontinue
liq	liquid, fluid
mEq	milliequivalent, a unit of measure of electrolytes (solutions which are conductors of electricity)
MR X 1 or mr x 1	may repeat one time
noc, noct	night
per, /	through, by, for each—*examples:*
	• Push fluids to 3000 cc/d means that the patient must have at least 3000 cc of fluid in 24 hours
	• Run IV at 100 cc per hour means the drip is regulated so the patient receives 100 cc of IV fluid every hour
	• Feed per NG tube means that the patient has a tube inserted into the nose and down to the stomach and a special formula will be dripped through the tube.
prn	when necessary or when patient requests
qs	quantity sufficient
Rx	prescription
$\bar{s}$	without
sos	if necessary
STAT	immediately, right now
U	unit, a determined amount of a medication
+	plus, acid reaction, positive
−	minus, deficiency, alkaline reaction
±	plus or minus; not exact but can vary one way or another
>	greater than
<	less than
≮	not less than
≯	not greater than
≠	not equal to
:	ratio, is to
⇌	denotes reversible reaction

Ba	barium; an element used in x-ray examinations to visualize internal structures clearly
Ca	calcium; element necessary for proper body function
C	carbon; element that is the basis of all organic matter
Cl	chloride; a salt of hydrochloric acid
CO_2	carbon dioxide; a gas found in the air; the body eliminates this gas in urine and perspiration; it is also exhaled by the lungs
Fe	iron; essential to life
Ga	gallium; a rare metal used in some examinations called scans
Hg	mercury; a metallic element used in thermometers, blood pressure reading instruments, and certain intestinal tubes
I	iodine; necessary for proper body function
K	potassium; essential for normal function of muscle tissue and conduction of nerve impulses
KCl	potassium chloride; given when a patient is K deficient
Mg	magnesium; mineral found in soft tissues, muscles, bones, and body fluids
Na	sodium; sodium salts are necessary for body function
NaCl	sodium chloride; common salt
$Na\,HCO_3$	sodium bicarbonate; an antacid
NS	normal saline; 0.9% solution of NaCl
O_2	a gas found in the air; essential for life
P	phosphorus; necessary for body function
Ra	radium, a radioactive element used in treatment of cancer
Rn	radon; a radioactive, gaseous element resulting from the breakdown of radium

You will need to memorize the symbols and abbreviations in order to understand physician's orders.

DRUG DOSAGE AND CLASSIFICATION

A **dose** of a drug is the amount of drug which will give a therapeutic (healing) effect. Factors that are considered when the doctor orders a medication are age, weight, the severity of the condition being treated, how the patient has previously reacted to drugs, and by what mode it should be given for that particular patient. Terms related to drug dosage are:

- **Minimal dose**—the smallest amount of the drug that will give a therapeutic effect
- **Maximal dose**—the largest therapeutic dose that can be given without being toxic (poisonous)
- **Toxic dose**—the amount of drug that will be poisonous
- **Lethal dose**—the amount of drug that will cause death

Drugs or medicines are classified according to their action. It is easier to remember the name of the drug and the action if the drug is studied in connection with the body system for which it is used. The majority of drugs will be presented in Section II after the discussion of the body system to which they relate. There are some classifications that are used for overall effect and may apply to all body systems. These are presented on pages 103 and 107 and include the mode or modes, the brand name, the generic name (in parenthesis) if that is often used, and the usual adult dose and/or the dosage range. If you are interested in generic names not given, consult the PDR.

Narcotics

The word narcotic is derived from the Greek word *narkotikos* meaning benumbing. Narcotics are given before surgery to relax the patient and after surgery to control pain. Patients with medical problems that cause pain will also need narcotics. Narcotics are always kept in the locked cabinet. The narcotics shown in Table 5-2 are usually a part of each hospital's stock supply.

Narcotic Antagonists

These are weak narcotics that exert an antagonistic action *only* when there is an overdose of narcotic. They cause depression when given alone.

- Nalline—SC, IM, IV—5 mg to 10 mg. May be repeated if respirations are not adequate.
- Lorfan—SC, IM, IV—one or more doses of 0.4 mg to 0.6 mg as needed. In acute morphine poisoning, 1 mg is given.
- Narcan—SC, IM, IV—0.4 mg. May be repeated at 2–3 minute intervals, according to response, for a total of three doses.

Hypnotics, Soporifics

These drugs produce sleep. The Greek word *hypnos* means sleep and the Latin word *sopor* means deep sleep. Hypnotics and soporifics are controlled drugs.

- Luminal (phenobarbital)—PO—30 mg q 3–4 hrs prn if patient is in need of prolonged, restful sleep. 30 mg to 60 mg if given HS for regular sleep.
- Sodium Luminal (sodium phenobarbital)—SC, IM—100 mg.

TABLE 5-2. NARCOTICS USUALLY STOCKED IN HOSPITAL

Brand Name*	Mode(s) of Administration	UAD and/or Dosage range**	Comments
Codeine	PO, SC, IM	30 mg (15 to 60 mg q 3–4 hrs prn)	Frequently used in combination with other drugs and in cough mixtures
Demerol (meperidine)	PO, SC, IM, IV	50 mg (50 to 150 mg q 3–4 hrs prn)	The mode may not be designated on post-op (after surgery) orders—check with the RN for the mode; it is usually IM because the patient is NPO.
Dilaudid (hydromorphone)	PO, SC, IM, IV Rectal supp	2 mg q 4–6 hrs prn 3 mg at HS	Give long-lasting relief
Innovar	IM IV	(0.5 to 2.0 ml) 1 ml/20 to 25 lbs	Before surgery Given in surgery by anesthetist Has a respiratory depressant action, chart should be labeled so nursing personnel may watch patient carefully.
Leritine	PO, SC, IM	25 mg (25 to 50 mg q 4–6 hrs prn)	
Dolophine (methadone)	PO, SC, IM	7.5 mg (2.5 to 10 mg q 3–4 hrs prn)	Individualized dosage for treatment of narcotic addiction
Morphine	PO SC, IM, IV	(30 to 60 mg q 4 hrs prn) 10 mg (5 to 15 mg q 3–6 hrs prn)	

Numorphan	SC, IM	(1 to 1.5 mg q 4–6 hrs prn)	
	IV	(0.5 mg q 4–6 hrs prn)	
	Rectal supp	(2.5 to 5 mg q 4–6 hrs prn)	
Pantapon	PO, SC, IM	(5 to 20 mg q 3–4 hrs prn)	
Percodan	PO only	tab ī q 6 hrs prn	May be given in higher dosages if other narcotics are not advisable.
Percodan-Demi	PO only	tab ī or īī q 6 hrs prn	Contains one-half the amount of narcotic as Percodan
Stadol	IM	(1 to 4 mg q 3–4 hrs prn)	
	IV	(0.5 to 2 mg q 3–4 hrs prn)	
Sublimaze (fentanyl citrate)	IM	(0.05 to 0.1 mg q 1–2 hrs prn)	Given pre- and postoperatively
	IV	(0.05 to 0.1 mg)	Given by anesthetist in surgery Chart should be labeled so patient is watched carefully as drug is a respiratory depressant.
Talwin (pentazocine)	PO	(50 to 100 mg q 3–4 hrs prn)	
	SC, IM, IV	30 mg q 3–4 hrs prn	

*Generic name in parenthesis
**Dosage range in parenthesis

- Nembutal (pentobarbital)—PO—100 to 200 mg, IM—150 to 200 mg, IV—100 mg, rectal supp—120 to 200 mg.
- Seconal (secobarbital)—PO, IM, rectal supp—100 to 200 mg
- Noctec (chloral hydrate)—PO, rectal supp—250 mg to 1 gm.
- Dalmane (flurazepam hydrochloride)—PO only—15 mg to 30 mg.

Analgesics

Analgesics relieve pain. Derived from the Greek word *an* meaning not and the word *algos* meaning pain.

- Ascriptin—PO—tab i̇ or i̇i̇ qid
- Aspirin (ASA) (acetylsalicylic acid)—PO—tab i̇ or i̇i̇ q 4 hrs prn. (tab = 5 gr) Supp mode supplied in 2 gr, 5 gr, 10 gr.
- Bufferin—PO—tab i̇ or i̇i̇ q 4 hrs prn, not more than 12/24 hrs.
- Ecotrin (Enteric ASA)—PO—40 gr to 80 gr a day in divided doses.
- Endecon—PO—tab i̇i̇ followed by tab i̇ or i̇i̇ q 4 hrs prn. Limit to 8 tabs/24 hrs.
- Empirin Compound—PO—tab i̇ or i̇i̇ q 4 hrs. Limit 6 tabs/24 hrs.
- Fiorinal—PO—tab i̇ or i̇i̇ prn. Limit 6 tabs/24 hrs.
- Midrin—PO caps—cap i̇ or i̇i̇ q 4 hrs. Limit 8 caps/24 hrs.
- Tylenol (acetaminophen)—PO—tab i̇ or i̇i̇ tid, qid, or q 4 hrs.
- Zomax—PO—50 mg to 100 mg q 4–6 hrs prn.

Analgesics with Narcotics

When Codeine is combined with an analgesic, the number after the name designates the amount of Codeine used.

- #1 = gr ⅛
- #2 = gr ¼
- #3 = gr ½
- #4 = gr 1.
- Empirin Compound c̄ Codeine #1, #2, #3, #4—PO—tab i̇ or i̇i̇ q 3 hrs. Limit 6 tab/24 hrs.
- Fiorinal c̄ Codeine #1, #2, #3—PO—cap i̇ or i̇i̇ prn. Limit to 6 cap/24 hrs.
- Percogesic c̄ Codeine—PO—tab i̇ or i̇i̇ q 4 hrs prn. Each tab contains 32.4 mg Codeine.
- Phenaphen c̄ Codeine #2, #3, #4—cap i̇ or i̇i̇ q 3–4 hrs prn.
- Tylenol c̄ Codeine #1, #2, #3, #4—PO—tab i̇ or i̇i̇ q 3–4 hrs.

Sedatives and Tranquilizers

These drugs provide a calming effect. Derived from the word *sedativus* meaning calming and *tranquilus* meaning agent to make calm. Some of the hypnotics may be given as sedatives by reducing the dosage and giving several times during the day as well as at bedtime. Phenobarbital is often given as a sedative.

- Atarax—PO—25 mg tid to 100 mg qid. IM—25 to 75 mg q 6 hrs.
- Endep—PO—10 to 25 mg tid.
- Elavil—PO individualized dose—tabs are 10 mg, 25 mg, 50 mg. Both Endep and Elavil are brands of amitriptyline.
- Pertofrane—PO—50 mg tid up to 200 mg/24 hrs. Caps are 25 mg and 50 mg.
- Phenergan (promethazine)—IM, IV—25 to 50 mg q 3–4 hrs prn. PO—12.5 to 25 mg tid or qid.
- Serax—PO—15 mg tid. Caps are 10 mg, 15 mg, 30 mg.
- Tofranil (imipramine)—PO—50 to 100 mg/24 hrs. Tabs are 10 mg, 25 mg, 50 mg. IM—individualized—2cc = 25 mg.
- Tranxene—PO—15 to 60 mg/24 hrs. Caps are 3.75 mg, 7.5 mg, 15 mg.
- Valium (diazepam)—IM, IV, PO—individualized dose. PO is usually 2 to 10 mg bid, tid, or qid. Tabs are 2 mg, 5 mg and 10 mg.
- Vistaril—PO—25 mg tid to 100 mg qid. IM—50 to 100 mg q 4–6 hrs prn.

Many times when a patient requests narcotics, hypnotics, analgesics, or tranquilizers more than is deemed necessary for their condition, a placebo will be ordered. Placebo is Latin for "I shall please." A **placebo** is an injection or capsule of an inactive substance. It is believed that they relieve pain by activating the brain to produce its own pain killing substances called endorphins. Placebos are also used in studies for new products.

Antinauseants

Nausea means a sick feeling as if you need to vomit. Anti- means against, so these drugs help prevent or control nausea.
- Atarax—IM—25 to 100 mg q 4–6 hrs prn. PO—25 to 100 mg tid ac.
- Compazine (prochlorperazine)—IM—5 to 10 mg q 3–4 hrs prn. PO—5 to 10 mg tid or qid.
- Dramamine (dimenhydrinate)—PO—50 mg q 4 hrs. IM, IV by weight and age. Supp 100 mg daily or bid.
- Emete-Con—IM—50 mg q 3–4 hrs.
- Phenergan—PO—12.5 to 25 mg tid ac or qid ac and HS. IM—25 mg q 4–6 hrs prn.
- Tigan—PO—Cap i̇ (250 mg) tid or qid. IM—200 mg q 6 hrs prn.
- Torecan—PO—tab i̇ (10 mg) daily or tid. IM—2cc daily or tid, 2cc = 10 mg. Supp 10 mg daily or tid.
- Wans—Supp No 1 q 4–6 hrs prn. Limit 4 supp/24 hrs.

The above examples do not mean that the drugs listed are all the drugs of that category. Drugs are listed in the PDR in various ways—Manufacturers' Index, Alphabetical Index, Drug Classification Index, Generic and Chemical Name, Product Identification, Product Information, and Diagnostic Products Information. Use the PDR.

REVIEW QUESTIONS

1. Identify the following abbreviations:

PO _____   Cl _____
subl _____   K _____
IT _____   q d _____
IVPB _____   qid _____
SC _____   tid _____
H _____   bid _____
IM _____   HS _____
IV _____   pc _____
Stat _____   ac _____
Na _____   c̄ _____

2. Define:

Sedative _____
Hypnotic _____
Narcotic _____
Analgesic _____
Antinauseant _____

3. Complete the following measures:

5 cc = _____ dr = _____ tsp
240 cc = _____ oz = _____ glass
1000 cc = _____ oz = _____ quart or liter
15 cc = _____ dr = _____ tbsp
gr ī = _____ mg

4. List eight narcotics and the UAD or dosage range for each.

_____
_____
_____
_____
_____
_____
_____
_____
_____

5. List four tranquilizers and the UAD or dosage range for each.

_____
_____
_____
_____

6. List five analgesics and the UAD or dosage range for each.

_____

_____

_____

_____

_____

7. List four antinauseants and the UAD or dosage range for each.

_____

_____

_____

_____

8. Define placebo _____

9. Controlled drugs are those _____

10. Define pharmacology. _____.

11. List ten ways in which drugs are prepared.

_____   _____

_____   _____

_____   _____

_____   _____

_____   _____

12. Why is accuracy so important in orders for drugs?

_____

_____

Situational Application

Apply the knowledge gained from this chapter to the following situations. Circle the letter for the most appropriate answer.

13. A patient is receiving a continuous IV and needs antibiotics. The doctor would order the antibiotic given by:
    a. IVPB
    b. IV push
    c. IV Heparin loc

14. A patient is having a great deal of pain. You would expect the doctor to order a:
    a. Hypnotic
    b. Tranquilizer
    c. Narcotic

15. An order is written ac qid. You would give the drug at:
    a. 0900-1300-1700-2100
    b. 0800-1200-1600-2000
    c. 0730-1130-1630-2200
16. A patient is admitted and states she has been vomiting. You would expect the doctor to order:
    a. An analgesic
    b. A soporific
    c. An antinauseant
17. A doctor is concerned with costs of medication for a patient who is going home and will require Home Health Care. Because of the cost concern, you would expect the medications to be:
    a. Given intramuscularly
    b. Given by mouth
    c. Given subcutaneously

Chapter 6 | Transcribing Physician's Orders

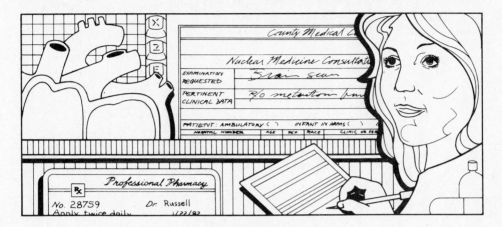

OBJECTIVES

Study of this chapter will enable you to:

1. Define transcription as it applies to Physician's Orders.
2. Discuss the use of computers in transcription.
3. List the information provided on medicine cards.
4. List the classifications of drugs that require renewal dates.
5. Identify abbreviations pertaining to treatments.
6. List and explain the types of doctor's orders.
7. Identify abbreviations for common IV solutions.
8. Explain the use of the kardex card.
9. List the rules for transcription.
10. Transcribe a set of orders.

The Latin word *transcribere* means to transfer in writing. Transcribing Physician's Orders means transferring what the doctor has written onto a departmental requisition, a computer screen, a card for nursing personnel, or a chart form and to a kardex card. Since different hospitals have different methods, this explanation will include computer use, Medical Administration Record (MAR) use, and use of medication cards.

COMPUTERS

The following information is reprinted with permission from *Patient Care Sys-*

tem (Pamphlet G520-3415-0) and *Patient Care at Good Samaritan Hospital* (Pamphlet GK20-1203-0) by International Business Machines Corporation. Screens are revised from *Health Care Support* DL-1, *Patient Care System* (OS-VS)—Pamphlet SH20-1955-0—published by IBM; permission given by IBM for use of the revisions.

The computer network operates much like a telephone system, except that messages are preserved in hard copy, and may be directed simultaneously to many locations.

Patient care data is entered into the system by staff professionals using video display terminals at nursing stations or in service departments. The system guides the terminal user through the steps of entering, updating or retrieving information on an individual patient. Data security may be assured by requiring that a staff identification code be entered before any patient information can be entered, modified, or retrieved.

The terminal user, who need not have any data processing experience or training, uses either a light pen or a typewriter-like keyboard to collect and display data. A light pen is a pencil-like instrument attached to the terminal by cable. The screen is touched by the tip of the pen at the appropriate spot and the button on the pen is pressed to register the item selected. When an entry is completed, data is displayed for the terminal user to verify all items entered or to make any necessary corrections. This information is then stored within the data base, where it is immediately available.

Both nurses and clerical personnel may enter orders. Orders entered by nurses become "active" immediately; orders entered by clerical personnel remain "inactive" until verified by a nurse. Only verified orders are transmitted to ancillary departments for processing. If necessary, a nurse may correct or delete an unverified order. In addition, outstanding orders or partially completed orders (such as a five-day medication order with three days yet to go) may be canceled if, for example, an attending physician requests a change in medication.

Nursing station displays perform other functions. They may be used to change an attending or consulting physician in a patient's data base record. Nurses may send messages to the dietary department, both in response to physician requests and to coordinate a patient's food service with scheduled radiology and other diagnostic services. Nursing station screens can also display a census of all patients currently assigned to a station, as well as a profile for each patient detailing status information, such as diagnosis, surgery date, and any allergies or isolation requirements.

A thrice daily (once-each-shift) working document for nursing stations that details information for each patient is printed.

Downtime means that a computer is not working. This means that the hospital must return to the manual paper back-up system. When the system is active again, all manual orders must be entered and the system updated. Therefore, you need to know the back-up system.

```
ROOM              PATIENT              DATE
545               _____, Marie   01–22–xx
               SELECT THE CATEGORY OF ORDER
Care & Treatment          Cardiology
Laboratory                Resp. Therapy
Radiology                 Physical Therapy
Dietary                   EEG
Nuclear Medicine          Home Health Care
Central Supply            Pharmacy

N ORD 17
```

Figure 6-1. Category Selection Screen.

```
ROOM              PATIENT
545               _____, Marie
                  REVIEW THE ORDER
              ORDER      FREQ       BGN DT      BGN TM
Hem 1         CBC        once       01–22       1400

PERFORMING LAB                END DT     END TM
Hematology                    01–22      1400

SPEC. COLLECTED BY            ORDERING DOCTOR
Lab                           Dr. Noel

WORDS OF THE ORDER                TEST INSTRUCTIONS
_____             ASAP
_____             _____
_____             _____

Review                Delete              Accept
```

Figure 6-2. Order Review Screen.

```
ROOM              PATIENT              DATE
545               _____, Marie   01–22–xx

TYPE ORDER        DOCTOR ORDERING      PERSON ORDERING
Pharmacy          Dr. Noel             M. Kopp, US

0001    Demerol          50–75 mgm      93hprn      IM
        (meperidine)
0002    Kefzol           250 mgm        q8h         IVPB
                         Accept: T. Beck, RN
```

Figure 6-3. Pharmacy Order Screen.

```
                    LABORATORY INTERIM REPORT

                 *****BLOOD CHEMISTRIES*****

                     CL    CO₂    K      NA    BUN   GLUC
                    MEQ/L  MM/L  MEQ/L  MEQ/L  MG%   MG%
   01–23  0630   CHEM  100    28    3.5    136    14    95

                 CHOL  BILI  LDH  SGOT  CREAT  T/P   ALB   CA   PHOS
                 MG%   MG%   IU    IU   MG%   GM%   GM%   MG%   MG%
   01–23  0630   CHEM  230   0.8  169   85    1.2   6.6   4.8   9.2   2.2


     Page 1                          _____, Marie RM 545
                                     026493
                                     Dr. Noel
                                     Adm: 01–22–xx
```

Figure 6-4. Laboratory Interim Report Screen.

TYPES OF DOCTOR'S ORDERS

A doctor may order a medication, a treatment, or some kind of therapy with different specifications for the length of time that order is to be considered current.

Standing Orders

Standing orders are those that remain in effect until the doctor discontinues them or changes the original order. Some examples are:

Tylenol tab ii q 4 hrs.
Physical Therapy to give whirlpool treatments daily.
Change dressing or operative wound once each shift.
Eggcrate mattress.

One-Time Orders

The doctor writes an order that is to be done only one time and then discontinued. If the order is a medication order, the card will have the stop date entered and the date will be the same as the start date. Orders of this category read like:

Valium 5 mgm now.
Give liquid diet this noon only.
Have patient in cast room at 11 A.M.
Will do spinal puncture at 8 A.M. tomorrow. Have tray ready.

Limited Time Orders

The doctor writes an order and specifies how many times the order is to be performed or how many hours the order is in effect. Limited time orders would read:

> *Give Demerol 50 mgm IM q 4 hrs for 24 hrs.*
> *Physical Therapy to get patient up twice today.*
> *Chart I & O for three days.*
> *Send to Radiation Therapy daily for 5 days.*

Standing PRN Orders

The doctor writes a standing order which is carried out on request of the patient or when deemed necessary by the personnel carrying for the patient. PRN means when necessary or as desired. Examples:

> *Alupent inhaler 2 whiffs qid prn.*
> *Tylenol tabs ii q 4 hrs prn for headache.*
> *IPPB c̄ Bronkosol ¼ cc in 3 cc 0.45 NS qid prn.*
> *Catheterize q 8 hrs prn.*

Combination Orders

The doctor writes an order for a one time medication or treatment followed by a prn or limited time. Examples:

> *Demerol 75 mg IM now and 50 mg q 4 hrs prn for pain.*
> *Physical Therapy to do whirlpool now and bid starting tomorrow.*
> *Incentive spirometer as soon as awake and q 1 hr for 8 hrs and then q 3 hrs.*
> *Change dressing now and q 4 hrs prn.*

Stat Orders

Any order containing the word stat must be carried out immediately. The word now means the same as stat. Examples:

> *Chest x-ray now.*
> *CBC stat and call results to me.*
> *Demerol 50 mg IV stat.*

MEDICATION ORDERS

Medication orders require the name of the medication, a dosage, a mode and a frequency. A doctor may omit the mode, assuming that it is understood which mode will be used. For instance, a patient is NPO following surgery and the order reads "Demerol 50 mg q 4 hrs prn pain" which excludes PO mode. You need to check with the nurse as to which mode, IM or IV, to enter on the card. Usually, IM mode is used but check with the nurse as she will know the doctors and their routines. Many medications that are ordinarily given PO will have the mode omitted on the order.

Medication orders are entered into the computer, written on the Medication Administration Record, or on medication cards. A card requires the patient's room number, the patient's name, the name of the doctor who wrote the order, the name of the medication, the dosage, the mode, the frequency, a start date, a stop or renewal date when applicable, times to correspond to the frequency, and initials of the desk RN.

Some medications may have automatic renewal dates set by the hospital. The common medications requiring renewal dates are narcotics, anticoagulants, and antibiotics. Your instructor will supply a list of drugs requiring renewal dates in your hospital and the renewal frequency.

Standing Medication Orders

Standing orders will not have a stop date as the medication will be given until the doctor writes an order to discontinue the medication or makes a change in the original order.

EXERCISE

Complete medication cards or enter into computer or enter on the MAR sheet the following: (Refer to Figure 6-5.)

1. *Tylenol tabs ïï PO q 4 hrs.*
2. *Lanoxin 0.25 mg IV daily.*
3. *Elavil 25 mg bid.*
4. *Kefzol 250 mg IM q 8 hrs.*

One Time Medication Orders

A one time order may be a stat, ASAP, or now order. Stat orders are completed *immediately*. ASAP orders are urgent and are completed as soon as possible. Now orders are the same as stat. On medication cards, there will be a stop date as well as the start date and both will be the same. Some hospitals have a rule that stat, ASAP, and now orders must be marked "given" on the Physician's Order Sheet and signed by the person giving the medication.

Other one time medication orders may read "today," "one time only,"or "this A.M." On medication cards, the general rule is to write the word or words in the order under the Time section of the card.

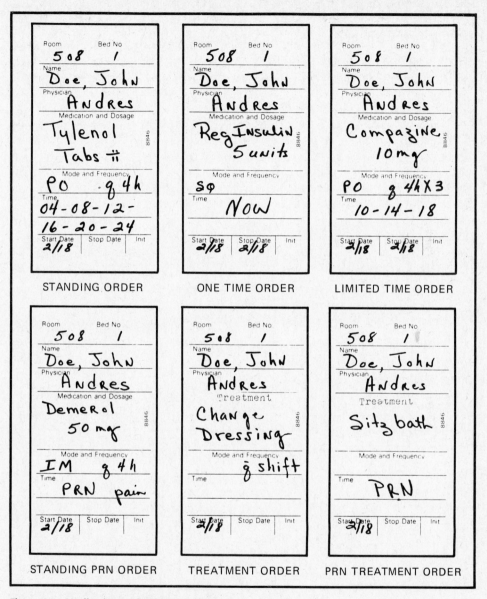

Figure 6-5. Medication and Treatment Cards.

EXERCISE

Refer to the cards in Figure 6-5 to complete medication cards, or enter on MAR, or enter into computer the following orders:

1. *Demerol 75 mg IM stat.*
2. *Dalmane 30 mg hs this evening only.*
3. *Valium 10 mg IM before changing the dressings.*
4. *Insulin for this AM, NPH 15 U and Reg. 5 U.*

Limited Time Medication Orders

A medication may be ordered for a certain number of times or repeated so many times or for a certain time period. Medication cards will have stop dates which may or may not be the same date as the start date. Be sure you have the card just as the doctor ordered and times correctly entered. A PRN medication may be ordered every so many hours for so many doses. Since the medication will be given only when needed, you have no way of knowing when the specified number of times will be completed. The general method is: in the time section of the card write doses and the numbers from one to the maximum times the medication is to be given; the nurse will cross off a number each time the medication is given so that the medication will be discontinued when all the numbers are crossed off the card. The frequency will be how often plus the number of times, such as q 4 hrs x 8 doses. The stop date would be p̄ 8th dose.

EXERCISE

Refer to Figure 6-5 and 6-6 to complete medication cards for the following orders or write them on the MAR sheet or enter into the computer:

1. *May have Demerol 50 mg IM q 4 hrs for 24 hrs.*
2. *Prednisone 5 mg daily for 6 days.*
3. *Benadryl 50 mg q 6 hrs x 3.*
4. *Lanoxin 0.25 mg IV today and tomorrow.*

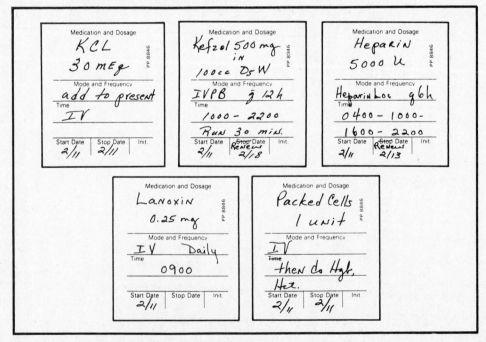

Figure 6-6. IV Medication Cards.

Standing PRN Medication Orders

The doctor writes an order for medication to be given at specified time intervals when needed. The order remains active until it is discontinued by the doctor or a change is made in the original order. Cards are completed with the time intervals in the frequency space and PRN under Time. The doctor may or may not specify why the medication is given, such as PRN for pain, for Temp over 101°, PRN for nausea, etc. When the reason is given, place it under Time with PRN. There are no actual times on PRN cards because it is not given routinely but only as needed.

EXERCISE

Refer to Figure 6-5 to complete the following orders on cards or enter on MAR sheet, or in the computer.

1. *Demerol 50 mg every 4 hrs prn for pain. May give PO or IM.*
2. *ASA gr x q 4 hrs for T > 101°.*
3. *Valium 5 mg q 6 hrs prn agitation.*
4. *Compazine 10 mg IM prn nausea.*

(Order #1 requires two cards, one for PO and one for IM in most hospitals as different colors designate modes. The two cards would be stapled back to back so the nurse could easily see the two colors and two modes.)

Combination Medication Orders

The doctor may order one dose of a medication stat and then every so many hours prn or routinely. This is actually two orders in one so it requires two cards, one for the stat and one for the rest of the order. The stat card would have a stop date the same as the start date, the other card would not have a stop date. If the order is prn, the card will not have specific times. If the medication is to be given routinely after the stat dose, enter times.

EXERCISE

Refer to Figure 6-5 and 6-6 to complete cards or MAR sheet or enter into computer the following orders:

1. *Valium 5 mg stat and then q 6 hrs, PO.*
2. *Demerol 50 mg IM now and then q 4 hrs prn for 48 hrs.*
3. *Tylenol tabs ii stat and q 4 hrs prn headache.*
4. *Vistaril 25 mg PO and q 6 hrs prn nervousness.*
5. *Ampicillin 500 mg IVPB stat and q 6 hrs.*

IV Solution Orders

Intravenous solutions supply nutrition when a patient is unable to take food orally or the digestive system is unable to function properly. Some of the solutions are composed of dextrose (a simple sugar) and water, others are a combination of elements the body needs. Common IV solutions and their abbreviations:

IV Solution	*Abbreviation*
5% Dextrose in 0.2% Sodium Chloride	D5/0.2NaCl or D5/¼NS
5% Dextrose in 0.45% Sodium Chloride	D5/0.45NaCl or D5/½NS
5% Dextrose in 0.9% Sodium Chloride	D5/NS or D5NS
5% Dextrose in Water	D5/W or D5W
5% Dextrose in Ringer's (Ringer's contains Na, K, Ca, and Cl.)	D5/R or D5R
5% Dextrose in lactated Ringer's	D5/LR or D5LR or D5/RL or D5RL
Lactated Ringer's or Ringer's lactated (Lactated Ringer's contains Na, K, Ca, Cl and lactate)	LR or RL
Normal Saline (0.9% Sodium Chloride)	NS, also known as physiologic salt solution
½ Normal Saline	½ NS or 0.45NS
10% Dextrose in Water	D10/W or D10W

Vitamins are often added to IV solutions. Electrolytes are added in the form of salts. If a patient needs sodium, sodium chloride is added; if a patient needs potassium, potassium chloride is added. These additives may change frequently on seriously ill patients according to the patient's blood evaluations.

Total Parenteral Nutrition (TPN), formerly called hyperalimentation, is a basic solution with added vitamins, electrolytes, and minerals. The additives change in accordance with the patient's blood evaluations.

IV solutions are prepared in 1000cc, 500cc, 250cc, 100cc, and 50cc glass bottles or plastic bags. The usual amount used is 1000cc. A doctor may specify the rate at which the solution is to be given instead of an amount. This means that a new bottle or new bag is hung as needed. If hospital policy dictates that you complete the IV solution requisition and the order reads "rate," consult with the nurse regarding amount of solution until you know solutions well and know how they are used.

IV solution orders are entered into the computer, on a special IV form for MAR users, or on cards.

Beck, Patricia 428-1	Beck, Patricia 428-1	Beck, Patricia 428-1
I.V. Card:	I.V. Card:	I.V. Card:
I.V. Solution: alternate 1000cc D₅W c̄ 1000cc D₅LR	I.V. Solution: 1) 1000cc D₅W 2) 1000cc D5 0.45 NaCl 3) 1000cc D₅W	I.V. Solution: D₅W
Medications added:	Medications added: to #2 only add 1 amp MVI	Medications added: 30 mEq KCl) each 1 Amp MVI / liter
Rate: 125 cc/h	Rate: 100 cc/h	Rate: 80 cc/h
Doctor: Elden	Doctor: Elden	Doctor: Elden
Misc. & or special precautions	Misc. & or special precautions	Misc. & or special precautions
Date: 2/11 Nurse:	Date: 2/11 Nurse:	Date: 2/11 Nurse:
P.P. 4731	P.P. 4731	P.P. 4731

Figure 6-7. IV Solution Cards.

EXERCISE

Refer to Figure 6-7 to complete the following orders on cards, or enter on IV sheet or enter in computer.

1. *1000cc D5W followed by 1000cc D5/¼NS at 100cc per hr.*
2. *D5W at TKO rate (TKO means to keep open)*
3. *D5/LR at 80cc/hr*

Blood and Blood Products

All blood and blood products are given IV and hospital policy dictates whether the card is a medication card or an IV solution card. The most common approach is to use a medication card since the time element is short compared to an IV solution.

Blood may be ordered as whole blood or packed red cells (PRC or PRBC). The patient must be typed (have their blood type determined) and cross-matched with the donor's blood before the transfusion may be given. A doctor may write an order for "2 U blood today" which means the patient will have to be typed and crossed (T&X or T&C) even though the order does not state the fact. You must remember to order the T&X if it was not previously ordered.

Blood is ordered in units and is obtained from the Blood Bank section of the laboratory. One requisition is needed to order the T&C, specify whole blood or PRC, and specify the quantity ordered. Another requisition is needed to pick up the blood or PRC. Your instructor will demonstrate the requisitions used in your hospital and the routine for picking up the product from the Blood Bank.

You may be required to order 250cc of IV Normal Saline and the blood tubing at the time you transcribe a transfusion order for unit personnel. Transfusions that are ordered to be held for OR would not include this duty. Normal saline is used to start the transfusion procedure to be sure the solution will flow smoothly and after the transfusion to flush the tubing to assure that the patient receives the entire unit. Your instructor will demonstrate the procedure used in your hospital.

Blood products include:

- **Plasma**—Fresh Frozen Plasma (FFP)
- **Albumin**—Salt Free Albumin (SFA); Salt Poor Albumin (SPA)
- **Thrombin**—a plasma constituent
- **Fibrinogen**—a plasma constituent
- **Cryoprecipitate**—antihemophilic component
- **Dextran**—plasma substitute obtained from the pharmacy
- **Dextran 40 or Rheomacrodex**—plasma substitute obtained from pharmacy
- **Platelets**—blood cells that aid clotting

EXERCISE

After your instructor has demonstrated the use of requisitions for the Blood Bank and procedure for transcription, practice with the following orders:

1. *Type and cross and hold for surgery in AM, 2U PRBC*
2. *Give 2 units PRCs today.*
3. *Give 4 units cyoprecipitate ASAP.*
4. *Give 2 units of platelets and then get platelet count.*

Changing Original Orders

Changing original orders can apply to any type of order. Changing a standing medication order will be used as an example. Transcribing a change in an order is a little different than transcribing an original order.

Example: the original order read "Demerol 50 mg IM q 4 hrs." The new order reads " ↑ Demerol to 75 mg q 3 hrs." The card does not have to contain the increase symbol, only the medication, the dosage, the frequency, and the times. The original card is torn and discarded after the nurse signs the orders. The mode is still IM even though the second order did not specify since it is a change in orders. Sometimes only the dosage is changed so you would use the frequency in the original order. Always refer to the original order on the Physician's Order sheet and not just the original card.

TREATMENT AND ACTIVITY ORDERS

Treatment is derived from the Latin word *tractare* which means to handle. Treatments include types of baths, enemas, douches, irrigations, dressings to wounds, heat or cold applications, positioning of the body or parts of the body and preparations for surgery. Activities refer to whether the patient is on bedrest, may use a wheelchair, may sit in a chair, or may walk around the unit.

Baths are to promote healing. A Sitz bath uses a special tub or a portable appliance to fit on a commode to soak the perineal area in very warm water. This promotes healing following surgeries like hemorrhoid surgery. Other baths are for skin problems and will have a medication or substance, such as oatmeal, added to the water.

Enemas are solutions introduced into the rectum and colon for cleansing purposes or medicinal purposes. A small rectal tip or colon tube is inserted into the anus, and the solution flows into the rectum and colon. Cleansing enemas are expelled, medicinal enemas are retained. Types of enemas are:

- **TWE**—tap water enema used for cleansing
- **SSE**—soap suds enema used for cleansing
- **Fleets** enema—pre-packaged solution in a plastic container. Used for cleansing when a patient is constipated or when the rectum and colon need to be clean for an examination.
- **Oil retention enema**—pre-packaged oil solution used to soften the stool. May be followed by a TWE in a specified period of time.
- **Medicinal enemas**—a medication dissolved in a small amount of solution; the solution is retained for absorption.

Douches are streams of a solution directed against a part of the body. The most common is the vaginal douche for cleansing, for surgical prep, or medicinal to treat a vaginal condition.

Irrigations are washings of a canal or wound by flushing with a solution. Irrigations may be applied to the bladder, throat, ear, colon, or wound.

Dressings may vary from a very simple dry, sterile dressing to a complex type. The patient may have an irrigation and then a dressing applied to a wound. Ointments may be applied before a dressing.

Heat and cold applications may be wet or dry. Hot wet packs may be used with a heavy wrapping and an electric heating pad on top of the wrapping. Heating pads are fixed to give a certain amount of heat; the high heat setting is eliminated to prevent an accidental burn. K-pads are used for moist heat and have water circulating inside a plastic pad. Heat may be applied by immersing a part of the body in warm water. Cold packs may be dressings soaked in ice water, use of an ice pack, or immersion of a part of the body in cold water for a short time. Ice packs for small areas may be made by filling a plastic glove with ice.

Surgical preparations include shaving an area, scrubbing an area with a bacteriostatic solution, showers, enemas, douches, and irrigations. Betadine is a popular preparation for scrubs. The doctor may specify the area to be prepared or the hospital may have standard preps for operations according to the area involved.

Tubes inserted into the nose and leading into the stomach or small intestines are explained in Chapter 13.

Catheters for urinary drainage are explained in Chapter 14.

Chest tubes may be inserted during thoracic surgery. Care of these tubes is a treatment. Orders will state the type of suction to the tube and the amount of pressure. One type of machine connected to the tube or tubes is an Emerson pump or suction.

Positioning may mean turning every so often, keeping a part of the body elevated to a specified degree or on pillows or special positions for comfort or for examinations. Types of positions:

- **Dorsal**—on back, legs straight
- **Fowler's**—semi-sitting, head of bed elevated 45°, knees flexed
- **Knee-chest**—kneeling with chest resting on thighs, head turned to the side
- **Lateral**—lying on a side
- **Lithotomy**—lying on back, feet out to the side and elevated above the hip; feet are usually in stirrups if an examination table is used
- **Prone**—lying face down
- **Recumbent**—lying on back, knees bent
- **Semi-Fowler's**—head elevated about 30°, knees flexed
- **Sim's**—lying on left side, knees bent with right knee and leg closer to the chest than the left leg, the left arm is extended behind the back
- **Trendelenburg**—the entire body is slanted so that the head is lower than the feet. Automatic beds are equipped to be placed in this position.

Abbreviations for Treatments

Abbreviation	*Meaning*
BLESS	patient may have a bath, laxative, enema, shampoo, shower, or shave prn.
bndg	bandage
chg, △	change
circ	circulation
ck or √	check
cont	continue, continuous
cxl	cancel
DSD	dry, sterile dressing
DB&C	deep breathe and cough
dc, D/C	discontinue, discharge
drge	drainage
drsg	dressing
irrig	irrigate, irrigation
isol	isolation
pt	patient
re	regarding
TCDB	turn, cough, deep breathe

U/O	urinary output
wd	wound
↑	increase
↓	decrease

Abbreviations for Activities

Abbreviation	*Meaning*
amb	ambulate, walk
BR	bedrest
BRP	bathroom privileges
BSC	bedside commode
OOB	out of bed

EXERCISE

Transfer the following orders to the card you will use for treatments and activities.
1. Ambulate with assistance bid
2. Irrigate abdominal wound c̄ NS and apply DSD q 8 hrs
3. Prep right groin for surgery in AM
4. Up in chair for meals

| NURSING OBSERVATION ORDERS

The orders written by the doctor involve some type of observation by the nurse. Some hospitals may consider these orders as treatment orders, they are usually carded in the same fashion as treatment orders.

- **I&O**—intake and output; the nurse records all the fluids taken *into* the body and the route and the nurse records all the fluids that *leave* the body and the route
- Checking for **circulation** or for specific signs. The order may read "Ck circ Ⓛ leg q hr."
- **Neuro signs** are discussed in Chapter 16.
- **VS**—temperature, pulse, respiration (TPR) with the blood pressure (BP).

The blood pressure may be ordered separately to be checked more often than the TPR. Pulses are of different types according to the area where they are taken:

- Radial pulse is at the wrist
- Pedal pulse is on top of the foot or the artery near the ankle bone

- Apical pulse is taken with a stethoscope at the apex of the heart
- Popliteal pulse is taken behind the knee.

Nursing observation orders may be written by the nurse on the Physician's Order Sheet if the nurse deems an observation is necessary. Hospitals have guidelines for these orders.

PREOPERATIVE ORDERS

The preoperative orders will be one time or limited time orders. The surgeon will write orders for the permit and the prep. The anesthesiologist writes orders for NPO (nothing by mouth) and what time the NPO begins, a hypnotic for that night, and a preoperative medication before surgery which will have a time specified or will be ordered on call. When a patient goes to surgery, all orders are canceled unless the postoperative orders state "resume all preop orders."

ORDERS REQUIRING CENTRAL SUPPLY ITEMS

Sterile examination trays, catheters, items for dressings, and comfort items are obtained as needed. Articles such as slings may be supplied from the Orthopedic Room, IV tubing and blood tubing may come from pharmacy. Therefore, it is better if your instructor gives you the CS requisition and demonstrates the procedure for ordering.

DEPARTMENTAL DIAGNOSTIC TESTS AND THERAPY ORDERS

Forms used for tests and therapy from departments were shown in Chapter 2. We will look at the types of orders for each department and requisitioning. Some of the information here may be repeated in Section II in the chapter concerning the system to which the orders apply. To perform transcription you need an overall view of orders.

Cardiology Lab

Cardiology is the study of the heart. This lab deals with the examinations which show how the heart functions and why the heart is not functioning correctly. Each test is explained in more detail in Chapter 11, but we will look at them briefly now.

- **ECG or EKG** (electrocardiogram) records the electrical activity of the heart.
- **Holter Monitor ECG** is a 12 or 24 hour EKG. Patient has a portable machine attached and goes about the usual activities.
- **Treadmilll exercise ECG** is a recording while the patient walks on a treadmill.
- **Echocardiogram** is a picture of the interior of the heart produced by ultrasound waves.
- **Heart catheterization** involves placing a catheter into the heart chambers. X-rays and blood samples are taken.
- **Pacemakers** are devices that supply an electrical charge to the heart to keep the heart rate steady.

EXERCISE

Use your classroom forms to order the following:
1. Routine ECG today
2. Holter monitor for 24 hours; try to start this AM.
3. Patient to cardiology lab at 1 PM today for pacemaker implant.

Dietary

Nutrition is an important part of recovery from an illness. The dietitians assist the doctor in the care of the patient. Types of diets are discussed in Chapter 13. The most common ones are clear liquids, full liquids, soft, ADA (diabetic), and regular.

EXERCISE

Using your classroom requisition, complete a diet order for:
1. Clear liquids for lunch, full liquids for evening
2. ADA 1500 calorie diet, have dietitian see patient
3. May have in-between meal snacks
4. Soft diet, give lunch before discharge

EEG Lab

Electroencephalograms record the electrical activity of the brain. The patient should be shampooed before the exam and told not to use any creams or sprays on the hair. EEG exams are discussed in Chapter 16.

EXERCISE

Using your classroom requisitions order an EEG without sleep deprivation on a patient who has had periods of vertigo for the past four months and whose coordination is decreasing.

Physical Therapy, Occupational Therapy

Chapter 2 discussed some therapy supplied by these sections of the Rehabilitation Department. The department needs to know the diagnosis of the patient, surgery, if any performed, and the exact order just as the doctor wrote it.

EXERCISE

Using your classroom requisitions order the following:
1. Cervical traction 5 lb tid for 30 min.
2. Teach 4 gait training, heel weight bearing
3. PT for whirlpool daily with debridement of burn areas and dressings
4. Devise exercise program for 15 yr old diabetic to assimilate everyday activities while he is in the hospital.

Laboratory

Chapter 2 discussed the divisions of the laboratory. Each division will have a requisition which lists the tests they performed. You will learn the different tests in Part 2 as you learn the body systems. All requisitions require the name of the doctor who wrote the order so when reports are called, the correct doctor will be contacted. The time the exam is to be performed will be specified by the doctor in most cases. If the time is not specified, the hospital will have rules about times. Some tests require that the patient be NPO after midnight, other tests require a certain length of time between the test and a medication. The lab manual on each unit will contain this information. Use the manual until you become familiar with tests. Appendix 1 of this text explains lab tests and if any preparation is needed.

Common tests are:

- **CBC**—complete blood count
- **H & H**—hemoglobin and hematocrit, components of the blood
- **C&S**—cultures and sensitivity, a study to determine what bacteria is present and what medication will kill the bacteria

- **Electrolytes**—the amount of sodium, potassium, chloride, and carbon dioxide in the blood
- **Urinalysis**—breaks down the urine into all normal components and shows if any abnormal components are present.

EXERCISE

Using your classroom requisitions, order the following:
1. CBC and UA (urinalysis) ASAP
2. H & H, electrolytes in AM; call results to Dr. Pearson

Radiology

All x-rays go to this department. Remember from Chapter 2 that the Ultrasound section does examinations ordered as ultrasound, sonograms, and echograms; the nuclear medicine section does scans which require administration of radioactive material.

Some x-rays require a dye and this type must be performed before barium (Ba) is given for other x-rays. X-rays requiring a dye:

- **Cholecystogram or Gallbladder Series (GB)**—dye given orally the night before; remember to schedule for the following day
- **Intravenous cholangiogram**—dye is given IV in x-ray; used to show the gallbladder and the bile ducts
- **Intravenous pyelogram (IVP)**—dye is given IV in x-ray. May be performed the same day it is ordered or may require a prep established by the radiology department.

The radiology department compiles a list of the order in which x-rays are to be performed. Your instructor will supply you with the list for the hospital where you will work. This varies in some hospitals—some will do several exams in one day and others will do only one exam a day. The x-ray manual will contain the prep used before certain x-rays. Special x-rays are explained in Part 2 with the system to which they apply.

EXERCISE

Using your classroom forms order the following:
1. AP & Lat chest stat
2. X-ray pelvis and both hips today
3. Skull series this AM
4. Sonogram of the pancreas
5. Bone scan to rule out metastasis from breast cancer

Respiratory Therapy

Chapter 12 explains all the therapy and tests performed by this department. Briefly they are:

- Oxygen therapy
- Pulmonary function tests to determine the condition of the lungs
- Incentive spirometry to assure deep breathing
- Nebulization treatments with medications to loosen secretions in the lungs, remove old air, and help the patient breathe easier
- Chest physiotherapy to loosen secretions and drain the lung or lungs; this is accomplished by a clapping of the cupped hands on the chest wall.

EXERCISE

Using your classroom requisitions, order the following:
1. O_2 at 2 l/m by nasal cannula
2. Incentive spirometer at bedside, instruct in use before surgery
3. Complete PFTs (pulmonary function tests) with blood gases in AM
4. Chest physiotherapy to left lower lobe qid

USE OF THE KARDEX OR PATIENT CARE CARD

Each hospital compiles a care card that is acceptable to the nursing staff. The card usually has printed items so you can easily see where each order should be entered. The cards fit into the holders (also called kardex) by room rotation. Whether pen or pencil is used for entries is an individual hospital preference. The most widely used approach is to use pencil so that orders may be erased when changed or discontinued.

The patient ID is entered on admission. Be sure to enter the name of the nearest relative and the telephone number so it will be readily available in an emergency.

Be sure to enter allergies if any are known or designate that none are known.

The kardex card shown has three divisions. The top portion includes typed entries. Circle the entry that corresponds to the order and enter the date ordered.

The underside of the top portion has spaces for diagnostic tests, the date to be done, and the date ordered. Complete all spaces for all entries. The night shift uses this section as a guide to hold breakfast or keep a patient NPO until a test is completed. The IV section is for IV solution orders and blood or blood products.

The medication section is for standing, limited time orders, and the IV orders for medications that are standing orders. All PRN medications are entered under the PRN section.

Treatments that are standing orders are entered under treatments. All PRN treatments are listed under PRN Treatments.

Keep the card neat as you transcribe. Orders that have been discontinued or are made obsolete by new orders are either erased or lined through with the DC date entered, whichever is hospital policy.

RULES FOR TRANSCRIPTION

If you transcribe in an orderly manner, the time to complete a set of orders is decreased. Your instructor may want you to use certain symbols as you transcribe. For this reason the symbols used in this book are minimal to allow for changes without a lot of confusion for you. The symbol / after an order means you have either made the card, entered the order on the MAR sheet or entered the order in the computer; ordered the test; or made the call necessary to carry out the order. An **X** means that you have kardexed the order as well as taken the steps to carry out the order. A step by step procedure follows:

1. Read all orders to see if there are any stats, nows, ASAPS. Do such orders first. If several charts contain new orders, look through all of them for items that need immediate action.
2. After all immediate action orders are completed, remove profiles (carbon copies) of Physician's Order sheets and send to pharmacy.
3. Work with one chart at a time. If not using computers, obtain all needed departmental requisitions for that chart and addressograph each. Check ID on chart and on order sheet with addressograph card. Be sure the addressograph is in the proper place.
4. Start with the first order. Enter in computer or complete requisition, card, or phone call. If the order is a DC, tear card or notify department. Make a slash mark on the right side of the order, far enough away from the doctor's writing so it does not interfere with reading the order. If order involves only a phone call, write called after the slash mark.
5. Enter order in kardex. One time orders are not entered in many hospitals. The order is now completed. Place another slash across the first one to make an X. These marks help you keep track of your place when you are interrupted.
6. Complete all orders in this manner.
7. When you are sure you have completed every order, draw a line down the right side of the order, sign your first initial, your last name, and St. for student. Under your name write the date and time you completed the orders.
8. Leave all cards and requisitions inside the chart for the RN to check. RN will sign cards, check requisitions for accuracy, and sign her name at the left side of the orders. RN will place cards and requisitions in designated places or ask you to do so.

9. If there is any question concerning an order and the RN at the desk or the head nurse cannot decipher the order, the doctor must be called for clarification. This may be stressful at times, but it must be done. There can be no guesswork when a patient's welfare is at stake. Secretaries usually do not take doctor's orders, hospital policy varies.

Figures 6-8 and 6-9 illustrate a set of orders with transcription symbols and a kardex with the orders. Look these over and refer to remarks for added clarification.

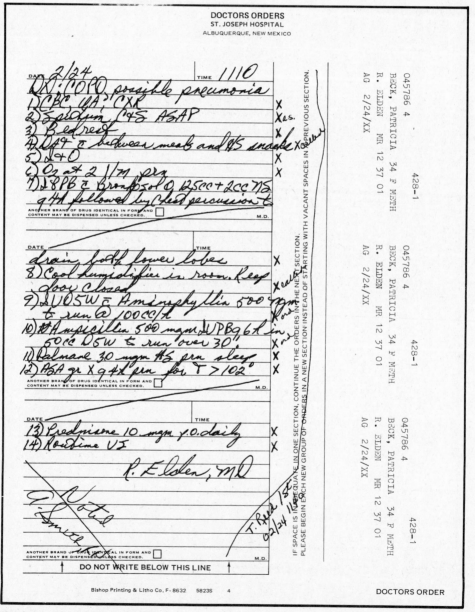

Figure 6-8. Physician's Order Sheet.

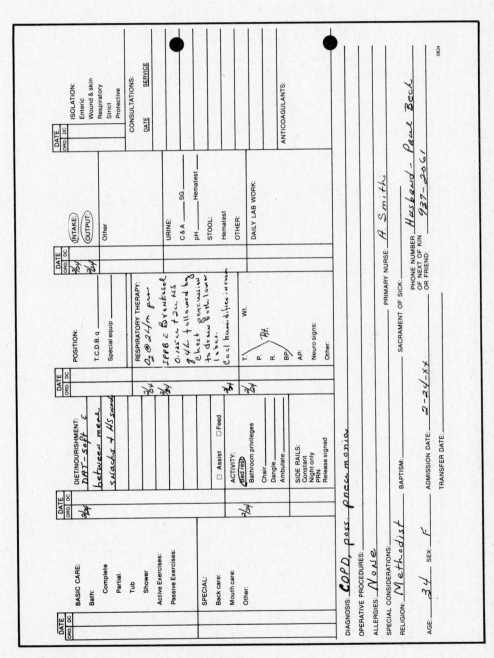

Figure 6-9a. Top Section of Patient Care Card.

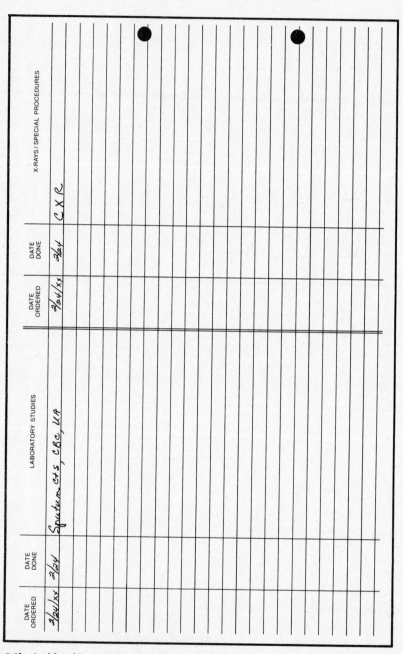

6-9b. Inside of Top Section of Patient Care Card.

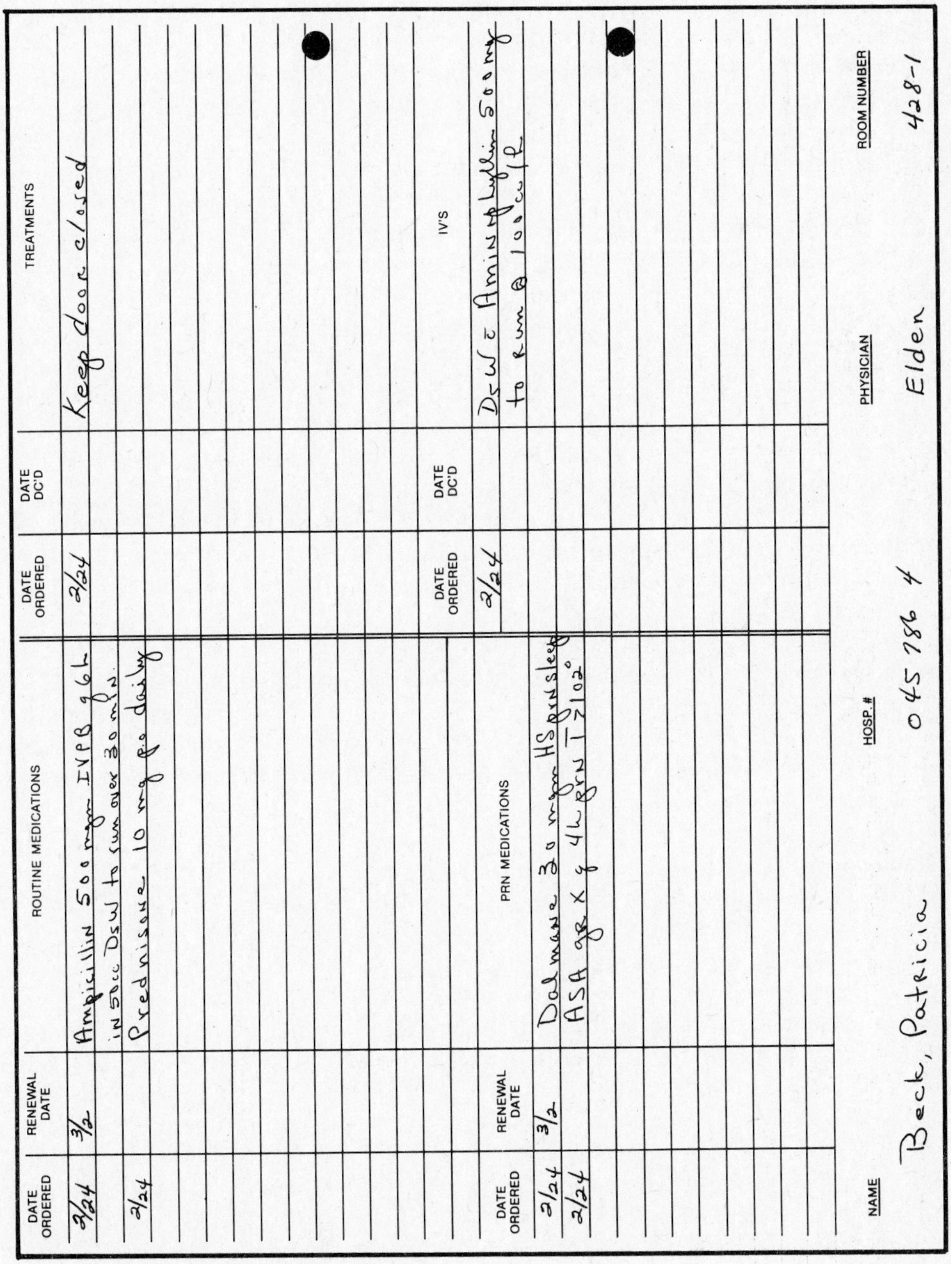

The card (rotated) contains:

ROUTINE MEDICATIONS

DATE ORDERED	RENEWAL DATE	ROUTINE MEDICATIONS	DATE ORDERED	DATE DC'D
2/24	3/2	Ampicillin 500 mg IVPB q6h in 50cc D5W to run over 30 min		
2/24		Prednisone 10 mg po daily		

PRN MEDICATIONS

DATE ORDERED	RENEWAL DATE	PRN MEDICATIONS	DATE ORDERED	DATE DC'D
2/24	3/2	Dalmane 30 mg po HS prn sleep		
2/24		ASA gr X po q4h prn T 7 102°		

TREATMENTS

TREATMENTS	DATE ORDERED	DATE DC'D
Keep door closed	2/24	

IV'S

IV'S	DATE ORDERED	DATE DC'D
D5W c̄ Aminophyllin 500mg to run @ 100 cc/h	2/24	

NAME Beck, Patricia

HOSP. # 045 786 4

PHYSICIAN Elden

ROOM NUMBER 428-1

6-9c. Bottom Section of Patient Care Card.

Transcription Comments

The set of orders illustrated in Figure 6-8 is for a new admission. Fill in the patient ID, name of doctor, name and telephone number of next of kin, age, sex, religion, admission date, and diagnosis on the kardex. Allergies may be noted after nursing returns the admission sheet to you.

Order #2 is an ASAP, complete it first. Either enter in computer or fill in requisition. This would be a Microbiology requisition. Check Culture-Routine and Sensitivity, enter sputum under Type of Specimen, write date under Date Ordered, and write date under Date/Time collected. RN will write in time when she collects the specimen. Write diagnosis in space provided, be sure requesting physician is the one who wrote the order, enter your initials, enter room, and bed number. Have RN check the order and give requisition to the RN for that patient so she may collect the specimen. Place / after order. Enter in kardex under Laboratory studies with date ordered and date done. Complete X. Send profile to pharmacy.

Go back to order #1. Enter in computer or fill in requisitions. Obtain requisitions for all tests on orders at same time and imprint with addressograph card. You need a Hematology requisition for CBC, a UA requisition for Urinalysis, CXR is a routine chest X-ray so you need a Radiology requisition, orders 6,7,8 are for Respiratory Therapy so you need an RT requisition, orders 9 and 10 may require special pharmacy order requisitions. Be sure the addressograph is placed correctly so the department receiving a requisition will not return it to you for correction.

Complete the Hematology requisition by checking CBC, write in date, Dx, requesting physician, your initials and patient's room number. Complete UA requisition in same manner. Complete x-ray requisition by writing in date to be done, name of exam (chest x-ray), pertinent information would be the diagnosis, how the patient can travel (by stretcher since bedrest was ordered) and write IV above so Escort Service will be sure to have an IV pole on the stretcher, complete the blanks for hospital number, age, sex, race, clinic or service, room number, height, weight, doctor requesting exam, attending physician. Place / after order when requisitions are complete. Enter in kardex in proper places with dates. Complete the X.

Order #3—enter in computer or complete a treatment card. Make / after order. Enter in kardex by circling bedrest and enter the date. Complete X.

Order #4—find out from the nurse what kind of diet patient will tolerate. Enter entire order in computer or call dietary since the diet sheet for noon has already gone to dietary. (If patient had been admitted early you would have written soft under New Admissions on diet sheet with patient's name and room # and placed between meals and HS snacks in the Special Requests section.) Place / after order and write called. On the kardex enter the date under Diet section and write DAT-soft-between meal and HS snacks. The RN will advance the diet as patient improves. Complete the X.

Order #5—enter in computer or place on treatment card you started in #3. Place an Intake and Output sheet in the chart. Place / after order. Enter in kardex by circling the words and entering the date. Complete the X.

Order #6—enter in computer or complete requisition. Call RT and read them order #6,7,8 so they may bring equipment to the room and start treatments at the same time. Write order #6 on RT requisition. Place / after order. Enter in kardex under Respiratory Therapy, enter date. Complete X.

Order #7—enter in computer or complete requisition. Write order on requisition exactly as doctor has written it. Place / after order. Enter in kardex under RT section with date. Complete X.

Order #8—enter in computer or complete requisition. Write order on requisition exactly as written. RT will bring humidifier and a card to place on the door stating "Keep door closed." The same requisition may be used for all RT orders. Make / after order and write called so RN will know the department was notified. Enter in kardex in RT section with date. Complete X.

Order #9—IV solutions usually require a special pharmacy order sheet. Enter in computer or complete pharmacy order and make an IV card or enter on IV record sheet. Cards are large enough for extensive orders. Write D5W under Solution, Aminophyllin 500 mgm under medications added, 100cc/h under rate, name of doctor and date. Remember to fill in patient ID on all cards. If space is not specified for this, place ID at top of card. Place / after order with ord to designate pharmacy order was completed. Enter in kardex under IV section with date. Complete X.

Order #10—enter in computer or complete pharmacy order sheet. Fill in IV medication card or record on MAR record. On card be sure to designate mode (IVPB), frequency q 6 h with times (each unit will have time schedule) to be given and notation to run 30'. Medication section reads—Ampicillin 500mgm in 50cc D5W. Place / after order with ord to designate that pharmacy order was made. Enter in kardex under routine Medications because it is given at routine times and is discontinued between doses. Enter date and renewal date if your hospital policy dictates. Complete X.

Order #11—enter in computer, on MAR record or on a medication card. HS is the frequency and PRN sleep is written in Time section. Pharmacy will send this from the profile, no special order is needed. Make / after order. Enter in kardex under PRN Medications with date. Complete X.

Order #12—enter in computer or MAR record or make medication card. Frequency is q 4h, PRN for T > 102°F goes under Time. Place / after order. Enter in kardex under PRN Medications. Complete X.

Order #13—enter in computer or in MAR record or make a card. Frequency is daily, place time under Time section (usually 0900). Place / after order. Enter in kardex under Routine Medications with date. Complete X.

Order #14—enter in computer or make treatment card. Use the card you started in order #3. Make / after order. Enter in kardex by bracketing T,P,R,BP and writing RT for routine, enter date. Complete X.

All orders are now completed. Draw a line down the left side of orders, write first initial, last name and St for student. Write date and time you completed the orders under your name. Leave all requisitions, cards, order sheets in chart for RN to check. The RN signs on the right side of the orders.

Transcription must be accurate. Hospitals have many check and countercheck procedures to insure safety. The profile to pharmacy is a check for orders sent to pharmacy as well as a record for pharmacy for each patient. The RN checking your orders is a countercheck for safety. There are many medications which are spelled similarly and it is easy to misinterpret. Having two persons check orders makes mistakes less likely. RNs or LPNs check kardexes against medication cards or computer printouts at the beginning of each shift. If the two do not correspond, the chart must be checked to ascertain the correct order. When a medication error occurs, an incident report must be made. The error may be due to incorrect transcription, wrong medication given for some reason, medication given at wrong time, wrong mode used, wrong dosage, or any number of reasons. These are reviewed by a committee at certain time intervals to see if one person is frequently involved or if the procedure needs changing for ease of administration. The two-person check system reduces the number of incident reports, but you are still legally responsible for your mistakes.

Accuracy can be increased by the use of the PDR or the Hospital Formulary to check dosages, modes and spelling until you learn medications. There are so many new medications every few months that all health care personnel depend on reference material and information from the pharmacy department. Do not hesitate to ask pharmacy for information if it is not in reference books. It takes a while for material to be included in books.

EXERCISE

Using your own forms and own kardex card, transcribe the set of orders in Figure 6-8.

REVIEW QUESTIONS

1. A kardex is _____
2. Give the meaning of the following abbreviations:
   BR _____
   BRP _____
   DSD _____
   TCDB _____
   U/O _____
   BLESS _____
   LR or RL _____
   D5W _____
   NS _____
3. There are several charts on the desk with orders to be transcribed. What do you do first? _____

4. Is speed or accuracy your first priority? _____

5. Explain the procedure for discontinuing a medication.

   _____

6. The use of the computer contributes to better patient care by

   _____

7. Computers serve many purposes. Name three. _____

   _____

8. State the type of order for each of the following:

   Tigan 250 mg tid _____

   Demerol 50 mg IM q 3–4 hrs prn for pain _____

   Sitz bath qid and prn _____

   Solu-Cortef 60 mg IVP q 6 h _____

   1000 cc D5LR to run 8 hrs then dc _____

   Give 2 units packed red cells today _____

9. List the rules for transcription.

   _____

   _____

   _____

   _____

   _____

   _____

   _____

10. Keeping a neat and up-to-date kardex is whose responsibility?

    _____

11. Transcription of Physician's Orders means _____

    _____

12. Medication cards contain what information?

    _____

    _____

13. What drugs usually require renewal dates?

    _____ .

Situational Application

14. The frequency of a medication order is written in such a way that it could be either qid or qd because of an unclear mark between the q and the d. The PDR supplies the information that the medication is

usually given qd but may be given qid. You would:

a. Transcribe the order as qd since that is the frequency most often used.

b. Ask the RN who is taking care of that patient to interpret the order.

c. Ask the desk RN and if she is not positive that the frequency is clear, call the doctor's office and tell the receptionist that _____ Hospital, (unit name) wishes to verify an order and to please have the doctor call.

d. Call the doctor and verify the order.

15. An order for a stat sputum specimen for culture and sensitivity states that RT may give one treatment if necessary to collect the sputum. You would:

a. Call RT to give a treatment stat.

b. Complete the requisition for C&S and give to the RN who is taking care of that patient.

c. Ask the desk RN what to do.

d. Consult the RN taking care of the patient to see if the RT treatment will be necessary. If it is, call RT for a stat treatment, complete a requisition for the C&S, have the desk RN check and initial the order, and give the requisition to the patient's RN.

16. An order for a medication states 100 mg and the PDR tells you that the usual dose for that medication is 10 mg. You would:

a. Call the doctor and receive an order change.

b. Show the order to the RN at the desk and then place a call for the doctor, when the doctor answers or returns the call have the RN take the change of order.

c. Mark through the 100 mg, write error and write 10 mg.

17. The doctor writes an order for a test that no one on the unit has heard of before, but they all think it is a laboratory test. The test is not listed in the laboratory manual. You would:

a. Write the order on a laboratory miscellaneous requisition.

b. Call the doctor to find out about the test.

c. Call the laboratory to determine if the test is a lab test, if there is any patient preparation, the purpose of the test, and what requisition to use. Inform the desk RN so she/he may relay the information to the head nurse and the test will be entered in the laboratory manual.

18. You are a student secretary on a unit and place a call for a doctor because a patient had requested a change in pain medication. The doctor returns the call and gives you an order for a new medication. You would:

a. Write the order, repeat the order for accuracy, and tell the desk RN of the order.

b. Ask the doctor to hold the line because you are not allowed to take doctor's orders and find an RN or LPN to take the order.

c. Write the order on the Physician's Order sheet and sign it "T.O. Dr. _____by (your name) ."

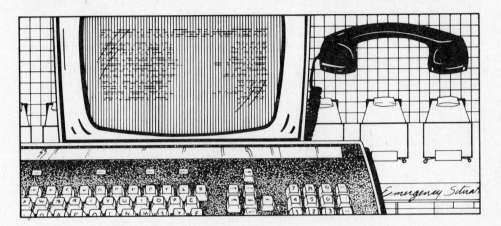

OBJECTIVES

Upon completion of study of this chapter, you will be able to:

1. List the steps of admission procedures.
2. List the steps of discharge procedures.
3. List the steps of transfer procedures.
4. List the steps of procedures following deaths.
5. List the duties of a secretary in isolation cases.
6. Discuss safety factors.
7. List the duties of a secretary in case of fire.
8. Complete routine reports.

ADMISSIONS

Patients are admitted to the hospital by a staff physician. Routine scheduled and unscheduled admissions are arranged by the physician's office. Emergency admissions are arranged by the patient's personal physician or the emergency room physician.

Scheduled Admissions

Patients scheduled for surgery or medical patients needing tests or care of a non-emergency nature are those scheduled for admission. The admitting office compiles a list each day and sends a copy to each unit. The steps of an admission follow.

1. The physician's office makes the arrangements with the hospital admitting office. If surgery is to be done, the physician's office schedules the surgery with the operating room before calling admitting.
2. The patient reports to admitting on the date and at the time specified by the physician's office. This is usually in the afternoon to give the units time to complete the discharges for that day and have rooms ready.
3. The admitting office completes the Patient Identification Sheet (shown in Figure 4-3, Chapter 4), the addressograph card, and the Identification bracelet.
4. According to hospital policies, admitting obtains patient consents. The majority of hospitals require an admitting consent for treatment while in the hospital and a consent to release information to the hospitalization insurance company listed on the Identification Sheet. The doctor may have called in the type of surgery and the surgical consent may be prepared by admitting personnel and signed by the patient.
5. Each hospital decides if certain laboratory exams are to be performed on each and every patient. If the hospital has established routine lab exams and a routine chest x-ray, these may be performed before the patient is taken to the unit if the patient's condition warrants. A notification of work already performed accompanies the patient to the unit.
6. Admitting personnel or a volunteer escorts the patient to the unit. The Identification Sheet, the ID bracelet, notice of x-ray, lab work performed, and an admission kit are given to the unit secretary. Admission kits ordinarily have a wash basin, an emesis basin, a box of tissues, mouthwash, lotion, soap, and a soap dish.

Unit Secretary's Duties for Scheduled Admission

1. Greet the patient in a manner that will put him/her at ease.
2. If the hospital policy dictates, escort the patient to the room assigned. Show the patient how to use the bed controls, the nurse call system, the television and radio controls. Volunteers may be allowed to assist the patient, and you will remain at the desk after greeting the patient.
3. The Admission Summary is addressographed and given to the NA or RN assigned to the room. The form is returned to the desk when completed. The NA or RN help the patient get settled. The RN will probably do a complete physical assessment.
4. All chart pages are addressographed and placed in the chart in the proper section. Dates are entered on appropriate forms.
5. Vital signs are entered on the Graphic Sheet and marked as the admission ones according to hospital policy.
6. A patient ID is placed in the slot of the chart back.
7. The patient's name is entered on the Census Sheet (see Figure 7-1).
8. A call is placed to the admitting physician's office for orders.
9. A patient ID card is made for the locator roster. The roster is a slotted rack where cards fit. The slots are numbered the same as the room numbers on the unit.

10. Patient's name is added to the TPR list, Patient's Condition Report, and the diet list. The type of diet is entered after orders are received.

BERNALILLO COUNTY MEDICAL CENTER

WARD CENSUS REPORT

(Forward one copy to the Admitting Office at 2400 hours)
(Prepare in duplicate: Original to Admitting Office, Copy remains on Ward)

Date	Ward No.	Bed Capacity	Previous Midnight Census Reported	Total Gain of Patients	Total Loss of Patients	Present Census	Available Beds
7-8-xx	4W	35	31	2	2	31	4

List every patient gained or lost during 24 hour period ending 2400 hours, above date

Hospital Number	Print Name (Last, First, MI.)	Room No. at 2400 Hours	Room Changes w/in Ward From	To	GAINS New Ad-missions	Interward Transfers From	From Pass	LOSSES Discharge From Hospital	Interward Transfers To	To Pass	SERVICE TRANSFERS From	To
096241	Smyth, William	403			X							
084349	Miller, Ruth	421	408	421								
062576	Jones, Susan	419						Death				
072431	Master, Lloyd	407						X				
090208	Starr, Vince	433				ICU						
043217	Bartlet, Maude	444									M	S

In event of loss other than stated above, please write in, i.e., Death, AMA, etc.

Totals: 1 | 1 | 2

Total Gains + 2   Total Losses – 2

Signature of Ward Nurse   Anne Koppe

Figure 7-1. Census Report.

11. A kardex card is started. Enter the patient's name in the space or spaces provided. Enter the name of the admitting doctor, the nearest of kin and their telephone number, the patient's diagnosis, and allergies. If no allergies are known, write NKA in the space. The hospital may want allergies written in red. The allergies are listed on the Admission Summary.

12. The chart is tagged if allergies are reported. Tags are self-adhesive, outlined in red with ALLERGIC in bold letters, and a space for entering the drugs or food to which the patient is allergic.
13. Physician's orders are transcribed.

Non-scheduled Admissions

The patient is seen by a physician or a telephone call to a physician determines the need for hospitalization. The physician's office notifies the Admitting Office. Admitting calls the unit and informs the unit of patient's name, age, diagnosis, and physician. The patient is usually taken to the unit and information for the Identification Sheet is obtained from a relative.

Unit Secretary Duties

1. Greet the patient. Escort patient to the room or have volunteer assist patient.
2. Write the patient's name on the Admission Summary if the addressograph card will not be completed until later.
3. Have an NA or RN admit the patient.
4. Orders may accompany the patient, otherwise call the physician's office for orders.
5. The chart is assembled as soon as the addressograph card arrives and all forms are imprinted.
6. Enter the patient's name on the census sheet, the TPR list, the Patient's Condition Sheet, and the diet list.
7. Place ID on chart back.
8. Start the kardex card.
9. Place ID card in roster.
10. Stat orders or ASAP orders may have to be handwritten in place of the addressograph as it may be some time before it is completed.
11. Transcribe the doctor's orders.

Emergency Admissions

The patient arrives by ambulance or is brought by car. The ER doctor determines if the patient is to be admitted to the unit or go directly to the operating room. The ER secretary notifies the admitting office who notifies the unit.

Unit Secretary Duties

1. Notify the head nurse of admission information.
2. If patient arrives on unit via the recovery room, the surgeon will have written the orders. If the patient arrives via the ER, the doctor who saw the patient may have written orders, or you may have to call the patient's private doctor.
3. Assemble the chart as you would for a new admission. The Emergency Room Report accompanies the patient and is a part of the chart.
4. Follow the same duties as for the routine admission.

EXERCISE

Your instructor will give you the forms for a new admission. Using the information on the Admission Summary shown in Chapter 4, go through the admission process. Once you have completed the process for a routine admission you will have no problem with the duties of a non-scheduled or an emergency admission.

You may want to do a role-playing type of practice to make the procedure more realistic.

DISCHARGES

Routine Discharges

Patients often think that when their doctor tells them they may go home that they can just leave. You will have patients asking for help to go to the car before you have received the chart with the discharge order from the doctor. Discharge orders need prompt attention so the patient does not have to wait. The doctor writes the order and admitting or the business office will tell you if the patient needs to stop by to make arrangements for their bill. The doctor may fill in a portion of the Discharge/Transfer Summary.

Unit Secretary Duties for Discharges

1. Transcribes the order for discharge by calling admitting or business office (whichever the individual hospital designates) and obtaining clearance for the patient. Some hospitals use a written form for notice of discharge and a copy goes to all departments caring for that patient.
2. Enter the patient's name on the Census Sheet, designate that the patient is discharged.
3. Clerical portion of the Discharge/Transfer Summary is completed. RN completes instructions portion. One copy is given to the patient after he signs it, one copy becomes a part of the chart. The NA or RN assist the patient in preparations for going home.
4. Follow-up appointments may be made by the secretary or by the patient according to individual hospital policy. The family makes arrangements for transportation home.
5. The secretary notifies Escort Service when the patient is ready to leave the unit. Patients should always be accompanied to the car.
   The RN writes a discharge note on the Nurse's Notes.
6. The chart is placed in discharge order as designated by the Medical Records department. There will be a list at each desk showing the

sequence of chart forms. Refer to this until you have memorized the sequence.

7. The roster card may be placed vertically in the slot as soon as the discharge is received from the doctor and then discarded when the patient actually leaves the unit.
8. Enter the patient's name on the diet list as a discharge.

UNIVERSITY OF NEW MEXICO HOSPITAL
BERNALILLO COUNTY MEDICAL CENTER
2211 Lomas Blvd. N.E.
Albuquerque, N.M. 87106
(505) 843-2111

DISCHARGE/ TRANSFER SUMMARY

Discharging Nursing Unit 5 W
Ext. 298

DISCHARGE INFORMATION DATE: 7-8-XX TIME: 9:45 AM GENERAL CONDITION: FAIR

Discharged:
X Via wheelchair
___ Ambulance
___ Ambulatory
___ Deceased
___ AMA
___ Release Signed
___ Release Not Signed
Staff Escort
Personal Belongings:
X Given
___ None present

Referral To:
___ VNS
___ Social Service
___ Other

Placement:
X Home
___ Transfer/Hospital
___ Extended Care
___ Other
Continued care by:
___ Referring physician
X Personal physician
___ Other
BCMC Clinic:
Date, Time, & Place of Appointment/s:

NURSING PLAN: (Completed by the R.N.)

Home Respiratory Care:
O_2@ 2 1/minute Continous ______, At night X and PRN X, Transport ______
Patient Instructions to:
Patient X, Family X, Other
By: Anne Koppe, RN
Booklets or Instructions given:
Medication Instructions: Slophyllin 250 mg — one capsule three times a day
Proventil Inhaler — two puffs when needed for shortness of breath
Home Diet: Regular
Activity Limitations: Move slowly
Home Treatments and Instructions: (ostomies, catheters, dressings changes, etc.)
Change dressing on chest wound daily.
Nutrition discussed with patient and wife by dietitian.
Teaching re: lab or x-ray studies:
Teaching re: Wound care: Cleanse with Normal Saline and apply dry 4x4. Use paper tape to hold 4x4 in place.
Teaching re: Equipment (walkers, crutches, commodes, etc.)
Patient Status: Allergy, skin condition, respiratory, bowel, bladder, pain, self care,
Patient able to take care of self except for wound dressing. Wife will do that. Oxygen while sleeping and as needed during day. Should walk some each day, slowly increase tolerance.
R.N. Signature: Anne Koppe, RN

SUMMARY OF HOSPITALIZATION (Completed by the physician):
Diagnosis: Bronchiectasis Medications to take home: Slophyllin - Proventil
Surgical Procedures: Thoracotomy - Resection RML and RLL
Complications: None
Clinical Summary and Lab: Chest X-ray Clear - CBC normal
ABG's borderline
Responsible House Officer: R. Westin Responsible Attending: B.T. Adson
Indicate here if continuation sheet is used: Yes ☐ No ☒

Physician's Signature: B.T. Adson
I have received a copy of my discharge instructions and understand them to my satisfaction.
DATE: 7-8-XX
PATIENT/GUARDIAN SIGNATURE: Matthew Saunders

0111

MEDICAL RECORDS

PATIENT
1-29664-2 WB
556789 S 01/01/01
SAUNDERS, MATTHEW

Figure 7-2. Discharge/Transfer Summary.

9. Remove the patient's name from the TPR list and the Patient Condition Report.
10. Medical Records usually compiles a list to be checked to make sure all the steps have been completed. This checklist is attached to the front of the chart. Each item is initialed and your full name is signed at the bottom. All discharge charts go to Medical Records where they may be microfilmed for future reference.

    Housekeeping cleans the rooms when the Census Sheet shows the actual time the patient left the unit or you notify them according to hospital policy.
11. The kardex card and addressograph card may be discarded or attached to the chart according to individual policy.
12. Remove the ID from the chart back and any tags that may have been placed on the chart.
13. Addressograph a Pharmacy Credit slip so the RN may credit unused medications.

Prior Preparation for Discharges

The doctor may write orders several days prior to the discharge for patient teaching of some type or family teaching. This is part of the Home Health Care (HHC) nurse's duties. You fill out the proper form and send to HHC. When teaching has been completed and the patient is ready to go home, HHC communicates that fact to the doctor by notes on the Progress Notes.

Orders may include dressings to be sent with the patient. These should be ordered and ready to go with the patient as soon as the discharge is written. Preparations that the nursing staff are responsible for are entered on the kardex.

Orders may be for the Physical Therapy department to start therapy and continue therapy on an out-patient basis. These arrangements are made by completing the departmental form and noting such on the kardex.

Examples of orders for prior preparation:

1. Have PT start leg strengthening exercises and arrange to see patient twice a week for five weeks, plan discharge in two days.
2. Home Health Care to teach patient how to give own insulin and teach family how to monitor blood sugar. Patient may go home when teaching is completed to HHC satisfaction.
3. Teach family how to care for wound. Send 2 dozen medium abdominal pads, 4 dozen 4×4's, and 2 rolls of silk tape. Send gloves if deemed necessary. Plan to discharge tomorrow or next day.
4. Have dietitian instruct patient and family on low salt, low sugar, low fat diet. Make sure family understands. Plan to discharge in 3 days.
5. Schedule for chest x-ray as out-patient in 2 weeks. Discharge tomorrow.

EXERCISE

Complete forms needed for all above orders according to your hospital's policies. Your instructor will supply the patient ID.

Against Medical Advice (AMA) Discharge

A patient may decide to go home even though the doctor has not completed treatment. The staff usually tries to convince the patient to stay but the patient cannot be detained against his/her will.

Unit Secretary Duties for AMA Discharge

1. Obtain a Release of Patient Against Advice of Physician form and complete the patient ID.
2. An RN or LPN should witness the patient's signature.
3. Place a call to the physician's office to notify him/her that the patient is leaving.
4. Notify Admitting that the patient is leaving AMA.
5. An RN records the AMA discharge on the Nurse's Notes.
6. Proceed as for a routine discharge.

| TRANSFERS

Intraunit Transfers

It is often necessary to move patients from one room to another. The patient's condition may make it necessary to move the patient closer to the nurse's station. Discharges may create several rooms with only one female so a female has to be moved in order to have an available male bed. Perhaps two patients are not compatible and have to be separated. Whatever the reason, you will find that playing "musical beds" is an everyday occurrence.

Unit Secretary Duties

1. Notify Admitting of the room change or changes.
2. Addressograph a Personal Belongings Checklist if one is used.
3. Notify the physician of the patient's move and new room number.
4. Transfer patient's chart to the correct chart back. Transfer chart back labels.
5. Enter patient's name on Census Sheet as intraunit transfer.
6. Enter change on the diet list, TPR list, and Patient Condition Report.
7. Change roster card to correct room.

8. Medication cards (if used) are changed to current room number.
9. Enter current room number on Physician's Order sheets that have already been imprinted.
10. Change kardex card to correct room number.
11. Change addressograph card to correct place in the rack.

Interunit Transfers

The patient is moved from one unit to another unit. A patient who was admitted as a medical patient may need surgery and will be transferred to the surgical unit from the recovery room. A patient may become critical and be moved to the intensive care unit. A patient may suffer a heart attack and be moved to the coronary care unit.

Unit Secretary Duties

1. Transcribes the physician's order for the transfer by calling Admitting and receiving the room number to which the patient will be moved.
2. The doctor writes complete new orders for the new unit. Only the orders that apply to period of time before the transfer are transcribed. The receiving unit transcribes remaining orders.
3. Addressograph a Personal Belongings Checklist if one is used.
4. Enter patient's name on Census Sheet as interunit transfer.
5. Remove patient's name from TPR list.
6. Enter patient's name on diet list as a transfer to room _____ and enter statement of transfer on Patient's Condition Report.
7. Assemble chart, kardex, roster card, addressograph card in one package. Chart is removed from chart back.
    The RN prepares the medication cards and medications for transfer.
8. Notify the receiving floor when patient is ready to be moved.
9. Notify Escort Service for the move when RN requests.

Receiving Unit Secretary Duties

1. Notify Team Leader of patient's arrival.
2. Place chart in chart back and place ID in slot.
3. Place roster card in roster and addressograph card in the rack.
4. Place kardex card in kardex holder.
5. Enter patient's name on Census Sheet, TPR list, and Patient's Condition Report.
6. Enter on diet list as a transfer.
7. Transcribe orders by checking the kardex card and medication cards and making any necessary changes. Change the room number on medication cards.

EXERCISE

Practice the routines of a transfer by actually going through the steps with a chart, a kardex, roster card, and all items. Your instructor may give you a set of Physician's Orders and one person can be the transferring secretary and one the receiving secretary. This would also give you practice with the telephone.

Transfers to Other Facilities

There are many reasons why a patient will be transferred from one institution to another. The most common is a move to a nursing home or extended care facility. Orders for the move are ordinarily written several days before and the HHC or social service worker will do the paper work necessary to transfer the patient. A form is used which has a section for the doctor to write orders and a section for the nurse to comment about the patient's care.

Unit Secretary Duties

1. Notify the proper individuals when the doctor writes the transfer order. Photocopy the specified parts of the chart as per orders.
2. Complete the clerical portion of the transfer form.
3. Note the pending transfer in the kardex card.
4. When patient leaves, be sure photocopies and transfer form accompany the patient.
5. Complete the steps of a routine discharge the day patient leaves.

PASSES

Long-term patients benefit from being away from the hospital for a few hours or overnight. A pass gives the patient and the family a chance to see how the patient can function in the home atmosphere and helps the doctor evaluate the patient's progress. The psychological benefits of being with the family in the home atmosphere are definitely advantageous. The doctor writes the order for the pass and specifies the time.

Unit Secretary Duties

1. Complete the necessary form.
2. Enter patient's name on the Census Sheet if the pass is overnight.
3. Notation is made on the Nurse's Notes when patient leaves and when patient returns.

4. Notation is made on Patient's Condition Report.
5. Enter name on diet list for meals to be omitted.
6. Enter name on Census Sheet when patient returns from overnight pass.
7. Chart is kept on unit even though patient is not counted in the census as being present.

EXERCISE

Complete a form for Robert Rescott to have a pass from 10 AM today (Friday) until 5 PM on Sunday.

DEATHS

This is always a difficult situation no matter how many times you are a part of the proceedings. The unit secretary helps the nursing staff in various ways besides doing the clerical work. Assist the family by taking them to the conference room, offering them coffee, and making them comfortable until the nurse or doctor can talk with them. Notify the Pastoral Care personnel so they may assist the family.

If the death is unexpected, be very careful of the information you give over the telephone. You may have to ask the family to come to the hospital. Tell the family that the patient's condition has changed and the nurse asked you to call the family and request that they come to the hospital. Answer questions by saying, "That is all the information I have at this time and the nurse is busy with the patient." News of a death over the telephone might cause someone to have an accident on the way to the hospital. Watch for the family and guide them into the conference room. The family is allowed as much time as they want with the deceased after the nurse prepares the body for viewing.

Unit Secretary Duties

1. Notify patient's doctor if he/she is not present. A doctor must pronounce the patient dead. An ER doctor may do this as a courtesy to the attending doctor if the doctor feels it is not necessary to speak personally with the family.
2. The time the doctor writes on the Progress Notes is the official time of death.
3. Certain deaths must be reported to the Medical Investigator's office. Your instructor will give you a list for the type of cases your area requires to be reported.
4. The doctor must obtain permission for an autopsy if one is to be performed. You may prepare the form for the doctor.

5. Requisition a Death Pack or Mortuary Kit from Central Supply.
6. Complete the ID tags in the Mortuary Kit.
7. The family makes the arrangements with a Mortuary. They may need some assistance.
8. The Mortuary picks up the body from the room if doing so within a short time period. If an autopsy is to be done, the Nursing Administration Office will notify the Mortuary when the autopsy is completed.
9. The nursing personnel take the body to the morgue if an autopsy is to be done. You prepare the ID for the morgue placement.
10. A written notice of death is sent to the admitting office, the switchboard, Nursing Administration, and the Pathology department or other departments according to hospital policy.
11. Enter the deceased's name on the Census Sheet and indicate that the patient expired and the time.
12. The chart is placed in discharge order and taken to the Pathology Department if an autopsy is to be performed. This may vary; your instructor may make a change in this part of the procedure.
13. The other duties are the same as for a routine discharge.

EXERCISE

Requisition a Mortuary Kit from Central Supply and complete the tags used for patient identification.

If time permits in your classroom, do a role-playing practice to capture some of the feelings you must deal with in a situation of this type. You cannot assist with the family if you cannot keep your own emotions under control. Role-playing may show you how to keep your emotions in check until you are free to express your feelings.

ISOLATION PROCEDURES

Each type of isolation requires a cart at the door of the room. The cart contains supplies needed in order to enter the room and to care for the patient. Isolation cases must be in a private room. The door of the room will be posted with instructions for the type of isolation. Visitors must check with the nurse before entering the room. The tray from dietary will be of disposable products so they may be discarded. Laboratory personnel will dispose of needles and syringes in a special container. Housekeeping will leave cleaning utensils in the room until the patient is moved from isolation into another room or is discharged; the utensils are then disinfected. Trash and used linens are placed in special bags.

Types of Isolation and Instructions

Enteric isolation for diseases transmitted by feces or urine.

1. A gown must be worn if direct contact with the patient will occur. To go into the room and hand the patient something without actually touching the patient or the bedclothes does not require a gown.
2. Gloves must be worn by anyone touching the patient or articles touched by the patient.
3. Hands must be washed before entering the room and upon leaving.

Respiratory isolation for patients with diseases that are airborn.

1. The door to the room must be kept closed.
2. Hands must be washed on entering and leaving the room.
3. Masks are worn by everyone who enters the room.
4. All articles with respiratory secretions must be disinfected.

Reverse isolation for protection of the patient from outside infection. The patient has a very low resistance due to a decreased white blood count or suppressed immune system.

1. The door to the private room must be kept closed.
2. Hands are washed before entering and upon leaving the room.
3. Gowns, masks, and gloves are worn by everyone entering the room.

Strict isolation for severe systemic infections.

1. The door to the private room must be kept closed.
2. Hands must be washed on entering and leaving the room.
3. Gowns, masks, and gloves are worn by everyone entering the room.
4. Articles that are not disposable must be wrapped and sent to central supply for sterilization.

Wound and skin isolation for infected wounds or skin infections.

1. Hands are washed on entering and leaving the room.
2. Gowns are worn by persons having direct contact with the patient.
3. Masks and gloves are worn when having direct contact with the infected area.
4. Techniques for changing the dressings are per each hospital's policies.
5. Instruments must be wrapped before being sent to central supply for sterilization.

Unit Secretary Duties

1. As soon as the order is written by the doctor or the nursing staff determines that isolation is needed, notify the admitting office. If the patient is in a ward or semi-private room, make arrangements just as you would for an intraunit transfer. A semi-private room may have to be used due to non-availability of a private room. The other bed would be blocked; admitting would not count it as an available bed and you would insert a card in the roster with the word "BLOCKED" so everyone on the unit will know a patient cannot be admitted to that room.

2. Notify housekeeping of the room number and type of isolation.
3. Obtain the cart for the supplies by notifying the designated department. Some hospitals designate Housekeeping and others designate Central Supply to furnish and maintain the carts.
4. Notify dietary.
5. Inform the personnel involved in any procedure that is ordered following the placement of the patient in isolation.
6. Any consultations that may be ordered following isolation must contain the information concerning isolation.
7. If Escort Service must transport the patient, be sure they know the type of isolation with which they will be involved.
8. When isolation is discontinued and the patient is moved to another room or the patient is discharged, notify housekeeping so that the disinfection of the room may be completed as soon as possible.

SAFETY PROCEDURES

The same precautions you might use in your own home apply to the hospital setting. You will probably be in an area where you can see the elevators and a large part of the hallway. Notify the housekeeping department immediately if anything is spilled or if any glass is broken in the halls. Have someone guard the area until it can be cleaned.

Electrical equipment on the unit should be kept in good condition. Never attempt to fix something yourself; notify the maintenance department.

Equipment in the patients' rooms require attention as soon as any malfunction is noted. The nurses will inform you of any problems in the rooms. Notify maintenance or engineering; be sure to complete the proper forms.

Keep your work area neat and free of excess equipment. If chairs at the desk are the roller type, be careful that the chair is not in motion when you start to sit down. Rolling around the nursing station in a chair can be disastrous. Stand up and walk, even if it is only a short distance.

The addressograph machine has been known to inflict injury on fingers, so be careful when using it. There are many kinds, and some are more dangerous than others. Be sure you know how to use the equipment before attempting to operate any machine.

Open-toed sandals invite trouble. With all the movement around the desk, people often step on each others toes. Wear comfortable shoes that allow ease in walking and provide protection.

Jewelry can become caught in equipment and cause damage to you. Most hospitals have rules concerning the wearing of any jewelry. Earrings interfere with the use of the telephone.

FIRE

Each hospital has a manual for procedures in case of fire. During your orientation to your job, this procedure will be explained. It is helpful to review the procedure from time to time so you can be sure of what to do if an actual fire does occur. Your duty will proboably be to close the fire doors and doors to all rooms, clear the halls of patients and visitors, then stay at the desk and answer the phone. Either you or the head nurse will be responsible for having a complete list of patients for checking purposes if evacuation of the unit is necessary. Fire drills are conducted at intervals to keep all personnel alert. Hospitals may provide classes in body mechanics to teach how to lift and carry patients in case of an emergency. Learn the location of the oxygen valve for the unit on which you will work in case maintenance needs assistance during an emergency.

COMPLETING REPORTS

Report of Patient's Condition

The nursing supervisors need to know the condition of the patients on the units they supervise. Reports are read by the supervisor going off duty to the one coming on duty. This gives each supervisor an indication of how busy each unit will probably be for the next eight hours and what problems to expect.

The format of this report varies a great deal. The common type is a computerized list of all rooms with the patient's name and name of the doctor for each patient. The unit secretary enters the diagnosis for each patient and may note if patient is going to OR that day or any scheduled tests. Each nurse fills in comments regarding the patients assigned to her/him. The reports are collected by the supervisors about an hour before the change of shift. It may be your duty to remind the nurses that the report needs to be completed as it is almost collection time.

Incident Reports

If a patient, a visitor, or an employee has an accident, a report must be completed to protect the individual and the hospital. You complete a report only if you witnessed the accident or are the person who had the accident.

Information needed on a patient incident report:

- Condition of the patient before the accident
- When and where the accident occurred
- Exactly what happened
- The equipment involved, if any
- Description of injury if an injury is apparent.

The doctor is notified and makes a notation on the form as to the physical findings following an examination of the patient and if any treatment is necessary. The report is sent to Nursing Administration. A committee reviews all incident reports at certain time intervals to see if any policies need to be changed to prevent such accidents.

A visitor who has an accident is asked to see the ER doctor to be checked. If they refuse, that information is entered on the report.

An employee who has an accident completes the incident report, has it signed by the head nurse on the unit or the nurse who is responsible for the unit for that day, and reports to the ER to be examined by the doctor. The report is taken to the Nursing Administration office.

OTHER ROUTINE DUTIES

Ordering Supplies

The Purchasing Department publishes a catalog of all the supplies kept on hand. The head nurse and the director of the purchasing department compile a list from the catalog of the supplies that particular unit will need to order at specified time intervals. The quantity is temporary until enough time has elapsed to establish the maximum quantity for the specified time interval. Once the maximum quantity has been established, that amount is entered into the budget for that unit and is changed only with the consent of the head nurse.

The list of supplies for that particular unit are photocopied so that you need only to enter the quantity when you order supplies. Any article that is not on your list will have to be ordered by a special requisition and signed by the head nurse.

The supplies are kept in a cabinet and brought to the nursing station as needed. The cabinet is usually locked and the key is either in the possession of the head nurse or the unit secretary. Routine supplies include all the departmental requisitions, medication cards and other cards the unit uses, chart forms of both the standard and supplemental kinds, kardex cards, kardex replacement inserts, chart dividers, pens, pencils, liquid ink eradicator for use on non-legal items, stationary, envelopes of various sizes, and other papers particular to that floor.

The ordering date is specified by the purchasing department and it is necessary to abide by the specification. If you are the permanent unit secretary on a unit, you should try to complete the requisition if your days off fall on the ordering date. Relief secretaries may not be aware of the needs of that particular unit.

Charting Vital Signs

The nursing staff may chart for the patients for whom they are responsible. The usual approach is to have a TPR list where the VS are entered, and the unit secretary transfers those VS to each patient's chart. There will be routine times for the nursing staff to take VS. The times are usually 8 AM and 4 PM with other times dictated by the doctor or by the patient's condition.

The majority of secretaries try to chart VS as soon as they are entered on the TPR list. If VS cannot be graphed before the doctors begin making rounds, you will continue to graph them when the unit activity is slow enough to allow the time. Mistakes on graphics are corrected in a specific manner. If the mistake is on the very first VS graphed, a new sheet may be used and the one with the mistake is discarded. Mistakes on subsequent graphing are corrected by circling the mistake, writing "error" above the mistake, and graphing the correct VS. Temperatures are ordinarily taken orally; if taken otherwise, designate so on the graph by placing the symbol R for rectal or the symbol Ax for axillary.

When you are responsible for graphing, practice the procedure enough so that you will be accurate and accomplish the task in a reasonable length of time.

Resupplying Chart Forms

The Physician's Order Sheet and the Progress Notes are the forms used most frequently. Charts are checked each morning to make sure these two forms, and all other forms, have adequate space and new ones are added as necessary. If a patient is due to go home that day or the next, do not add sheets since they will probably not be used. Once your are on a unit and become familiar with the routines of the doctors you can anticipate fairly accurately the discharge time for the patients.

Patient's Valuables

More and more people are realizing that nothing of value should be taken into the hospital. There will be times when a patient has valuables and there is no family to take them home. The valuables are placed in an envelope that has been addressographed with the patient's ID and has a portion to be torn off and given to the patient as a receipt. A list of the valuables placed in the envelope is recorded on a form and a copy given to the patient and a copy placed inside the envelope. The envelope is taken to the business office and locked in the safe. The patient may claim the valuables at any time. A notation is made on the chart that the valuables are in the safe. The admitting office questions the patient about valuables and either has a relative take them or processes the forms for placing the valuables in the safe. The person admitting a patient also asks about valuables and takes the necessary steps. A patient going to surgery is asked about valuables and may have a wristwatch that needs to be in the safe until the patient is fully recovered from anesthesia. You will be responsible for addressographing the envelope and the form for listing the valuables. The nursing staff is responsible for the listing and care of the valuables.

Filing Chart Forms

The routine for this varies from hospital to hospital. The various departments may do their own filing, you may receive forms through the messenger service, or forms may be tubed to your unit. Filing by unit secretaries is usually performed at one time when the activities of the unit permit. The afternoon shift may be responsible for all the filing. Forms must be checked for the patient ID and be placed in the correct chart in the correct section. If a form is found in the wrong chart, place it in the correct chart. A form may be found during discharge procedures when placing the chart in order and will be placed in the correct chart. A doctor may need to be notified of the error—the form may be a test result that would give incorrect information for that particular patient. Any forms found that are for a patient that has been discharged previously are sent to Medical Records to be incorporated into the correct chart.

ESTABLISHING ROUTINES

The unit secretary needs to set routines as much as possible so work progresses in an orderly fashion and confusion is at a minimum. You need to be in control of the activity in your work area. There may be times when you feel that the nursing staff is taking over your space and interfering with your work. The head nurse will work with you to resolve such problems.

Example of a routine for the morning shift (7 AM to 3:30 PM)

1. Listen to shift report if that is an acceptable policy of the hospital. This gives you information as to the condition of each patient and enables you to communicate accurately with the patient and the patient's family.
2. Check all charts for orders that may have been overlooked. You can recognize orders that have not been transcribed as there will be no transcription symbols and no signatures of a unit secretary and/or an RN.
3. Resupply Physician's Order Sheets and Progress Notes as you check for orders.
4. Make an assignment list to tape to the top of your desk so you have a quick reference when needing to locate a staff member.
5. Compile a list of patients having tests in other departments for the day if the blackboard is not used for this purpose. This serves as a quick reference when Escort Service arrives for a patient.
6. Start graphing the VS.
7. Doctors are arriving by this time and transcription duties will continue throughout the day.
8. Answer telephones as soon as possible and refer calls to the proper person or department.
9. There may be calls or appointments that the evening or night shift was unable to complete. Complete these as offices and departments open for business.

10. Laboratory reports that are called to the unit or received by computer may need to be called to doctor's offices. Show the reports to the nurse and call the doctor as soon as possible after receiving the report. If several tests were ordered and different sections of the laboratory are involved, wait until all results are reported before contacting the doctor unless directed otherwise by the nurse. Laboratory reports may be quoted to the receptionist in the doctor's office, record the name of the person receiving the report and the time on the report sheet.
11. Duties such as ordering supplies, replenishing station supplies, putting new supplies in the cabinet etc. are performed as time permits.

ESTABLISHING PRIORITIES

It is very important to the functioning of the unit that you, the unit secretary, recognize the importance of sequence of tasks. Transcription takes precedence over ordering supplies, patient's requests take precedence over telephoning for an appointment, and Stat orders should be completed before leaving the unit to photocopy chart forms to go with a patient to another facility.

Incoming telephone calls are completed in the order of importance. A call from OR to give the preop medication to a patient must be relayed to the Team Leader or nurse giving medications immediately. If another caller is on hold, leave them on hold while you take care of the call from OR.

Notification from the admitting office that a patient is coming from the ER must be relayed to the head nurse or Team Leader at once.

Calls from RR to give report on a patient to be returned to the unit require immediate attention or ask if a nurse may return the call in a few minutes. Be sure the message is delivered.

Stat, ASAP, and now orders always command immediate attention.

REVIEW QUESTIONS

1. The _____ is a record of admissions, discharges, overnight passes, deaths, and transfers.
2. The graphic sheet is started by obtaining the vital signs from the _____ _____ .
3. Charts are placed in discharge order and sent to the _____ department.

4. The volunteer bringing a routine admission patient to the unit will also bring _____ _____ .

5. Emergency cases may come to the unit via the _____ or the _____ .

6. Admissions, discharges, transfers, deaths and passes are entered on the _____ for the supervisors.

7. Autopsy permits are obtained by the _____ .

8. Patients to be autopsied are taken to the _____ .

9. Admission to a hospital is arranged by a _____ .

10. Incident reports may involve a _____ , a _____ , or an _____ .

11. When a patient insists on leaving the hospital before treatment is completed, the discharge is called an _____ .

12. Name the five types of isolation.

_____   _____

_____   _____

_____

13. List four safety precautions you would use in the hospital.

_____

_____

_____

_____

14. In case of fire, your duties would be _____ _____ _____

15. List your duties when a patient is ordered in isolation.

_____

_____

_____

Situational Application

16. You have three admissions within five minutes. One is a routine admission, one is an unscheduled admission with ASAP orders for some tests, one is from ER with orders for surgical consent, a pre-op medication on call, and a surgical prep. The orders read "before surgery" and surgery is scheduled to follow the case the surgeon is operating

on at the present time. You would:
a. Complete the ASAP orders first
b. Consider the before surgery order as a stat one and take care of those orders first so the patient will be ready when OR calls; then complete the ASAP orders followed by the routine admission
c. Complete the orders in the rotation in which patients arrived.

17. A death occurs about 30 minutes after the wife leaves the hospital. The daughter is with the patient. The nurses need some assistance. You would:
a. Call the wife and then take the daughter to the conference room
b. Call Pastoral Care to help with the daughter and then call the wife
c. Escort the daughter to the conference room and offer to call the wife; stay with the daughter until the wife arrives.

18. A volunteer is helping on your unit. Three tasks need to be completed:
a. Some forms need to be xeroxed
b. Supplies need to be placed in the cabinet
c. VS need graphing.
You would ask the volunteer to do which tasks—a, b or c?

19. Escort Service arrives to take a patient to the OR, a patient tells you he is ready to go home, and a doctor asks you to call the lab for a report. You would:
a. Ask the patient to wait in his room and you will call the Escort Service, find an RN to help with the surgical patient, call the lab and obtain the report for the doctor, and then call Escort Service for a wheelchair for the discharged patient
b. Have Escort Service and the patient wait while you call the lab for the doctor
c. Call the lab, assist Escort Service, and then help the patient

SECTION II

Section II presents the body systems, the diseases and disorders of each system, the terminology, and the general treatment of the diseases and disorders. It also includes the laboratory examinations, x-ray examinations, surgical procedures, and medications related to each system. Physician's Orders are given for each system so you can practice transcription procedure.

Your communicaation skills will become more effective and you will find the work more interesting as you learn about the body systems. The body structure and function presented give you the information needed to understand what is happening to the patient. Read each one of the chapters for information and then use the objectives for concentrated study.

The treatments described here for diseases and disorders are very general. Each patient is an individual who reacts differently to a disease process and will be treated according to his/her needs. The treatments are given to acquaint you with different procedures so that when you go into the clinical area you have a better idea of what to expect and how to go about your work.

You need to know how to spell the diseases and disorders in order to be able to readily write down information when the admitting office or ER call you regarding a new patient that is to be admitted.

The Physician's Orders are typed for ease in reading. After you have mastered the transcription procedure, your instructor may give you some handwritten orders from your area. You may find both milligram abbreviations, mgm and mg, are used in one set of orders. That is the way orders will come to you in the actual work situation. Do not expect every order to be clear-cut. The RN assigned to the desk will help you with orders that are not immediately clear.

The laboratory examinations are explained in Appendix II so that you may easily refer to the appendix after reading each of the chapters. Some examinations are used for all systems while others are highly specialized. You need to become familiar with the examinations and their results in order to efficiently record results given over the telephone.

Chapter 8 | Introduction to the Body

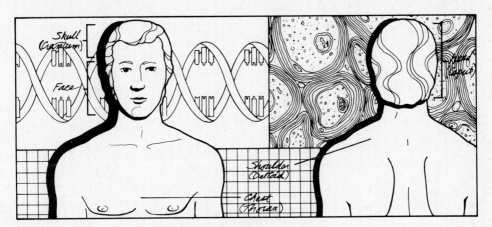

OBJECTIVES

After careful study of this chapter, you will be able to:

1. Identify word elements pertaining to the study of the body and give the meaning of each.
2. List the planes of the body.
3. List the terms for areas of the body.
4. Define a cell.
5. Define DNA.
6. Define chromosome.
7. Define gene.
8. Define cancer.
9. List the categories for cancer treatment.
10. Define tissue.
11. Define organ.
12. Define system.
13. Transcribe Physician's Orders relating to cell and tissue diseases and disorders.

To understand the structure and function of the body, you must first understand the terminology related to the body. Professionals sometimes forget that the average non-medically-oriented person does not understand medical lingo. This can lead to problems in patient care. Learn the terminology well, but be careful how and when you use it.

You probably remember from English classes that words have different parts called elements. A **root element** is a simple word or word form. A **prefix** is an element added at the beginning, a **suffix** is an element added at the end of a word. A **combining form** is a root plus a vowel. Words are formed by various combinations of the different elements:

- A root (man) plus a root (kind) constructs the word mankind.

- A prefix plus a root: The prefix *dis* means without, and the root *ease* means comfort. Combined they form *disease,* meaning without comfort.
- A root plus a suffix: The root *tonsil* is the name for the mass of tissue on each side of the throat, and the suffix *ectomy* means removal of. Together they form *tonsillectomy,* meaning the removal of the tonsils.
- A root plus a prefix and a suffix: The prefix *poly* means many, the root *cyst* means sac, bag, or pouch, and the suffix *ic* means consisting of. Together they form *polycystic,* which means consisting of many cysts.
- A prefix plus a suffix: The prefix *hemi* means half, and the suffix *plegia* means paralysis. Together they form *hemiplegia,* which means paralysis of one-half of the body.
- A combining form and a suffix: The combining form *pneumono* means air or lungs, and the suffix *itis* means inflammation. Together they form *pneumonitis,* which means inflammation of the lungs.

The list of word elements on pages 167 to 171,their meanings, and examples is reproduced from the book *Being a Ward Clerk* with permission of The Hospital Research and Educational Trust.

WORD ELEMENT	REFERS TO OR MEANS	EXAMPLE	
A-, AN-,	without, lack of, absent, deficient	asepsis anorexia	a/SEP/sis, an/or/EX/i/a
AB-, ABS-	from, away	abnormal abscess	ab/NORM/al ABS/cess
AD-	near, toward	adrenal	ad/RĒN/al
ADENO	gland	adenopathy	ad/en/OP/a/thy
AERO	air	anaerobe	an/Ā/er/obe
ALB	white	albumin	al/BŪ/min
-ALGIA, -ALGESIA	pain	analgesia	an/al/GĒ/si/a
AMBI-	both	ambidextrous	am/bi/DEX/trous
ANGIO	vessel (blood or lymph)	angioma	an/gi/O/ma
ANO	anus	anoscope	A/no/scope
ANTE-	before	antenatal	an/te/NĀT/al
ANTI-	against	antiseptic	an/ti/SEP/tic
ARTERIO	artery	arteriosclerosis	ar/ter/i/o/scler/O/sis
ARTHRO	joint	arthroplasty	Ar/thro/plas/ty
-ASTHENIA	weakness	myasthenia	my/as/THĒ/ni/a
AUTO-	self	autonomic	au/to/NOM/ic
BI-	two, twice	biweekly	bi/WEEK/ly
BRADY-	slow	bradycardia	brad/y/CAR/di/a
BRONCHO	bronchus	bronchitis	bron/CHĪ/tis
CARDIO	heart	myocardium	my/o/CAR/di/um
-CELE	tumor, swelling, hernia, sac	enterocele	EN/ter/o/cēle
-CENTESIS	puncture	thoracentesis	tho/ra/cen/TĒ/sis
CEPHALO	head	hydrocephaly	hy/dro/CEPH/a/ly
CHOLE	gall	cholelithiasis	chol/e/lith/i/a/sis
CHOLECYSTO	gall bladder	cholecystectomy	cho/le/cys/tect/o/my
CHOLEDOCHO	common bile duct	choledochostomy	chol/ed/o/CHOS/to/my
CHONDRO	cartilage	chondroma	chon/DRŌ/ma
-CIDE	kill	germicide	GERM/i/cide
CIRCUM-	around	circumcision	cir/cum/CI/sion
-CISE	cut	excise	ex/CISE
COLO	colon	colitis	co/LĪ/tis
COLPO	vagina	colporrhaphy	col/POR/rha/phy
CONTRA-	against	contraception	con/tra/CEP/tion
COSTO	rib	intercostal	in/ter/COS/tal

WORD ELEMENT	REFERS TO OR MEANS	EXAMPLE	
CRANIO	skull	craniotomy	cra/ni/OT/o/my
CYANO	blue	cyanotic	cy/an/OT/ic
CYSTO	urinary bladder	cystogram	CYS/to/gram
CYTO	cell	monocyte	MON/o/cyte
DE-	down, from	decubitus	de/CŪ/bi/tus
DENTI	tooth	dentistry	DEN/tis/try
DERMO, DERMATO	skin	dermatology	derm/a/TOL/o/gy
DI-	two	diataxia	di/a/TAX/i/a
DIA-	through, between, across, apart	diarrhea	di/a/RRHĒ/a
DIS-	apart	dissect	dis/SECT
DYS-	painful, difficult, disordered	dysmenorrhea	dys/men/o/RRHĒ/a
ECTO-	outer, on the outside	ectoparasite	ect/o/PAR/a/site
-ECTOMY	surgical removal	prostatectomy	pros/ta/TEC/to/my
-EMESIS	vomiting	hematemesis	hem/at/EM/e/sis
-EMIA	blood	leukemia	leu/KĒ/mi/a
EN-	in, inside	encapsulated	en/CAP/su/la/ted
ENCEPHALO	brain	encephalitis	en/ceph/a/LĪ/tis
ENDO-	within, inner, on the inside	endometrium	en/do/MĒ/tri/um
ENTERO	intestine	enteritis	en/ter/I/tis
EPI-	above, over	epigastric	ep/i/GAS/tric
ERYTHRO	red	erythroblast	er/yth/RŌ/blast
-ESTHESIA	sensation	paresthesia	par/es/THĒ/si/a
EX-	out	excretion	ex/CRĒ/tion
FEBR	fever	afebrile	a/FEB/rile
FIBRO	connective tissue	fibroid	FĪ/broid
GASTRO	stomach	gastro-intestinal	gas/tro-in/TEST/in/al
-GENE, -GENIC	production, origin	neurogenic	neu/ro/GEN/ic
GLOSSO	tongue	glossalgia	glos/SAL/gi/a
GLUCO, GLYCO	sugar, sweet	glycogen	GLY/co/gen
-GRAM	record	myelogram	MY/e/lo/gram
-GRAPH	machine	electro-encephalograph	e/lec/tro/en/CEPH/al/o/graph
-GRAPHY	practice, process	ventriculography	ven/tri/cu/LOG/ra/phy
GYNE	woman	gynecology	gy/ne/COL/o/gy

WORD ELEMENT	REFERS TO OR MEANS	EXAMPLE	
HEMA, HEMATO, HEMO	blood	hematology	hem/at/OL/o/gy
HEMI-	half	hemiplegia	hem/i/PLĒ/gi/a
HEPA, HEPATO	liver	hepatitis	hep/a/TĪ/tis
HERNI	rupture	herniation	her/ni/A/tion
HISTO	tissue	histology	his/TOL/o/gy
HYDRO-	water	hydronephrosis	hy/dro/neph/RŌ/sis
HYPER-	over, above, increased, excessive	hypertension	hy/per/TEN/sion
HYPO-	under, beneath, decreased	hypotension	hy/po/TEN/sion
HYSTER	uterus	hysterectomy	hys/ter/ECT/o/my
-IASIS	condition of	psoriasis	psor/I/a/sis
ICTERO	jaundice	icterus	IC/ter/us
ILEO	ileum (part of small intestine)	ileitis	il/ē/I/tis
ILIO	ilium (bone)	iliosacrum	il/i/o/SĀ/crum
INTER-	between	intercellular	inter/CELL/u/lar
INTRA-	within	intramuscular	in/tra/MUS/cu/lar
-ITIS	inflammation of	appendicitis	ap/pen/di/CĪ/tis
LAPARO	abdomen	laparotomy	la/par/OT/o/my
-LEPSY	seizure, convulse	narcolepsy	NAR/co/lep/sy
LEUKO	white	leukorrhea	leu/ko/RRHĒ/a
LIPO	fat	lipoma	lip/O/ma
LITH	stone, calculus	lithotomy	lith/OT/o/my
-LYSIS	loosen, dissolve	hemolysis	hem/OL/y/sis
MACRO-	large, long	macrocyte	MAC/ro/cyte
MAL-	bad, poor, disordered	maladjusted	mal/ad/JUST/ed
-MANIA	insanity	kleptomania	klep/to/MĀN/ia
MAST	breast	mastectomy	mas/TEC/to/my
MEGA-	large	acromegaly	ac/ro/MEG/a/ly
MEN	month	menstruation	men/stru/A/tion
MESO-	middle	mesentery	MES/en/ter/y
-METER	measure	thermometer	ther/MOM/e/ter
METRO	uterus	metrorrhagia	met/ror/RHĀ/gia
MICRO-	small	microscope	MĪC/ro/scope
MONO-	single, one	monocyte	MON/o/cyte
MUCO	mucous membrane	mucocutaneous	mu/co/cū/TĀ/ne/ous

WORD ELEMENT	REFERS TO OR MEANS	EXAMPLE	
MYELO	spinal cord, bone marrow	myelomeningocele	my/el/o/men/IN/go/cele
MYO	muscle	myopathy	my/OP/a/thy
NARCO	sleep	narcotic	nar/COT/ic
NASO	nose	nasopharynx	nas/o/PHA/rynx
NECRO	death	necropsy	NEC/rop/sy
NEO-	new	neoplasm	NĒ/o/plasm
NEPHRO	kidney	nephritis	ne/PHRĪ/tis
NEURO	nerve	neuralgia	neu/RAL/gi/a
NON-	no, not	nontoxic	non/TOX/ic
OCULO	eye	oculist	O/cū/list
-OLOGY	study of	bacteriology	bac/ter/i/OL/o/gy
-OMA	tumor	carcinoma	car/ci/NO/ma
OOPHOR	ovary	oophorectomy	ō/ophō/REC/to/my
OPHTHALMO	eye	ophthalmoscope	oph/THAL/mo/scope
-OPIA	vision	diplopia	dip/LŌ/pi/a
ORCHI	testicle	orchipexy	ORCH/i/pex/y
-ORRHAPHY	to repair a defect	herniorrhaphy	her/ni/OR/raph/y
ORTHO-	straight	orthopedics	orth/o/PĒD/ics
-OSCOPY	look into, see	esophagoscopy	e/soph/a/GOS/co/py
-OSIS	condition of	neurosis	neu/RŌ/sis
OSTEO	bone	osteoporosis	os/tē/o/por/O/sis
-OSTOMY	surgical opening	colostomy	col/OST/o/my
OTO	ear	otolith	OT/o/lith
-OTOMY	incision, surgical cutting	gastrotomy	gas/TROT/o/my
PARA-	alongside of	paraplegia	par/a/PLĒ/gi/a
PATH	disease	pathology	pa/THOL/o/gy
PED (Latin)	foot	pedicure	PED/i/cure
PED (Greek)	child	pediatrics	pē/di/AT/rics
-PENIA	too few	leukopenia	leu-ko/PĒN/i/a
PERI-	around, covering	pericarditis	pe/ri/car/DĪ/tis
-PEXY	to sew up in position	nephropexy	NEPH/ro/pex/y
PHARYNGO	throat	pharyngoplasty	pha/RYN/go/plas/ty
PHLEBO	vein	phlebitis	phle/BĪ/tis
-PHOBIA	fear, dread	photophobia	pho/to/PHŌ/bi/a
-PLASTY	operative revision	rhinoplasty	RHĪ/no/plas/ty
PLEGIA	paralysis	quadriplegia	qua/dri/PLĒ/gi/a

WORD ELEMENT	REFERS TO OR MEANS	EXAMPLE	
-PNEA	breathing	orthopnea	or/thop/NĒ/a
PNEUMO	air, lungs	pneumonia	pneu/MO/ni/a
POLY-	much, many	polyuria	po/ly/U/ri/a
POST-	after	postpartum	post/PAR/tum
PROCTO	rectum	proctoscopy	proc/TOS/co/py
PRE-	before	preoperative	pre/OP/er/a/tive
-PTOSIS	falling	nephroptosis	neph/rop/TŌ/sis
PYELO	pelvis of kidney	pyelonephritis	py/el/o/neph/RĪ/tis
PYO	pus	empyema	em/py/Ē/ma
PYRO	heat, temperature	pyrexia	py/REX/i/a
RENAL	kidney	suprarenal	su/pra/RĒ/nal
RETRO-	behind, backward	retrosternal	ret/ro/STER/nal
-RHAGE	hemorrhage, flow	hemorrhage	HEM/or/rhage
-RHEA	flow	diarrhea	di/a/RRHĒ/a
RHINO	nose	rhinopathy	rhi/NOP/a/thy
SALPINGO	oviduct	salpingectomy	sal/pin/GEC/to/my
SEMI-	half	semicircular	sem/i/CIR/cu/lar
SEPTIC	poison, infection	septicemia	sep/ti/CĒM/i/a
STOMATO	mouth	stomatitis	sto/ma/TĪ/tis
SUB-	under	subacute	sub/a/CUTE
SUPER	above	suprapubic	su/pra/PŪ/bic
-THERAPY	treatment	hydrotherapy	hy/dro/THER/a/py
-THERMY	heat	diathermy	DĪ/a/therm/y
THORACO	chest	thoracotomy	thor/a/COT/o/my
THROMBO	clot	thrombosis	throm/BŌ/sis
THYRO	thyroid gland	thyroxin	thy/ROX/in
TRANS-	across	transfusion	trans/FŪ/sion
URO	urine	uremia	u/RĒ/mi/a
-URIA, -URIC	condition of, presence in urine	glycosuria	gly/co/SŪR/i/a
UNI	one	unicellular	u/ni/CELL/u/lar
VASO	blood vessel	vasoconstriction	vas/o/con/STRIC/tion

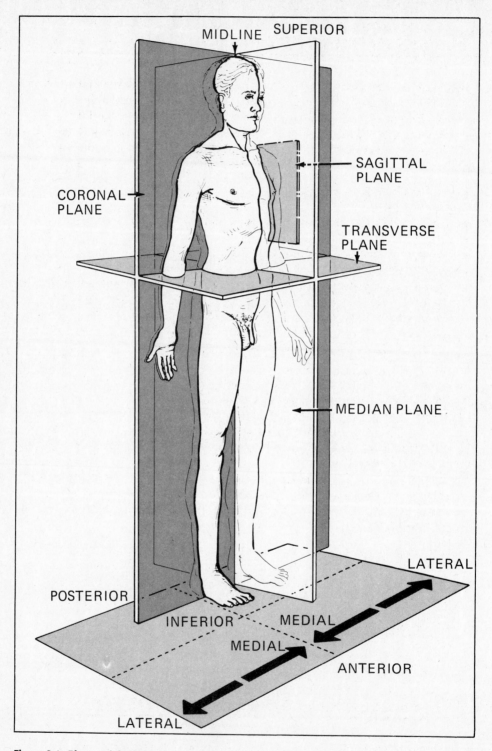

Figure 8-1. Planes of the Body.

PLANES OF THE BODY

A **plane** is a flat surface derived from cutting an imaginary line through the body or a part of the body. The planes of the body are determined by the anatomical position—the body is erect with the face toward the observer and the arms at the side with the palms of the hands turned toward the observer. Diagnostic and treatment machines use planes for their calculations of body parts and positions.

- The **frontal or coronal plane** is upright and divides the body into front and back portions.
- The **horizontal or transverse plane** is across the body and divides the body into upper and lower portions.
- The **medial plane** is front to back and divides the body into two equal parts. Medial refers to middle.
- The **midsagittal plane** is vertical and divides the body into equal right and left halves. It is the same as the medial plane.
- The **sagittal plane** is vertical and divides the body into unequal right and left sections.

CAVITIES OF THE BODY

A **cavity** is a hollow space. The two primary cavities of the body are the **dorsal cavity** and the **ventral cavity.**

The *dorsal cavity* is in the back of the body and consists of the **cranial cavity,** which houses the brain, and the **spinal cavity,** which encases the spinal cord.

The *ventral cavity* is in the front of the body and is filled with organs. It consists of three sections:

1. The **thoracic** or **chest cavity** contains the heart, two lungs, the thymus gland, the windpipe, the esophagus, blood vessels, and nerves.
2. The **abdominal cavity** contains the stomach, the intestines, the kidneys, the adrenals, the liver and gallbladder, the pancreas, and the spleen.
3. The **pelvic cavity** contains the urinary bladder, some of the intestines, and the internal organs of reproduction.

TERMS RELATING TO AREAS OF THE BODY

Abdominal refers to that section between the last rib and the pubic area. If a horizontal line is drawn through the navel, the abdominal area is divided into quadrants (four sections):

- The **right upper quadrant** (RUQ)
- The **left upper quadrant** (LUQ)
- The **right lower quadrant** (RLQ)
- The **left lower quadrant** (LLQ)

The abdomen is divided into nine regions by drawing a line across the body at the level of the tip of the hip bone, drawing another horizontal line just above the bottom of the rib cage, and drawing two vertical lines from inside the nipples to the pelvic bone:

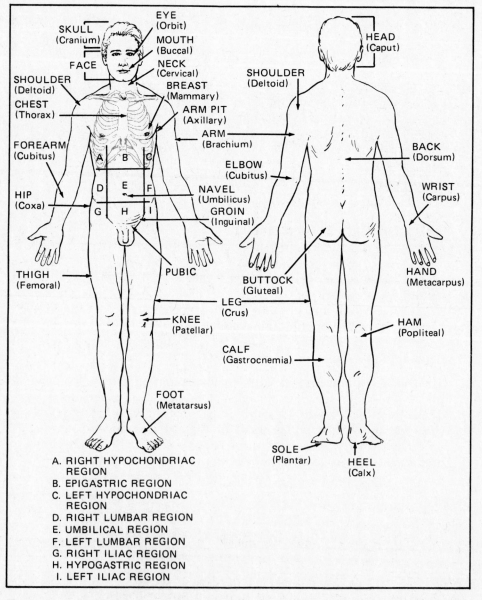

A. RIGHT HYPOCHONDRIAC REGION
B. EPIGASTRIC REGION
C. LEFT HYPOCHONDRIAC REGION
D. RIGHT LUMBAR REGION
E. UMBILICAL REGION
F. LEFT LUMBAR REGION
G. RIGHT ILIAC REGION
H. HYPOGASTRIC REGION
I. LEFT ILIAC REGION

Figure 8-2. Areas of the Body.

- The **umbilical region**—the central area containing the navel.
- The **epigastric region**—just above the umbilical region.
- The **hypogastric region**—just below the umbilical region.
- The **right** and **left hypochondriac regions**—upper side sections.
- The **right** and **left lumbar regions**—middle side sections.
- The **right** and **left iliac** or **inguinal regions**—lower side sections.

- **Anterior or ventral**—front.
- **Caudal**—lower "tail-end" of the spinal column.
- **Cervical**—neck.
- **Cranial**—skull.
- **Distal**—farthest from the center.
- **Facial**—face.
- **Inferior**—lower, beneath.
- **Lateral**—side.
- **Posterior or dorsal**—the back.
- **Proximal**—nearest to the center.
- **Sections**—
  A **cross-section** is a portion obtained by cutting an organ or body horizontally from front to back.
  An **oblique section** is cut diagonally from front to back.
  A **longitudinal section** is cut vertically from top to bottom.
- **Superior**—higher, over, above.
- **Thoracic**—chest.

THE CELL

The **cell** is the basic unit of life. The **cell membrane** is extremely thin and cannot be seen with the ordinary microscope. The membrane selects the material which may enter or leave the cell. The membrane varies according to the function of the cell. Some have long projections called **flagella,** some have short projections called **cilia** or **microvilla.** Cells have the ability to move and the projections aid in movement.

The living matter inside the membrane is called **protoplasm,** the chemical life of the cell. Protoplasm contains proteins, fats, carbohydrates, and inorganic substances. Many of the proteins are **enzymes,** which aid in the chemical reactions without any change in their own composition. Some enzymes contain vitamins. Enzymes are specific in their actions and are influenced by the temperature and the pH of substances with which they come in contact. The **pH** is the degree of acidity or alkalinity of a substance.

- On the pH scale, the number 7 denotes neutrality
- Numbers from 7 to 0 signify increased acidity
- Numbers 7 to 14 signify increased alkalinity.·

Each number on the scale represents a tenfold change—a pH of 8 is ten times more alkaline than a pH of 7, a pH of 9 is 100 times more alkaline than a pH of 7.

Organelles are structures in the protoplasm which perform individual functions. Together they produce digestion, respiration, secretion, and excretion. The **nucleus** is the largest organelle and is surrounded by a two-layered membrane. The protoplasm outside the nucleus is called **cytoplasm.**

The nucleus contains **chromatin,** which is the physical basis of heredity. During cell division, the chromatin breaks up into chromosomes which contain **genes,** the unit of heredity. Each gene is composed of **deoxyribonucleic acid** (DNA), the chemical basis of heredity that carries genetic information. DNA provides the blueprint for construction of a new individual. Genes produce **ribonucleic acid** (RNA) which has the ability to leave the nucleus. DNA cannot leave the nucleus so it instructs the RNA to carry the genetic code to the place

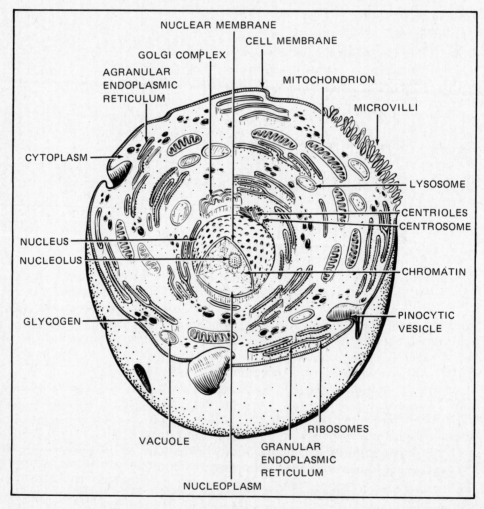

Figure 8-3. Structure of a cell.

in the cell where protein synthesis occurs. Spheroid bodies inside the nucleus, called nucleoli, are mostly RNA.

Somatic cells (all body cells except germ cells) duplicate themselves by a process called mitosis during which the chromosomes duplicate themselves and become two sets. The cell divides into two daughter cells which contain exactly the same materials as the mother cell. The number of chromosomes, 23 pairs in all somatic cells, is kept constant. There are many types of somatic cells.

Germ cells (reproductive cells) are for the specific function of reproducing a like organism. Germ cells in the female are called eggs or ova, and male germ cells are called sperm cells or spermatozoa. Germ cells have 23 chromosomes, one of which is a sex determiner. The meeting of two germ cells, a female and a male, results in the 23 pairs of chromosomes. The female sex chromosome is X; the male chromosome is either Y or X. Two X chromosomes produce a female; one X and one Y chromosome produce a male.

Hereditary Disorders

Hereditary disorders result from some abnormality of a cell. Genetic counseling helps determine hereditary risks.

Diabetes Mellitus is an endocrine system disorder which has a familial tendency. Chapter 15 discusses the disorder.

Down's Syndrome (mongolism) occurs most often in a baby when the mother is over 30 years of age. The child has mental retardation, poor muscle tone, slanted eyes, a large tongue, and abnormal handprints and footprints.

Fibrocystic disease or cystic fibrosis is a disease of the exocrine glands, especially the lungs. Chapter 12 discusses the disease.

Galactosemia is an enzyme deficiency which results in eye cataracts and damage to the liver and brain. If diagnosed early, a diet excluding all milk and milk products relieves the symptoms.

Hemophilia occurs when the clotting factor in blood is absent. The disorder is discussed further in Chapter 11.

Muscular dystrophy causes degeneration of the muscles. Chapter 10 discusses the disease.

Tay-Sachs disease, a disorder of fat metabolism, causes death in children between the ages of three and five. The hereditary condition is confined almost exclusively to Jewish children whose families are of Eastern-European descent. One of every 30 Eastern-European Jews is a carrier.

Genetic Engineering

Recombinant DNA technology is a powerful new tool in medical research and industry. The recombinant DNA technique is a method used by scientists to combine genetic material from separate organisms, a way to shuffle hereditary information. Bacteria can be engineered to manufacture human protein, for example. Some genetically engineered microorganisms help in the manufacture of synthetic pharmaceuticals at a greatly reduced cost.

Someday, we will probably see the creation of artificial genes to correct genetic defects and the creation of a method to alter the DNA of tumors to eradicate cancer.

The National Institutes of Health (NIH) published guidelines for research of recombinent DNA in 1975 and updates them at regular intervals to assure that the technology is used only for valid scientific purposes.

TISSUES

A **tissue** is a group of similar cells which perform a special function. There are four different kinds of tissue: connective, epithelial, muscular, and nervous.

Connective tissues are the most abundant; they unite and support all the other tissues of the body. In connective tissue, the cells are widely scattered with a large amount of fluid in the intercellular material.

Epithelial tissue consists of closely packed cells with very little intercellular material or fibers. It provides protection, filtration, secretion, and absorption. Epithelial tissue regenerates itself very well. It lines body cavities and organs and covers all body surfaces.

Muscular tissue consists of highly specialized cells with four qualities: they receive and respond to stimuli (irritability); they stretch (extensibility); they thicken and shorten when stimulated (contractility); and they return to their original shape after being stretched (elasticity). Muscular tissue enables the body to move.

Nervous tissue contains two types of cells, neurons and neuroglia or glial cells. Neurons conduct impulses from one part of the body to another. Glial cells form a supportive network and destroy microbes and waste products.

Organs are groups of tissues that perform complex functions. The heart, liver, and lungs are some of the body's organs.

Systems are groups of organs that perform highly complex functions. A system is the largest structural unit of the body.

TERMINOLOGY

Word	Definition
Cytocide	Any material that destroys cells
Cytogenesis	The origin and development of a cell
Cytoid	Resembling a cell
Cytology	The study of the structure and function of cells
Cytolysis	The breaking up or destruction of living cells

Cytopathology	The study of the changes that occur in a cell during a disease process
Cyturia	The presence of cells in urine
Histo	The prefix for tissue
Histology	The study of microscopic structure of tissue
Histolysis	The disintegration of tissue
Histoma	A tumor composed of tissue
Patho	A combining form that indicates disease
Pathogen	A microorganism or some material capable of producing a disease
Pathologist	A doctor who specializes in diagnosing the changes in tissues and examines tissues removed during surgery and performs autopsies
Tumor	A new, abnormal growth of tissue which forms a mass. It is also called a neoplasm

- Benign tumors are mild, non-recurrent growths that are confined to one area.
- Malignant tumors invade surrounding tissue, are harmful, and are resistant to treatment. They are also called cancers.
- Metastasis means that cancer cells travel from one part of the body to another and develop another growth.

DISEASES AND DISORDERS

Abscesses are localized areas of inflammation with pus formation which may occur in any tissue. **Tx:** Antibiotics according to C&S results, warm soaks if area permits, surgical incision and drainage. Central supply has a heating pad with circulating water for moist heat. It is called a K-Pad, comes in various sizes, and must be ordered by the physician.

Cancer, which literally means crab, is a disease that spreads in a crab-like fashion. Some characteristics of cancer are:

1. Growth may be rapid in comparison to benign tumors.
2. Cancers invade surrounding tissue (i.e., malignant tumor)
3. Cancer cells are not like the normal cells of the tissue of origin.
4. Recurrent growth
5. Cancer cells spread to other parts of the body (i.e., metastasis).
6. Growth of cancer cells cause tissue destruction.
7. The growth causes death if not controlled.

According to the American Cancer Society, the warning signs of cancer are:

1. Unusual bleeding or discharge
2. A lump or thickening in the breast or other parts of the body
3. A sore that does not heal
4. Change in bowel or bladder habits
5. Hoarseness or cough
6. Indigestion or difficulty in swallowing
7. A change in a wart or mole

Tx: Surgical removal, radiation therapy, chemotherapy, hormone therapy. Treatment may be any single type or a combination of two or more, depending on the type of cancer and the stage of development when first diagnosed. Each cell has its own type of cancer. Many cancers have a high cure rate if diagnosed early and treated promptly.

Cellulitis is a spreading inflammation of tissues. **Tx:** Bedrest, application of warm, moist dressings, elevation of the part of the body involved, if possible. Depending on the results of the C&S, antibiotics may also be given.

Lupus erythematosus is a connective tissue disease (CTD), with an unknown cause usually occurring in women during their 20s.

- The **cutaneous type** involves only the skin. Exposure to sunlight may trigger lesions of a red, scaly, butterfly pattern over the nose and cheeks. **Tx:** Avoiding sunlight, sunscreen preparations, topical corticosteroids, antimalarial therapy in some cases.

- The **systemic type** (SLE) may occur suddenly or gradually with episodes of fever, malaise, and joint pain. Lesions may occur anywhere on the body. All systems are eventually affected. **Tx:** Salicylates and corticosteroids to control inflammation, individual treatment as symptoms arise. There is no cure.

Scleroderma, a collagen tissue disease with an unknown cause, causes thickening and rigidity of the skin. It frequently involves the digestive, respiratory, circulatory, and urinary systems. Women are more susceptible to the disease. **Tx:** Corticosteroids, physiotherapy for muscle involvement, treatment of symptoms as they arise.

Disease-Causing Organisms

- Staphylococci
- Streptococci
- Clostridia

SURGERIES AND PROCEDURES

Biopsy of lesions, tissues, or tumors are often performed. A frozen section is often done in the pathology department immediately after removal of the tissue to determine if more extensive surgery is required. Surgery personnel take the specimen to the pathology section of the lab, and the report is phoned to the OR in just a few minutes.

Incision and Drainage (I&D) is a procedure in which the affected area is incised and drained. The incision may be closed with a drain placed in the wound or may be left open for more drainage. Penrose drains are often used for drainage.

LABORATORY TESTS

- Aldolase
- ANA
- ANA Profile
- Creatine phosphokinase (CPK)
- Cultures of skin lesions and abscesses
- ESR
- LE prep
- RA Latex
- Serum globulin

RADIOLOGY AND NUCLEAR MEDICINE EXAMS

CT or CAT (computerized axial tomography) scan visualizes cross-sections of the body and aids in locating tumors and abscesses.

MEDICATIONS

Corticosteroids reduce inflammation and decrease allergic symptoms.

- Aristocort, Kenacort (triamcinolone)—PO—initial dose of 8 mg to 20 mg daily in divided doses. Maintenance dosage individualized.

- Aristocort, Acetonide, Kenalog (triamcinolone acetonide) for topical use as directed by physician. Available in 0.1% cream, lotion, and ointment.
- Prednisone—PO—60 mg/d then reduce to minimal dose for control of inflammation according to individual response.

Analgesics relieve pain.

- ASA—PO—0.6 gm PO q 4 hrs. (0.6 gm = 600 mg = gr x)
- Tylenol—PO—tab ī or īī tid or qid or q 4 hrs prn.

Analgesics with narcotics relieve severe pain.

- Empirin CMPD c̄ Codeine—PO—# 1, 2, 3, 4—tab ī or īī q 3 hrs prn.
- Tylenol c̄ Codeine—PO—# 1, 2, 3, 4—tab ī or īī q 4 hrs prn.

Antibiotics inhibit the growth of or destroy bacteria.

- Common ones are penicillin, erythromycin, tetracycline, Kefzol.

EXAMPLES OF PHYSICIAN'S ORDERS

Dx: Cellulitis

1. IV TKO D5/0.2 NS
2. Kefzol 1.0 gm IVPB q 6 hrs
3. Elevate ® hand on 2 pillows
4. K-Pad to ® hand
5. ASA gr × PO q 6 hrs prn for fever > 101° (0) or for pain
6. Routine lab

Next day:

1. Betadine dressing to ® hand. Change q 6 hrs wet to dry then place hand in splint and hold with Kling wrap.

Dx: SLE

1. ESR, SMA-20, ANA profile, LE preps × 2, UA, CBC
2. EKG
3. IV D5/W q 12 hrs
5. DAT
5. Tigan 200 mg IM q 6 hrs prn for N
6. Tylenol tab īī q 4 hrs prn for discomfort if no N
7. Demerol 50 mg IM q 6 hrs prn severe pain
8. Prednisone 10 mg qid
9. Dalmane 30 mg q HS prn

REVIEW QUESTIONS

1. The planes of the body are based on the body being in the _____ position.

2. The _____ plane is vertical and divides the body into front and back portions.

3. The _____ plane is horizontal and divides the body into upper and lower portions.

4. _____ means back.

5. _____ means front.

6. _____ means above, higher.

7. List the two main cavities of the body and their divisions.

   _____

   _____

8. _____ is the living matter inside the cell membrane.

9. pH is the degree of _____ or _____ of a substance.

10. _____ is the chemical basis of heredity.

11. A _____ is the unit of heredity.

12. Define tissue and list the four main types.

    _____

    _____

13. Define organ. _____

14. Define system. _____

15. Define cancer. _____

16. List the main categories for cancer treatment.

    _____

    _____

17. Define a cell. _____

18. Define a chromosome. _____

Chapter 9 | The Skin

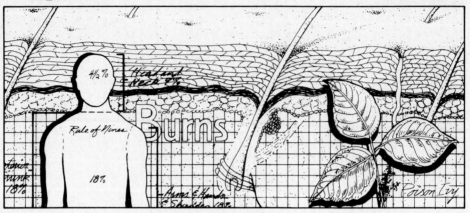

OBJECTIVES

1. List the layers of the skin.
2. List the functions of the skin.
3. Identify terms relating to the skin.
4. List diseases and disorders of the skin.
5. List medications used in diseases and disorders of the skin.
6. Transcribe Physician's Orders relating to skin diseases and disorders.

The skin is the largest organ of the body. The skin and its appendages, hair and nails, are often called the **integumentary system,** the covering. We usually think of the skin as just a cover that holds the body together, but it does much more than that. The skin protects the body against bacterial invasion and the harmful rays of the sun, helps tissues from becoming dehydrated, aids in regulation of body temperature, eliminates wastes through sweat, stores food and water, receives stimuli from the environment, and manufactures Vitamin D from sunlight.

LAYERS OF THE SKIN

The skin consists of two layers, the **epidermis** and the **dermis,** which are connected to a subcutaneous layer of tissue.

Epidermis

The outer most layer, the epidermis, is composed of layers of cells. There are five layers on the palms of the hands and the soles of the feet and four layers on most of the rest of the body. Cells of the epidermis are continually shed and replaced.

Melanin, a pigment ranging from yellow to black, is found in the various layers of the epidermis. Exposure to ultraviolent radiation increases the amount and darkness of melanin.

Dermis

The dermis is composed of connective tissue containing lymph vessels, blood vessels, sebaceous and sweat glands, papillae, nerves and nerve endings, and elastic fibers.

Sebaceous glands are connected to the hair follicles and secrete an oily substance called **sebum.** The sebum keeps the hair from drying out, prevents excessive loss of water from the skin, and keeps the skin flexible and soft. Sebaceous glands on the face, neck, and upper chest are larger than those on the rest of the body.

Sweat glands are also called sudoriferous—*sudor* meaning sweat and *ferre* meaning to bear, glands. The gland is comprised of a coiled structure that lies

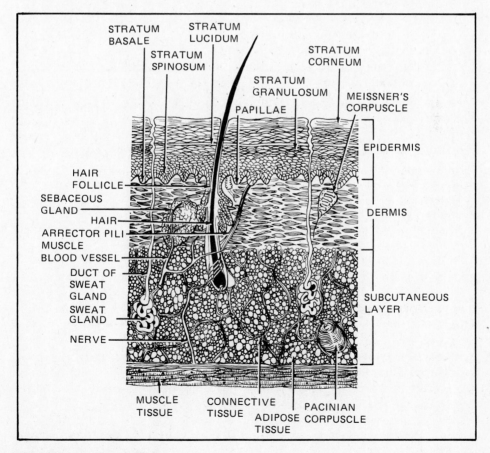

Figure 9-1. Structure of the Skin.

in the dermis or the subcutaneous layer and a tube that leads through the dermis and epidermis to end in a pore on the surface of the skin. The mixture of water, salts, and wastes produced by sweat glands is called sweat or perspiration.

Papillae are small projections in the upper part of the dermis that extend into the epidermis causing ridges. These ridges produce distinct, individual fingerprints.

Subcutaneous Layer of Tissue

The subcutaneous layer of tissue is often referred to as the superficial fascia. This layer contains the hair follicles, sweat glands, nerves, blood vessels, and adipose tissue.

Hair follicles begin in a bulb-like structure containing blood vessels that supply the hair with nourishment and cells that produce new hair when the old hair is lost.

Arrector pili, a smooth muscle, is attached to the side of hair follicles and pulls the hair erect when a person is frightened or cold.

| TERMINOLOGY

Cyst—an abnormal sac or pouch containing fluid, semi-fluid, or solid material
Derma—the true skin
Dermatoid—resembling skin
Dermatologist—a physician who specializes in diseases and care of the skin
Dermatology—the study of the skin and its diseases
Dermatoplasty—a restoring operation of the skin, skin grafting
Dermatorrhea—excessive secretion of the sebaceous glands
Erythema—redness of the skin
Excoriation—a scraped area of the epidermis due to trauma, burns, chemicals, or other causes
Keratosis—a formation of horny growths on the skin
Macule—a small spot or colored area on the skin with no elevation or depression present
Multiform or polymorphous—when there is more than one kind of skin lesion present
Papule—a solid, red elevation of the skin
Pustule—a blister filled with pus
Telangiectasia—a permanent dilatation of superficial blood vessels producing a colored area—may be a birthmark
Universal—the entire skin is affected
Vesicle—a blister filled with clear fluid
Wheal—an area of transitory edema in the skin; usually caused by an allergic reaction
Zosteriform—a linear arrangement of a rash or lesions along a nerve.

DISEASES AND DISORDERS

Acne is a common skin disorder of adolescents and young adults. The exact cause is unknown, but the increased activity of certain endocrine glands at puberty is thought to trigger the sebaceous glands to secrete large amounts of oil. Acne may be non-inflammatory with only blackheads, whiteheads, which are caused by plugged follicles, and a few pimples. The inflammatory type will have many pimples and pustules, abscesses, cysts, and scarring. Cleanliness does not prevent acne, and frequent scrubbings may irritate the skin and cause more pustules. **Tx:** Benzoyl peroxide topically, salicylic acid, and sulfur.

Alopecia means loss of hair and occurs after febrile diseases, severe emotional trauma, and radiation and chemotherapy of certain cancers. This is usually temporary, and the hair growth is resumed when the illness or treatment is no longer present. Ordinary baldness is largely due to hormones or hereditary factors and is not treatable.

Angiomas or birthmarks are benign tumors of the blood and lymph vessels that involve the skin. Those with flat, violet-red patches are called **port-wine stains;** those with raised, bright red nodular lesions are called **strawberry.** The strawberry angiomas usually disappear spontaneously. Laser treatment is the therapy of choice for port-wine stains.

Burns are a great threat to life because of their systemic effects, effects that occur throughout the body. Burns may be caused by heat, electrical, radioactive, or chemical agents. Burns kill cells by changing the protein substance of cells. The total body surface area (TBSA) involved in a burn injury is estimated by dividing the body in multiples of nine. The head is 9%, each arm is 9%, each leg is 18%, front of the trunk is 18%, back of the trunk is 18%. **First degree burns** produce redness of the burned area. **Second degree burns** cause damage of the epidermal and dermal layers with blister formation. Hospitalization is required if the burn covers a large area. **Third degree burns** destroy the full thickness of the skin and may involve fat, muscles, and bone. If the patient survives, disabling and disfiguring scars are frequent. Shock, infection, circulatory problems, and kidney problems make treatment difficult. Hospitals with special burn units give these patients a better chance of recovery. **Tx:** Keeping the burn wounds free from infection, monitoring electrolytes to replace body fluids that are lost, controlling pain, and grafting skin to cover wounds.

Cancer of the skin is usually caused by the ultraviolet rays in sunlight. The appearance of skin cancer varies: it may be a dry, scaly patch; it may be a pimple that never heals; it may be a reddened area with a crusty center; it may be a pale, wax-like, pearly nodule which ulcerates. The most common types are **basal cell epithelioma** and **squamous cell carcinoma.** Exposed parts of the face, neck, forearms, and backs of the hands are common sites. **Tx:** Excision with tissue studies. Radiation therapy may be needed if the lesion extends beyond the skin.

- A pigmented tumor, called **melanoma,** is the leading cause of death for individuals with skin diseases. There are five types of melanomas and all have irregular color, irregular borders, and irregular surface. **Tx:** Complete excision with biopsy. If diagnosed early, surgical excision may be a complete cure. Radiation therapy is used in other cases. Each case is treated according to the extent of the lesion, the individual's condition, age, and history.

Decubitus is a bedsore caused by pressure from a bony prominence. Preventive measures are frequent turning of the patient, good skin care, special mattresses (the eggcrate or floatation mattress), and sheepskins under pressure points for bedridden patients. **Tx:** Since the breakdown of tissue begins inside and the red, swollen area with ulceration develops later, the best treatment is prevention. Once the bedsore is an open wound, treatment centers around prevention of infection; skin grafts may be needed.

Dermatitis is an inflammation of the skin with redness, oozing of fluid, crust formation, and scales.

- **Contact dermatitis** is an inflammation caused by a substance coming in contact with the skin. This may involve all of the body or only a particular area. The appearance of the lesions, the distribution of lesions, and a history of what the patient has been in contact with may establish the cause. Patch testing may be necessary to establish the allergen. **Tx:** Remove the offending agent. Wet compresses relieve burning, itching, and inflammation and have a soothing, cooling effect. Therapeutic baths containing medications aid in removal of crusts and scales and relieve itching. Steroids, topical and systemic, relieve inflammation.
- **Atopic dermatitis** is a chronic superficial inflammation of the skin. The patient usually has a history of an allergic disorder such as hay fever or asthma. Testing shows allergic reaction to numerous inhalants and food. Itching is usually the only symptom. Secondary infections may occur due to scratching. The condition will subside and reappear periodically. **Tx:** Topical corticosteroids, antihistamines, cautious use of systemic corticosteroids, change in climate to a warm, sunny area.

Erysipelas is an acute streptococcal infection of the skin with well defined, red, swollen areas. The patient will have a fever and a vague feeling of discomfort. **Tx:** Culture lesions, penicillin or erythromycin, cold compresses to relieve discomfort, ASA or analgesic with codeine for pain.

Fungus infections usually involve the superficial layer of the skin, the nails, and hair.

- **Tinea corporis** is ringworm of the body. **Tx:** Specific antifungal medications, antibiotics.
- **Tinea pedis** is a ringworm of the feet, commonly called Athlete's Foot. Preventive treatment is good foot hygiene, use of a drying powder, and light footwear that prevents sweating. **Tx:** Foot soaks of warm potassium permanganate followed by corticosteroid lotion, antifungal medications.
- **Tinea capitis** is ringworm of the scalp and is contagious. **Tx:** Hair is cut short and shampooed frequently. Antifungal medication is prescribed orally and topically. Brushes and combs require isolation for patient's use only. A stockinette cap should be worn at night.
- **Tinea barbae** is ringworm of the beard. **Tx:** Antifungal medication orally and topically.

Furuncles and carbuncles are staphylococcal infections around a follicle with pus formation. Furuncles are commonly called boils. Carbuncles are a group of adjacent furuncles, each furuncle having a core or central, firm accumulation of pus and dead tissue. These usually develop on the back of the neck but can also appear on the body. **Tx:** Moist heat, antibiotics, culture to be sure of organisms' susceptibility, surgical incision to remove core or cores.

Herpes simplex (fever blister, cold sore) is a viral infection on the face or lips causing blisters or clusters of blisters on an inflamed base. **Tx:** Drying agents such as Blistex.

Hyperhidrosis is excessive perspiration due to overactivity of the sweat glands. It may involve general or specific areas. It may be a condition in itself or be caused by another condition. **Tx:** Determine and treat any underlying disease. Where none exists, treatment includes cooling baths, drying powders, mild astringents prn, reduction of emotional distress, anticholinergic drugs.

Hypertrichosis, or hirsutism, means heavy growth of hair in areas normally free of hair. If not due to a familial or a racial tendency, this may be due to an endocrine system disturbance. **Tx:** Treat any endocrine disorder. Electrolysis is an effective but tedious process of hair removal. Depilatories can be used but may cause skin irritations.

Impetigo contagiosa is a skin infection caused by staphlococci or streptococci. It is contagious only in children and young adults. Pustules form, then rupture, and crusts form. Fatal systemic infection may occur in infants. **Tx:** Removal of crusts with soap and water followed by topical antibiotics. Compresses of warm, normal saline may be needed to remove crusts. Severe cases require systemic antibiotics.

Keloids are benign growths of fibrous tissue at a scar from surgical incision or a scar from trauma. **Tx:** Corticosteroids injected into area, radiation therapy.

Nevi are skin tumors composed of specialized epithelial cells containing melanin. Commonly called moles or birthmarks, they usually cause no problems. **Tx:** Surgical removal if at a point of frequent friction or for cosmetic purposes. If there has been any change in size or appearance, a wide excision is necessary to rule out melanoma. All nevi removed should be studied histologically.

Pediculosis is an invasion of the skin and hair by lice, a parasite.

- **Pediculosis capitis** occurs on the scalp, eyelashes, eyebrows, and beard. It can be transmitted by combs, brushes, hats, and personal contact.
- **Pediculosis corporis** is inhabitation of clothing by body lice that feed on the skin.
- **Pediculosis pubis** is an infestation of crab lice on the hair in the anogenital region primarily, but it may involve hair under the arms, etc. **Tx:** All pediculi infestations are treated with specific antiparasitic shampoos, lotions, creams, and sprays. Personal items such as combs, hats, and clothing along with mattresses, bedding, and furniture are sprayed with an insecticide. Objects that cannot be dry cleaned or washed should be sprayed.

Pemphigus is a serious, debilitating disease of unknown cause. Normal appearing skin and mucous membranes suddenly have fluid-filled blisters which break and crust. The patient is extremely uncomfortable, and the lesions have a foul odor. **Tx:** High doses of corticosteroids, diminishing as lesions disappear. Good nutrition to maintain normal protein levels; protection of skin against secondary infections; wet dressings or antiseptic lotions; therapeutic baths. Antibiotics if infection from bacteria occurs.

Pruritus is itching, which may be secondary to a skin disease, may be a symptom of a systemic disease, or may be caused by drug or food allergies. **Tx:** Therapeutic baths, specific antipruritic preparations, antihistamines, corticosteroids. Discontinue medication if possible to rule out allergic reaction.

Psoriasis is a chronic disease of the skin with well defined red papules or plaques covered with shiny, overlapping scales. The disease has periods of remission and recurrences. Biopsy can differentiate the disease from others with similar lesions. **Tx:** Photochemotherapy is an interaction of light and drugs to produce a beneficial effect on disease.

Scabies is commonly called the itch. The itch mite, Sarcoptes scabiei, is a parasite that burrows into the skin and lays eggs along the tunnel. This causes intense pruritus and the scratching usually causes secondary inflammation. Personal contact transmits the disease; sometimes an entire family is infected. **Tx:** Scabicides, thorough cleansing of clothing and skin, starch baths for pruritis, antibiotics if infection present.

Sebaceous cyst forms when a sebaceous gland duct becomes plugged. These tumors grow slowly. **Tx:** Surgical removal, injection of steroids into the cyst if inflammation is present.

Seborrhea is hyperactivity of the sebaceous glands, usually of the forehead, nose, and scalp. Skin appears greasy and may develop thin, gray scales. Dandruff is a form of seborrhea. **Tx:** Special shampoos, sulfur and salicylic acid preparations, corticosteroid creams.

Warts are benign tumors caused by a virus. If not numerous or bothersome, no Tx. **Tx if necessary:** Freeze with liquid nitrogen, apply Compound W or 40% salicylic acid plaster topically, inject Bleomycin into base of wart.

Disease-Causing Organisms

Bacteria

- Staphylococci
- Streptococci
- Pseudomonas aeruginosa
- Proteus vulgaris

Fungi

- Epidermophyton (ringworm of skin and nails)
- Microsporum (ringworm of skin, hair, nails)
- Trichophyton (ringworm of skin, hair, nails)

Parasites

- Pediculus humanus capitus (head louse)
- Pediculus humanus corporis (body louse)
- Phthirus pubis (crab louse)
- Sarcoptes scabiei (itch mite)

| SURGERIES AND PROCEDURES

Biopsy of a lesion or growth is done to examine its cells and determine what treatment is needed.

Skin graft is a procedure in which a piece of tissue is removed from its normal position and transferred to another area.

- **Autografts** are tissue transfers or transplants from the same person.
- **Homografts** are tissue transfers or transplants from one person to another person.
- A **flap** is a portion of tissue cut away to cover another area.
- A **pedicle** is the stem of tissue that connects the flap to the body.
- A **split thickness skin graft** (STSG) is used to cover an area too large to close by suturing the two sides together. An STSG is about 0.015 inch or 0.4 mm thick. The donor site heals quickly.
- A **full thickness skin graft** (FTSG) includes all of the epidermis.

| LABORATORY TESTS

- CBC
- C&S of skin lesions or exudate
- Electrolytes
- Hgb, Hct
- Histology studies of biopsied tissue
- SMA-20

| MEDICATIONS

Antiacne

Benzoyl peroxide in a 5% or 10% solution applied once or twice a day to the point of mild dryness. Benzoyl peroxide preparations:

- Benoxyl
- Oxy-5
- Oxy-10
- Persadox
- 5-Benzagel
- 10-Benzagel

Antibiotics

Topical:

- Betadine ointment—to affected areas as needed.
- Betadine surgical scrub—to clean area before surgery.
- Polysporin ointment—apply 2 to 5 times a day.
- Silvadene Cream and Sulfamylon Cream for burns. Clean and debride area, apply cream with a sterile, gloved hand once or twice daily; reapply if rubbed off.

Systemic:

For skin and soft tissue infections caused by strains of staphylococci and streptococci.

- Bristamycin (erythromycin)—PO—250 mg q 6 hrs.
- Cefadyl—IM or IV—500 mg to 1 gm q 4 to 6 hrs.
- Ilosone (erythromycin)—PO—250 mg q 6 hrs.
- penicillin V—PO—250 mg to 500 mg q 6 hrs.
- Polymox (amoxicillin)—PO—250 mg q 8 hrs.
- Velosef—PO—250 mg q 6 hrs or 500 mg q 12 hrs, IV—500 mg to 1 gm q 6 hrs for severe infections.

Antihistamines:

These drugs reduce itching and reduce allergic reactions.

Topical:

- Caladryl lotion or cream—apply to affected areas tid or qid.
- PBZ (pyribenzamine) Cream—apply gently to affected areas 3 or 4 times a day.
- Ziradryl lotion—cleanse affected areas and apply liberally 3 or 4 times a day.

Systemic:

- Atarax—PO—25 mg tid or qid.
- Benadryl—PO—50 mg tid or qid. IM or IV—10 mg, 50 mg or 100 mg as a one time dose, if necessary to repeat do not exceed 400 mg/d.
- Chlortrimeton—PO—Repetabs 2 mg q 8 to 10 hrs. One dose at HS may be enough. SC or IM or IV—10 to 20 mg once.
- Forhistal—PO—Lontabs 2.5 mg—dosage individualized.
- Phenergan—PO—12.5 mg qid or 25 mg at HS.

Antiseborrheas

Antiseborrheas decrease oil secretion. The following shampoos are used as directed by the physician:

- DHS Zinc dandruff shampoo
- P & S shampoo

- X-seb shampoo
- X-seb T shampoo

Astringents

Astringents check secretions or give tone to the skin.

- Acno astringent—saturate cotton pad and clean areas bid or tid.
- Counter Balance Pore Lotion—cleanse oily areas.
- Deep Mist Mild Skin Freshener—apply to dry or very dry skin to provide toning.
- Tucks Premoistened Pads—specifically designed for perianal and perineal pruritus and irritation, use in addition to toilet tissue or apply to area for 15 to 30 minutes.

Coal Tar and Sulfur

These substances treat itching, scaling, and erythema.

- Alphosyl Lotion or Cream—cleanse areas and apply 2 to 4 times daily, massage into lesions. When condition is controlled, use 2 to 3 times weekly.
- Lavatar—add to bath water as directed by physician.
- Tar-Doak Lotion—apply as directed by physician.
- Sebutone Liquid or Cream—massage shampoo into wet scalp for 5 minutes then rinse out and repeat procedure, use as needed for itching and scaling.

Corticosteroids

Corticosteroids reduce inflammation and relieve itching.

Topical:
Some topical agents contain an antibiotic.

- Acticort Lotion—apply to affected areas tid or qid.
- Cort-Dome ⅛%, ¼%, ½%, 1% Cream or Lotion—apply tid or qid to affected areas.
- Cortisporin Cream or Ointment—start with tid or qid applications and gradually decrease.
- Cyclocort Cream—apply light film to affected areas bid or tid and rub gently until it disappears.
- Kenalog Cream, Lotion, Ointment—apply bid to qid as directed, may be covered with a pliable nonporous film dressing.
- Maxiflow Cream 0.05%—gently massage a small amount into affected areas bid to qid.
- Racet Cream—apply tid or qid.
- Valisone 1% Cream, Lotion, Ointment—apply as directed by physician.

Systemic

All systemic dosages are individualized.

- Celestone—PO—tablets 0.6 mg.
- Celestone Phosphate—IM, IV.
- Decadron Phosphate—IM, IV.
- Decadron tablets—PO—0.25 mg, 0.5 mg, 0.75 mg, 1.5 mg and 4 mg tablets.
- Kenocort (triamcinolone)—PO—tablets of 2 mg, 4 mg, 8 mg.
- Medrol—PO—tablets of 2 mg, 4 mg, 8 mg, 16 mg, 24 mg, 32 mg.
- Prednisone—PO—tablets of 5 mg, 10 mg, 20 mg, 50 mg.

Fungicides

Fungicides are medications used to kill fungi.

Topical:

- Costellani Paint—apply to affected areas once or twice a day.
- Fungoid Creme—apply to affected areas tid.
- Fungoid Tincture—for ringworm of the nails—apply bid.
- Mycolog Cream and Ointment—rub cream into areas bid or tid, apply thin film of ointment bid or tid.
- Mycostatin Cream and Ointment—apply liberally twice a day.
- Tinactin 1% cream or Solution—apply sparingly to each lesion and massage gently until it disappears, twice a day.

Systemic:

- Fulvicin P/G (griseofulvin)—PO—250 mg daily.
- Fulvicin U/F (griseofulvin)—PO—500 mg daily.
- Grifulvin V (griseofulvin)—PO—500 mg daily.

Keratolytics

Keratolytics are used to soften dry, horny layers of the skin.

- Elaqua XX—apply bid or tid when skin is moist after washing.
- Keralyt Gel (salicylic acid)—after bathing and complete drying, apply to affected areas at night and cover. Wash off in the morning.
- Salactic Film—apply once daily as directed.

Pediculocides

Pediculocides are used to kill pediculi (lice).

- A-200 Pyrinate Liquid or Gel—apply enough to thoroughly wet the area. Leave on no longer than 10 minutes and wash out thoroughly. Remove lice and eggs with fine comb.
- Kwell Cream or Lotion—cover only the affected area and surrounding hairy areas. Rub in and leave for 12 hrs. then wash areas.

- Kwell shampoo—thoroughly wet hair and skin of infested and surrounding areas. Add small quantities of water until lather forms and shampoo for four minutes. Rinse thoroughly.
- Li-Ban Spray and R & C Spray—Use as directed on container for killing lice on bedding, mattresses, furniture, and inanimate objects.

Scabicides

Scabicides kill the itch mite.

- Eurax Cream and Lotion—massage into skin of body from chin down, repeat in 24 hrs. Cleansing bath 48 hrs after last application.
- Kwell Cream or Lotion—apply after bath and thorough drying to entire body from neck down, leave on 8 to 12 hrs, and then remove with shower or bath.

Wart Medications

- Compound W—as directed by physician.
- Cantharone—as directed by physician.
- Salicylic Acid Plaster 40%—as directed by physician.
- Blenoxane (bleomycin)—used only by physician, injected into base of wart.

Sunscreens

Sunscreens are used to protect the skin from ultraviolet rays.

- Block-Aid—apply liberally to exposed areas before going into sunlight
- Pabanol Lotion—apply evenly and allow to dry before exposure
- Presun 8 Lotion, creamy lotion, and gel—apply liberally one hour before exposure
- RVPaque—apply in thin film
- Super Shade 15—apply before exposure
- Total Eclipse—apply before exposure.

LASER THERAPY

Laser is an acronym for light amplification by stimulated emission of radiation. Lasers give an intense beam of consistent radiation. They are a valuable surgical tool, partly because of their well-controlled hemostatic effect. Lasers are used to remove some birthmarks and tattoos and are used in many other surgeries.

PHOTOCHEMOTHERAPY

Longwave ultraviolet light (UVA) exposure plus oral administration of **psoralen** (PUVA) results in photobiologic reactions that lead to improvement of psoriasis.

UVA is administered via a small room where glass walls have built-in ultraviolet lights. The length of time for exposure requires individual calculations.

Psorolens are compounds activated by UVA to produce phototoxic reactions. Some psorolens are:

- 8-Methoxypsoralen—PO—0.6 mg/kg two hours before exposure to UVA.
- Oxsoralen (8-MOP) 10 mg capsules—PO—two capsules two to four hrs before UVA exposures.
- Trisoralen 5 mg tablets—PO—two tablets daily before UVA exposure.

Medium wave ultraviolet (UVB) radiation is used with tar derivatives. UVB is the type of ultraviolet light that causes typical sunburn. This treatment, like PUVA, is performed in a hospital. It may be called the "Goeckerman regimen" after the doctor who developed it.

EXAMPLES OF PHYSICIAN'S ORDERS

Dx: Dermatitis, cause unknown

1. Tepid starch bath BID
2. Remove crusts and scales following baths.
3. Cortisporin Cream to lesions BID p̄ baths and cleaning
4. Ice packs prn to areas of discomfort
5. Ilosone 250 mg q 6 hrs PO
6. TPR q 4 hrs
7. Tylenol gr X for T greater than 101°
8. High protein diet
9. Force fluids—at least 2000 cc/24 hrs.
10. Prednisone 5 mg BID
11. Valium 5 mg PO HS

Dx: Pilonidal Cyst (A dermoid cyst containing hair—usually a prenatal development defect.)

1. CBC, UA, SMA-20, chest x-ray on admission
2. Liquid diet this PM
3. NPO p̄ midnite.
4. Permit for excision of pilonidal cyst
5. Shower this PM and in AM
6. Betadine scrub to pilonidal area in AM following shower
7. Dulcolax supp early AM

REVIEW QUESTIONS

1. The outer layer of the skin is the _____.
2. The layer under the outer layer is the _____.
3. The dermis is connected to a _____layer.
4. Hair and nails are _____of the skin.
5. _____ is produced by sebaceous glands.
6. Perspiration is produced by _____.
7. Port-wine stains are treated with _____therapy.
8. Define acne. _____
9. Why are burns a serious type of trauma? _____
   _____
10. _____ is the skin cancer that is the leading cause of death in all skin diseases.
11. A bedsore is a _____.
12. What medication is in antiacne preparation? _____
13. Pruritus is _____.
14. Corticosteroids decrease _____and _____.
15. The functions of the skin are _____
    _____.
16. Sunscreens help prevent _____.
17. Photochemotherapy is _____
    _____.
18. STSG means _____.
19. FTSG means _____.
20. Astringents are used for what purpose? _____
    _____

Chapter 10 | Musculoskeletal System

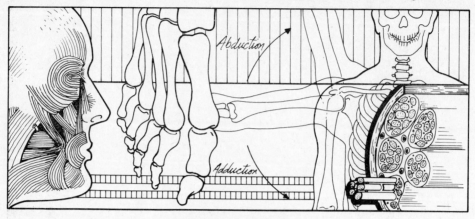

OBJECTIVES

Upon completion of study of this system, you will be able to:

1. List the functions of the skeletal system.
2. List the functions of muscles.
3. Define terms related to the musculoskeletal system.
4. List some diseases and disorders of the musculoskeletal system.
5. List some diseases and disorders of muscles.
6. Recognize the surgeries performed on the musculoskeletal system.
7. List some medications used in treating diseases and disorders of the musculoskeletal system.
8. Transcribe Physician's Orders relating to the musculoskeletal system.

MUSCULAR SYSTEM

The muscles of the body make movement possible, maintain posture, and produce heat. **Voluntary** or **skeletal muscles** are attached to bones and can be made to contract by conscious control. **Involuntary** or **smooth muscle** forms an important part of the walls of blood vessels and some internal organs; therefore, it is also referred to as **visceral muscle. Cardiac muscle** is an involuntary muscle that forms the walls of the heart.

Voluntary muscles are well supplied with nerves and blood vessels. They need large amounts of oxygen and nourishment in order to have the energy to contract. They also need a stimulus from a nerve in order to contract. Voluntary muscles contract individually. Connective tissue wraps around voluntary muscle to provide protection, divides the muscles into bundles for strength, and attaches the muscle to other structures of the body.

Involuntary muscles that act individually are located in blood vessels, in arrector muscles attached to hair follicles, and in the inside of the eye. Those in viscera contract in a wave, one after another. Involuntary muscles contract and relax at a slower rate than do voluntary muscles.

Cardiac muscle contracts continuously in a rapid, rhythmic pattern. Stimulation is provided by specialized conducting tissue within the heart rather than by nerves.

The names of all the muscles and all their locations are not important in your work. The ones you will be most likely to use are listed below:

- **Deltoid**—triangular muscle that covers the shoulder
- **Biceps**—muscles in the arm and thigh
- **Pectoralis major**—a large, triangular muscle of the anterior chest
- **Trapezius**—a triangular muscle of the posterior neck and shoulder
- **Gluteus maximus**—the largest muscle of the buttocks
- **Quadriceps** (quads)—a muscle of four parts that acts on the knee joint
- **Intercostals**—muscles between the ribs
- **Oblique**—muscles of the abdomen
- **Triceps**—arm muscles

If you are interested in learning more, consult the table of muscles in the appendix of *Taber's Cyclopedic Medical Dictionary*.

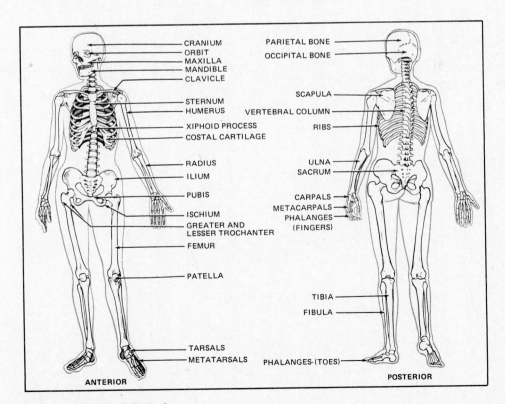

Figure 10-1. Bones of the Body.

SKELETAL SYSTEM

Bone and cartilage form the skeletal system which supports and gives shape to the body, protects internal organs, provides movement, stores mineral salts, and produces blood cells.

Bone is connective tissue and is also called **osseous tissue**. Mineral salts, calcium phosphate and calcium carbonate, give hardness to bone. Vitamins A, C, and D are needed for the body to utilize calcium and phosphorus for normal bone growth. Hormones also play a part in bone growth and maintaining homeostasis. Bone and skin have the unusual feature of replacing themselves throughout the adult life of an individual. There are 206 bones in the body.

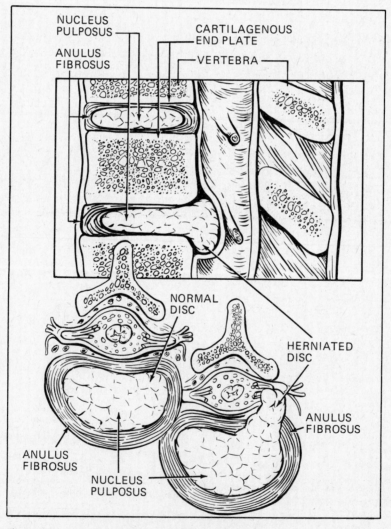

Figure 10-2. Normal and Ruptured Intervertebral Discs.

TABLE 10-1. BONES OF THE HUMAN BODY

	Bone	No.	Location
CRANIAL	Frontal	1	Forehead and upper eye sockets
	Parietal	2	Bulging topsides of cranium
	Temporal	2	Lower sides, contain ear structure
	Occipital	1	Back of skull, contains hole called *foramen magnum* thru which spinal cord enters skull
	Sphenoid	1	Central part of floor of skull, depression *sella turcica* contains pituitary gland
	Ethmoid	1	Floor of skull, side walls and roof of nose
FACIAL	Nasal	2	Upper bridge of nose
	Maxillary	2	Upper jawbones
	Zygomatic	2	Cheek bones
	Mandible	1	Lower jawbone
	Lacrimal	2	Small, medial wall of eye socket and side wall of nasal cavity
	Palatine	2	Back part of roof of mouth
	Inferior Turbanates	2	Side wall of nose
	Vomer	1	Lower and back portion of nasal septum
NECK	Hyoid	1	U-shaped bone at base of tongue
EAR (1 in each ear)	Malleus (Hammer)	2	
	Incus (Anvil)	2	
	Stapes (Stirrup)	2	
VERTEBRAL COLUMN (BACKBONE)	Cervical	7	Neck, 1st one is Atlas on which skull sits 2nd one is Axis on which skull rotates
	Thoracic	12	Chest, ribs attach
	Lumbar	5	Small of back

Category	Bone	Number	Description
THORAX	Sacrum	1	Broad last portion (5 in child, fuses into 1 in adult)
	Coccyx	1	Tail bone (3 in child, fuses into 1 in adult)
	Intevertebral discs		Pads of fibrocartilage filled with a gelatinous pad called nucleus pulposus
	True ribs	14	Upper 7 pair, attached to sternum
	False ribs	10	Lower 5 pair, last 2 pair called-floating ribs
	Sternum	1	Breast bone, cartilage at end called Xiphoid process
UPPER EXTREMETIES AND SHOULDER GIRDLE	Clavicle	2	Collarbone
	Scapula	2	Shoulder wing bones
	Humerus	2	Arm bone
	Radius	2	Smallest forearm bone
	Ulna	2	Largest forearm bone
	Carpal bones	16	Form the wrist
	Metacarpals	10	Form framework of hands
	Phalanges	28	Finger bones
PELVIC BONES	Innominate	2	Form hip girdle, has three divisions: • Ilium—upper flared portion • Ischium—lower back portion • Pubis—lower front portion NOTE: The female innominate bone is broader than the male's to accommodate the birth of a baby.
LOWER EXTREMITIES	Femur	2	Thigh bone
	Patella	2	Kneecap
	Tibia	2	Shin bone, largest of leg
	Fibula	2	Smallest of leg
	Tarsals	14	Form ankle
	Metatarsals	10	Form foot
	Phalanges	28	Form toes

TERMINOLOGY

Muscular System:

Abduction—movement away from the center of the body

Active exercises—exercises the patient does alone or with little help

Activities of daily living (ADL)—taught by the physical therapy and occupational therapy departments to enable patients to adjust to activities and do tasks even though they may have limitations

Adduction—movement toward the center of the body

Bursa—a small sac of connective tissue filled with fluids, found near joints to decrease friction

Contraction—a shortening of a muscle

Contracture—a permanent shortening of a muscle

Convulsion—an alternating contraction and relaxation of involuntary muscles, may involve some or all of the muscles of the body

Cramp—a painful contraction of a muscle

Dystrophy—progressive wasting and weakening of the muscles

Extension—movement that increases the angle between two bones

Fibrillation—rapid contraction of a muscle

Flexion—movement that decreases the angle between two bones

Gangrene—death of tissue due to an inadequate blood supply

Hernia—a rupture, the bulging out of an organ through the wall of the cavity in which it lies

Insertion—the place a muscle attaches to the bone so that it can move

Isometric—a contraction without movement, an increase of the tension in the muscle

Isotonic—a contraction produces movement

Ligaments—hold bones together at joints

Myology—study of muscles

Myomalacia—softening of muscles

Myopathy—an abnormality or disease of the muscle

Myosclerosis—a hardening of muscles

Origin—the more fixed attachment of muscle to bone

Paralysis—muscles have lost their ability to produce voluntary movement

Passive exercise—since the patient cannot help, the body part is moved by someone else

Range of motion (ROM)—refers to all the movements a joint can make

Rotation—the circular motion of a ball and socket joint

Spasm—a sudden, involuntary contraction of a muscle

Sprain—trauma to a joint causing pain and disability with injury to ligaments

Synovial fluid—lubricates the joints

Synovial membrane—lines the capsule of a joint and secretes synovial fluid

Tendons—white glistening bands or cords of tissue that attach muscles to bones

Tension—stretching or the state of being stretched

Tone of a muscle—the normal tension of the muscle.

Skeletal System:

Acetabulum—the cavity on the innominate bone that fits around the head of the femur

Ankylosis—a stiff joint

Aponeuroses—flat bands of connective tissue which connect muscle to muscle or muscle to bone

Articulation—the joining of bones, a joint

Cartilage—gristle which gives shape, support, and flexibility

Cavities—hollow spaces

Condyles—rounded bulges at the end of a bone forming a joint

Crests—narrow ridges of bones

Dislocation—the bone is displaced from its normal position in the joint

Fissure—a narrow slit in bone or tissue

Fontanels—the soft spots between the cranial bones in infants

Foramen—a hole in a bone to allow vessels or nerves a passageway

Fossa—a depression in a bone

Fracture (Fx)—a break in a bone

Joints—the places where two bones join together

Marrow—the soft tissue in the medullary cavities of long bones

Meatus—a canal or tubelike passageway

Mucus—in orthopedics refers to a clear jelly seen in certain cysts

Ossification—the process of bone formation

Periosteum—membrane that covers bones except at the joints

Processes—projections on bones

Pubic symphysis—the point where the pubic bones join anteriorly

Spongy—refers to bones that have many large spaces filled with marrow

Subluxation—incomplete or partial dislocation of a bone in a joint

Traction—force applied in two directions to regain normal position and alignment of bones and muscles

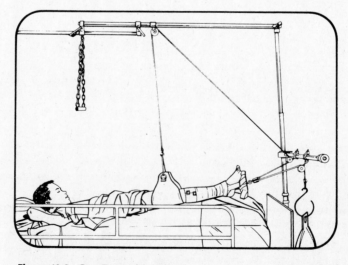

Figure 10-3. One Type of Traction.

DISEASES AND DISORDERS

Ankylosing Spondylitis (Marie-Strümpell Disease) is a chronic, progressive disease with inflammation and stiffness of the sacroiliac, the intervertebral and the costovertebral joints, and the hip and shoulder joints. **Tx:** Exercises for maintaining posture, braces. Salicylates, phenylbutazone, and indomethacin can control the disease in about 90% of the cases, but there is no cure.

Arthritis is an inflammation in a joint. The terms rheumatism and rheumatic disease are sometimes used to designate arthritis. There are numerous types of arthritis; the two main ones are discussed below.

- **Rheumatoid arthritis** is a chronic disease with inflammation that destroys joint cartilages and the joint surfaces of bones and causes deformities. **Tx:** Rest, complete bedrest during the acute stage, good nutrition, salicylates, specific antiarthritic drugs, corticosteroids, exercise with the help of a physical therapist, surgery for deformities. Finger joints, hip joints, and knee joints can be replaced.
- **Osteoarthritis** is a degenerative joint disease which causes the loss of joint function. **Tx:** Obese patients should lose weight; very active people should limit activities. Analgesics can be taken to control pain. Surgery using artificial joint implants is successful in the majority of cases.

Back pain in the lower back is one of the most common complaints of man. In about 80% of the cases, the pain is due to underexercised muscles and tension which causes muscle weakness. The other 20% are due to organic problems. **Tx:** An exercise program geared to the individual, traction to decrease muscle tension, surgery for some organic problems.

Bursitis is an inflammation of the bursa resulting in excess fluid which causes movement to be painful. **Tx:** Rest, physical therapy, removal of any infection elsewhere in the body, aspiration of the excess fluid.

Cleft lip and cleft palate are congenital defects resulting in a fissure remaining in the lip and palate tissues. **Tx:** Plastic surgery.

Curvatures are exaggerations of the normal curves of the spine. The cervical and lumbar curves are normally inward anteriorly. The thoracic curve and the sacral curve are normally outward anteriorly. **Tx:** Exercises, braces, surgery in some cases. Abnormal curvatures are:

- **Kyphosis**—an exaggerated thoracic curve which results in a hunchback condition
- **Lordosis**—exaggerated inward curve of the lumbar region causing a swayback
- **Scoliosis**—a side to side curvature of the spinal column. **Tx** for scoliosis: Surgical fixation of the spine in a straight line. The Harrington Rod and Dwyer instrumentation are metal fixation devices.

Fibromyositis is an inflammation of fibromuscular tissue which causes pain. The condition may be caused by infections, trauma, poisons, or exposure to damp or cold environment. Types include:

- **Lumbago**—involvement of the back muscles
- **Torticollis**—involvement of the neck muscles
- **Pleurodynia**—involvement of the muscles of the shoulders and thorax. **Tx:** Heat, massage, rest, salicylates, and use of bed boards.

Fractures are breaks in bones. There are several types of fractures:

- **Simple**—the bone is broken, but there is no damage to tissues. **Tx:** Bone is placed in alignment, and a cast is applied.
- **Complete**—the bone is broken all the way through. **Tx:** The bone is replaced in normal position and a cast is applied.
- **Incomplete**—the break is not completely through the bone, only a line or fissure is present. **Tx:** Splint or cast.
- **Compound**—the bone is broken and pushed through the skin. **Tx:** The bone may be replaced in position and the wound closed surgically, or surgical replacement of the bone may be needed with the use of pins, wires, nails, plates, etc. to maintain alignment; traction may be used after surgery.
- **Comminuted**—fragments of bone are in the open wound. **Tx:** Surgery to cleanse the wound and replace the bone, fixation devices, casts, traction.
- **Greenstick**—an incomplete fracture with a curve in the bone. **Tx:** Splints, casts. Physical therapy is usually required after the removal of any cast to restore the muscle to good condition.

Ganglion cyst is a mucus cyst on a tendon or aponeurosis. It is often located on the wrist. **Tx:** Aspiration of contents several times may eliminate the cyst, surgical removal.

Gout, a metabolic disease, causes acute inflammation of the joints with intense pain. **Hyperuricemia** (excessive uric acid in the blood) is the cause resulting in deposits of sodium urate crystals in and around joints, on the ears, and on the knuckles. **Tx:** Corticosteroids, colchicine for acute attacks, probenecide, and allopurinol are specific medications. The dietitian should instruct the patient in a low purine diet, a diet that produces little uric acid.

Hallux valgus (bunion) is a condition in which the great toe is displaced toward the other toes, and the bursa of the great toe joint is inflamed. **Tx:** Properly fitted shoes, surgery.

Hernia (rupture) is a tear in a muscle or organ which may occur anywhere in the body. The most common ones are **umbilical** (navel) and **inguinal** (groin). **Tx:** Surgical correction.

Herniated disc is a ruptured intervertebral disc. The nucleus pulposus leaks out causing pressure on the adjacent nerve which causes pain. **Tx:** Traction, surgery, chymopapain injections.

Internal derangement of the knee occurs when ligaments are torn. The semilunar cartilages (menisci) may be torn or torn from their attachment to the bone. **Tx:** Surgical removal of the injured cartilage.

Muscular dystrophy is an inherited disease which causes progressive weakness and degeneration of muscles. **Tx:** Exercises to help maintain muscle strength, braces. There is no cure.

Osteomyelitis is a bone infection caused by a microorganism, usually the staphylococcus aureus. The infection may originate in another part of the body and be carried by the bloodstream, or it may occur after fractures or trauma. **Tx:** Antibiotics, high caloric diet, immobilization of affected area.

Osteoporosis decreases new bone formation and causes the bone to be less dense leading to a loss of strength. Many post-menopausal women have the condition. **Tx:** Encourage activity, back braces, calcium, and estrogen.

Paget's disease (osteitis deformans) is a chronic, slowly progressive disorder in which there are periods of decalcification and softening of long bones, followed by hypertrophy and bowing, and thickening with deformities of flat bones. The most common sites of lesions are the skull, vertebrae, femur, tibia, and pelvis. Fractures are frequent. The disorder usually develops after the middle 30s. **Tx:** No specific therapy. X-ray therapy may relieve the pain. Elevated alkaline phosphatase levels and **hypercalciuria** (excessive calcium in the urine) are reduced by **estrogens** (female hormones) and **androgens** (male sex hormones).

Rickets results from a lack of Vitamin D. The deficiency causes disturbances in calcium and phosphorus metabolism with resulting abnormal shapes and structures of bones. Rickets is a disease of children; the same process in adults is **osteomalacia. Tx:** Vitamin D, exposure to sunlight, and a well-balanced diet.

Slipped disc occurs when an intervertebral disc is pushed out of position causing the vertebra above the disc to tilt and put pressure on the spinal nerve. **Tx:** Traction, bed boards (solid or slats joined together and placed between the mattress and springs), muscle relaxants.

Spurs, small projections of bony growth on a bone, may or may not involve ossification of muscular attachments. Spurs are most common on the heel of the foot and the neck of the femur. They are painful and may cause inflammation of nearby tissues. **Tx:** Corticosteroids injected into the site; surgery according to the location of the spur, the amount of disability, and the response to the corticosteroids.

Synovitis, inflammation of the synovial membrane of a joint, is usually caused by an injury. The knee is the most common joint to be involved. Increased fluid in the joint capsule (water on the knee) causes pain. **Tx:** Aspiration of fluid from the joint, pressure bandage, rest the area, and apply heat to the area.

Tendinitis and tenosynovitis, inflammation of a tendon, involves the synovial sheath. Therefore, the terms are interchangeable. **Tx:** Corticosteroids injected into the space between the tendon and the synovial sheath, heat to the area, anti-inflammatory drugs. Antibiotics are used if an infection is proven by a culture and sensitivity test of aspirated fluid.

Tumors are abnormal growths of any of the skeletal tissues. Diagnosis depends on biospy and tissue study. Tumors may be benign or malignant.

- **Benign tumors:**

    Osteomas are tumors of bone-forming connective tissue, usually found on the surface of bones. **Tx:** Surgical removal.

    Chondromas are tumors of cartilaginous tissue. **Tx:** Surgical scraping of lesion or complete excision.

    Giant-cell tumors (osteoclastomas) destroy the spongy portion of the bone. They involve the ends of long bones, the pelvis, and the spine.

Tx: Surgical removal, radiation therapy if surgery is not possible.
- **Malignant tumors:**
  Osteogenic sarcoma originates in bone-forming connective tissue and is usually found in long bones. It occurs most frequently in young persons and spreads to the lungs rapidly. **Tx:** Amputation through or above the next joint, chemotherapy, radiation in some cases.

  Chondrosarcoma originates in the cartilaginous tissue. **Tx:** Surgical removal.

  Ewing's sarcoma originates in the cells which form the connective tissues. It usually occurs in adolescents and young adults but may occur in children. It may involve any part of the skeleton. Survival rate is low. **Tx:** Chemotherapy and radiation.

  Malignant giant-cell tumors (osteoclastoma) have the same involvement as the benign giant-cell tumors. About one-sixth of all osteoclastomas are malignant. **Tx:** Surgical removal.

  Multiple myeloma originates in blood forming cells, occurs most frequently in males over 40 years of age, and causes changes in the blood as well as multiple skeletal lesions. **Tx:** Chemotherapy, adrenocorticosteroids, androgens, radiation to reduce pain, and physical therapy.

  Metastatic tumors are those that originate in some other organ and spread to the bone. Primary tumors that most frequently metastasize are those of the breast, lungs, prostate, kidneys, and thyroid. **Tx:** Chemotherapy and radiation.

Disease-Causing Organisms

- Gonococci
- Mycobacterium
- Pseudomonas Aeruginosa
- Staphylococci
- Streptococci

SURGERIES AND PROCEDURES

Amputation means removal of a part or all of a limb. The permits for surgery specify which limb. Leg amputations are above the knee (AKA) or below the knee (BKA). Postoperatively, the patient may complain of pain in the amputated limb; this is called "phantom pain." If the patient's general condition permits, the stump may have a cast applied in the operating room with an artificial limb **(prosthesis)** fitted. This allows the patient to be up and bear weight on the stump after 24 hours, which reduces or eliminates phantom pain. Physical therapists play a large part in the convalescence of these patients.

Arthrodesis is the surgical fixation of a joint, most often performed to correct deformities.

Arthroplasty is the surgical repair of a joint.

Arthroplasty with total hip replacement (THR) places an artificial socket in the cleaned out space of the worn socket. The worn femur head is removed, and a steel ball and stem are inserted into the shaft of the femur. The surgical bone cement fits into all the spaces between the bone and the artificial parts to lock the pieces in place.

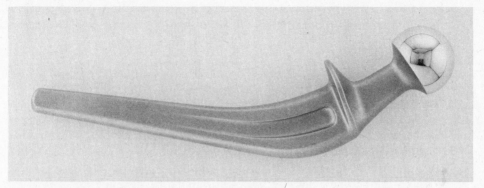

Figure 10-4. Harris HD*2® Total Hip *(Courtesy of Howmedica, Inc., Orthopaedics Division).†*

Arthroplasty with total knee replacement (TKR) is the insertion of artificial plastic and stainless steel parts to replace the ends of the femur and tibia.

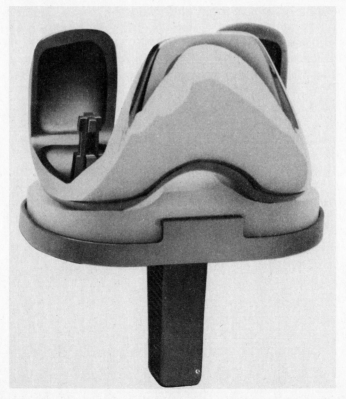

Figure 10-5. Howmedica® Kinematic™ Condylar Total Knee System, Posterior Cruciate Retention *(Courtesy of Howmedica, Inc., Orthopaedics Division).†*

---

†Howmedica and HD*2 are registered trademarks of Howmedica, Inc.

†Howmedica® Kinematic is a trademark of Howmedica.

Arthroscopy is the removal of injured cartilage **(meniscus),** through a special scope which has light fibers, surrounded by a telescope, that fit into a water sleeve. The incision is small, recovery is quick, and physical therapy begins soon after the patient returns to the room on the unit.

Arthrotomy with menisectomy is removal of the meniscus through an incision into the knee joint. A longer recovery period is required than with the arthroscope.

Bunionectomy is the removal of inflamed bursa and straightening of the great toe. Casts may or may not be applied after surgery.

Chymodiactin (chymopapain) injection is a procedure in which the extract from papaya, a tropical fruit, is surgically injected into the nucleus pulposus of a ruptured disc. Chymopapain is an enzyme which dissolves the nucleus pulposus, thus relieving the pressure on the nerve.

Closed reduction indicates setting of a broken bone without a surgical incision. Casts, splints, or traction are applied to maintain proper alignment.

Laminectomy is the removal of the nucleus pulposus in a ruptured disc to eliminate the pressure on the involved nerve. The spine must be kept straight until healing occurs, so patients are turned from side to side by a method called "logrolling." Laminectomies are performed by an orthopedic surgeon or a neurosurgeon.

Open reduction with internal fixation is a surgical incision made to set a broken bone. Wires, screws, or pins are used to maintain alignment. Traction may be used following surgery. Pins are removed when complete healing has occurred, and the patient may be hospitalized overnight or may be in the ambulatory surgery unit.

Plastic surgery is the reconstruction of an area. Reconstruction may be needed for deformities acquired because of an illness, for congenital defects, or for injuries due to trauma.

Repair of a hernia (herniorrhaphy) involves repairing a ruptured muscle with replacement of organs in their proper position. A mesh support is sometimes sutured over the impaired muscle for extra strength. Repair of an inguinal hernia and an umbilical (navel) hernia are two types.

Spinal fusion connects several vertebrae so they are immobile. The procedure may involve grafting bone from another area into the spinal column. A laminectomy may be combined with a spinal fusion.

Tendon lengthening or shortening corrects deformities to allow normal movement.

LABORATORY TESTS

- Acid phosphatase
- ACT
- Alkaline phosphatase
- Histology studies
- IgM, IgG
- Pro Time, PT

- C&S of wound exudate
- Calcium, serum and urine
- CBC
- ESR
- Hgb & Hct

- PTT
- Spinal fluid analysis
- Type and crossmatch (T&X or T&C)
- Uric acid

RADIOLOGY AND NUCLEAR MEDICINE

Vertebrae are designated on requisitions by a capital letter and a number. The third cervical vertebra would be C-3, the sixth thoracic vertebra would be T-6, the fourth lumbar vertebra would be L-4, etc.

Arthroscopy examines a joint through an arthroscope (different from the surgical arthroscope) with x-rays taken during manipulation of the joint.

Bone scans visualize the entire skeletal system. Radioactive material is given by injection and concentrates in abnormal bone tissue so that growths are visible on x-ray film. Bone scans are valuable in determining if a newly diagnosed cancer has metastasized to any bone.

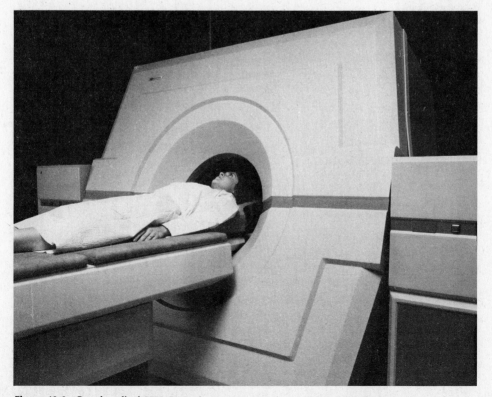

Figure 10-6. Omnimedical 6000 CT Body Scanner *(Courtesy of Omni Medical).*

Epidural venogram aids in determining the cause for acute back pain and in ruling out the presence of tumors. The **dura,** a membrane that covers the brain and spinal cord, extends to the second sacral vertebrae. The epidural space contains veins, connective tissue, and nerve roots. Dye is injected into this space via a catheter inserted into the femoral vein and on into presacral veins to show the entire network of veins and the surrounding space.

Myelograms show if a disc is ruptured or if there are any abnormalities of the spinal cord. A spinal puncture is performed by placing a needle between two vertebrae into the space of the spinal canal that contains spinal fluid. Some fluid is removed and replaced with a radiopaque oil which is visible on x-rays and outlines the area. When the x-rays are completed, the oil is removed.

Tomograms may be of any part of the system. This type of x-ray gives pictures of a single selected plane with the outline of structures in other planes eliminated so that a particular structure is more clear.

X-rays are routinely used to study fractures, to examine the results of surgery, and to determine the extent of injury or damage caused by a disease. The doctor will specify which bone is to be visualized.

MEDICATIONS

Antiarthritics

Antiarthritics reduce the inflammation and pain of arthritis.

- Ascriptin A/D—PO—tabs īi or īīi qid.
- Azolid (phenylbutazone)—PO—supplied as 100 mg tabs, dose is individualized. Used for short-term relief in acute arthritis, ankylosing spondylitis, and painful shoulder due to bursitis, tendinitis, or arthritis.
- Butazolidin and Butazolidin-Alka—PO—dosage determined by age and weight, average is 400 mg daily in 3 or 4 divided doses
- Clinoril (sulindac)—PO—150 to 200 mg bid c̄ food
- Feldene (piroxicam)—PO—20 mg/d. Supplied in 10 mg and 20 mg
- Motrin—PO—300 to 400 mg tid or qid
- Nalfon—PO—300 to 600 mg tid or qid
- Naprosyn—PO—250 mg to 375 mg morning and evening
- Tandearil—PO—400 mg daily in divided doses, reduce when improvement is noted
- Tolectin—PO—400 mg tid

Antibiotics

- Amikin—IV, IM—not to exceed 15 mg/Kg/d and should be divided into 2 or 3 equal doses

- Cefadyl—IV, IM—500 mg to 1 gm q 4–6 hrs
- Garamycin (gentamicin)—IV, IM—1 mg/Kg q 8 hrs
- Keflex—PO—250 mg q 6 hrs
- Keflin—IV, IM—500 mg to 1 gm q 4–6 hrs
- Kefzol—IV, IM—250 mg to 500 mg q 8–12 hrs. For severe cases, 500 mg to 1 gm q 6–8 hrs
- Staphcillin—IM—1 gm q 4–6 hrs, IV—1 gm q 6 hrs. Treatment of osteomyelitis may require several months of therapy.

Antigout

Antigout drugs are analgesic, uricosuric (increase uric acid elimination), or inhibit uric acid production.

- Anturane—PO—200 mg to 800 mg daily, individualized; urocosuric action
- Colbenemid—PO—tab ī daily for 1 week then tab ī bid, may be increased to 4 tab/d according to uric acid levels; urocosuric action
- Colchicine—PO—Tab ī or īī q hr till pain subsides or N/V, diarrhea occur. IV—2 mg then 0.5 mg q 6 hrs till acute pain subsides, up to 4 mg/ 24 hrs; analgesic action
- Indocin (indomethacin)—PO—50 mg tid until pain subsides, then reduce gradually until none is given; analgesic and anti-inflammatory action
- Zyloprim—PO—200 mg to 600 mg daily, individualized; inhibits the formation of uric acid

Corticosteroids

These drugs reduce inflammation.

- Aristospan (triamcinolone)—2 to 20 mg injected into joints q 3–4 weeks according to response. For bursitis, synovitis, arthritis.
- Celestone—Parenteral and PO preparations. Dosage individualized
- Decadron (dexamethasone)—PO, IM, IV, intra-articular—dosage individualized
- Kenalog 10—intra-articular or intrabursal—2.5 mg to 15 mg
- Kenalog 40—IM, intra-articular, individualized dosage
- Prednisone—PO—5 mg at HS for rheumatoid arthritis

Hormones

Androgens are substances produced by the male sex glands. They affect the storage of inorganic phosphorus, sulfate, sodium, and potassium. They prevent atrophy in bones from disease and promote healing of wounds. Type and dosage depend on disease, extent of disease, and response needed. Testosterone, Durabolin, Nilevar are names of preparations.

Estrogens are substances produced by the ovaries. They decrease alkaline phosphatase and hypercalciuria. Some preparations are Diethylstilbestrol, TACE, Estrace. Dosages and preparations are according to disease and response needed.

Muscle Relaxants

- Flexeril—PO—10 mg tid
- Lioresal—PO—5 mg tid and increase to 20 mg qid, individualized
- Norflex—PO—tab i̇ bid, AM & PM. IM, IV—60 mg q 12 hrs
- Paraflex—PO—tab i̇ (250 mg) tid or qid
- Parafon Forte—PO—tabs i̇i̇ qid
- Quinamm—PO—tab i̇ HS. If necessary, add tab i̇ after evening meal.
- Valium—PO—2 mg to 10 mg bid or qid. IM or IV—2 mg to 10 mg as ordered.

Vitamins

- Vitamin D—PO—60,000 units a day for rickets
- Calciferol (contains Vitamin D_2)—PO—50,000 to 1,000,000 units a day for rickets
- Hyalex—combination of minerals and vitamins. PO tabs i̇ or i̇i̇ c̄ each meal. For minor pain of arthritis, bursitis.

ELECTROTHERAPY

Electrostimulation promotes bone healing. Electrical nerve stimulation reduces pain and allows free mobility. The patient can control the amount needed.

A low-frequency, low-intensity electromagnetic field over a fracture area helps fractures heal.

Orthofuse is an implanted bone growth stimulator. It is a solid state, constant current generator designed for use in cases of posterior spinal fusion. It is removed at approximately 24 weeks in the outpatient surgery department.

TENS—transcutaneous electrical nerve stimulation—is used to control pain, surgical and non-surgical. The physical therapist will apply the external electrode tapes to the skin in the area of pain in non-surgical cases and teach the patient how to use the device. Thin wires lead from the electrodes to a battery powered stimulator with a control. Surgical cases have the electrodes applied to the skin surrounding the incision while still in surgery. The patient is taught the use of the device the day before surgery, if possible. Stimulation is usually continuous for 72 hrs post-op and then the patient can turn it on whenever pain occurs.

EPC—electronic pain control is another form of stimulation. It works the same as TENS.

EXAMPLES OF PHYSICIAN'S ORDERS

Dx: Acute back (admission orders)

1. Reg diet
2. BRP
3. BLESS
4. UA, CBC, SMA—20
5. 10# bilateral pelvic traction
   (The orthopedic technician sets up the traction and helps doctors with cast applications, splinting, and cutting casts.)
6. Parafon Forte ̈ii qid
7. Dalmane 30 mg q HS prn
8. Stadol 2 mg IM q 3–4 hrs prn pain
9. Consent for epidural venogram

Next day:

1. Tomograms of sacrum
2. Consent for lumbar myelogram
3. Valium 10 mg tid
4. Pericolase ̇i q d

Next day:

1. Consent for laminectomy and three-way fusion
2. Prep back
3. T&X × 3 units PRBCs

Anesthesiology orders:

1. NPO p̄ MN
2. Demerol 100⎫
   Vistaril 100 ⎬ mg @ 0645
   Robinul 0.2 ⎭

Post-op:

1. Con't slow IV 5%/½ NS q 12 hrs
2. Kefzol 500 mg IVPB q 12 hrs
3. M.S. gr ¼ IM q 3–4 hrs prn pain
4. DAT
5. Log roll in bed
6. Cath q 6 hrs prn
7. Dalmane 30 mg HS prn

Dx: Total hip replacement, Left

Post-op:

1. VS q 15 min till stable
2. Hg & Hct @ 1800 today then qod × 3

3. Demerol 25 mg IV q 2 hr prn pain
4. Tigan 200 mg IM q 6 hr prn N
5. Liquids as tol
6. Keep IV open c̄ D₅ Ringer's lactate
7. I & O
8. Cath × 1 if patient uncomfortable and cannot void

3rd PO day:

1. DC IV
2. May sit up, cushion between legs
3. Reg diet
4. Valium 10 mg q 4 hrs prn

4th PO day:

1. Ask P.T. to see, start ambulation.
2. DC valium
3. Lioresal 10 mg tid

Examples of P.T. orders

1. Teach crutch walking, no wt. bearing on (R or L) leg
2. Ambulate c̄ walker
3. Straight leg raises
4. Quad exercises
5. Whirlpool (WP) daily
6. Passive exercises. Paraffin bath to hand bid
7. Hot packs to lower back bid. Teach patient muscle strengthening exercises.

REVIEW QUESTIONS

1. Name the three types of muscles. _____,
   _____, _____

2. List the functions of muscles. _____
   _____

3. List the functions of skeletal system. _____
   _____
   _____

4. Name three diseases and disorders of the muscular system. _____,
   _____, _____

5. The membrane that covers bone is the _____.

6. Intervertebral discs are _____
   _____

7. Define:
   Contraction _____
   Dystrophy _____
   Hernia _____
   Paralysis _____
   ROM _____
   Spasm _____
   Cartilage _____
   Cavity _____
   Fracture _____
   Traction _____
8. Name three abnormal curvatures of the spine and define each. _____
   _____
   _____
   _____
   _____
   _____

9. Name five diseases and disorders of the musculoskeletal system.
   _____ , _____ ,
   _____ , _____ ,
   _____

10. Name four medications for arthritis. _____ ,
    _____ , _____ , _____

11. Name three medications for gout. _____
    _____ , _____

12. Name three muscle relaxants. _____
    _____ , _____

13. Name three types of electrotherapy. _____
    _____ , _____

Chapter 11 | The Circulatory System

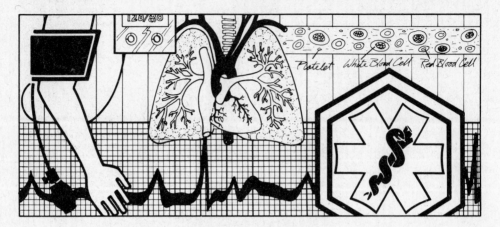

Platelet   White Blood Cell   Red Blood Cell

OBJECTIVES

Upon completion of study of this chapter, you will be able to:

1. List the structures that make up the circulatory system.
2. List the functions of blood.
3. List several diseases and disorders of the blood.
4. List the functions of blood vessels.
5. List diseases and disorders of blood vessels.
6. List the functions of the heart.
7. List diseases and disorders of the heart.
8. List the functions of the lymphatic system.
9. List diseases and disorders of the lymphatic system.
10. List the functions of the spleen.
11. List and classify medications used to treat the diseases and disorders of the circulatory system.
12. List several examinations that aid in diagnosing circulatory system diseases and disorders.
13. List surgeries performed on the circulatory system.
14. Transcribe Physician's Orders relating to the circulatory system.

The circulatory, or cardiovascular, system consists of the heart; blood vessels and blood; lymph nodes, ducts, and vessels; the spleen; and an accessory organ, the thymus.

The dictionary defines circulation as movement in a circular course. The circulatory system has two circular courses. Blood moves through the right side of the heart to the lungs and back to the left side of the heart to establish the **pulmonary circulation**. Blood moves from the left side of the heart to all the tissues of the body and back to the right side of the heart to create the **systemic circulation**. Circulation in the unborn child, the fetus, does not flow through the lungs. Circulation through the lungs begins at birth.

Every cell of the body depends on the functions of the circulatory system for survival. Oxygen from the lungs and food from the digestive system are carried to all cells. Carbon dioxide and other waste materials are transported from tissues to the excretory organs (kidneys, lungs, skin). Hormones produced by the endocrine system are delivered to the organs they effect. The circulatory system also aids in the regulation of body temperature and in protecting the body against disease.

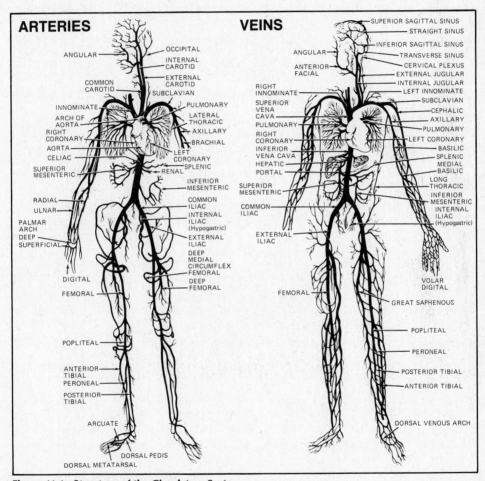

Figure 11-1. Structure of the Circulatory System.

BLOOD

Blood is a combination of fluid and cells. It moves through the circulatory system delivering food, oxygen, and hormones and picking up waste products for excretion. Blood is about five times thicker than water, is slightly sticky to the touch, has a salty taste, and has a slightly alkaline pH value. Blood is composed of water, cells, gases, nutrients, proteins, mineral salts, protective substances, hormones, non-protein nitrogen solutes, and plasma.

Plasma

Plasma and **serum** are the fluid part of blood. Plasma is obtained by removing the cells with a machine called a **centrifuge**. Serum is the liquid remaining after blood has clotted. When a doctor writes an order for a blood component test and puts the word serum in front of the component, you do not specify that on the lab requisition; instead you check the component. This is often confusing, so remember that serum is a part of the blood and that the lab must draw a blood specimen. The average person has about five or six quarts of blood, and plasma constitutes about 55% of that volume. Plasma is nearly 90% water, the other 10% is solutes.

Solutes in Plasma

Proteins aid in the transport of lipids (fats), help keep the pH of blood at a normal level, and aid in maintaining the **viscosity** (stickiness) of blood. Proteins are classified as albumin, globulins, and fibrinogen.

- **Albumin** gives the gummy texture and keeps the water concentration low so that water moves readily from the tissues into the blood.
- **Globulins** transport other proteins and form antibodies which help fight disease-causing organisms. Globulins are sub-divided into groups called alpha-1, alpha-2, beta-globulin, and gamma globulin.
- **Fibrinogen** is essential for the clotting of blood.

Mineral salts maintain a balance between calcium and potassium, keep the pH normal, regulate the pressure in cells and body fluids so that material may be transmitted back and forth to maintain an adequate water level in the tissues, and regulate the excitability of the nervous and muscular tissues of the body. Sodium, potassium, calcium, and magnesium are minerals in the form of salts in the blood.

- **Sodium** (Na) maintains a balance between calcium and potassium, aids in pH balance, and assists in keeping water in the tissues.
- **Potassium** (K) aids in pH balance, helps maintain pressure to allow exchange of fluids between cells and tissues, assists in the transport of oxygen and carbon dioxide, and is necessary for nerve conduction and muscle contraction.
- **Calcium** (Ca) is necessary for bone and teeth formation, for keeping the excitability of nerve endings at a normal level, and for the clotting of blood.
- **Magnesium** (Mg) is needed to build proteins, to help in body temperature regulation, to aid in enzyme activity, and to aid in the conduction of nerve impulses.

Glucose (sugar) is a nutrient derived from food, stored in the liver as glycogen, and converted into glucose as the body needs it to supply energy.

Lipids (fats) are nutrients which supply energy, are necessary for growth and development, and provide transportation for fat-soluble vitamins. The types of fats are triglycerides, phospholipids, and cholesterol.

Non-protein nitrogen solutes

- **Amino acids** are necessary to build protein. Some are produced by the body and some are derived from food. Those from food are called **essential amino acids.**
- **Creatinine** (Cr) is a normal alkaline component of blood and urine.
- **Urea** is formed in the liver when proteins are broken down by the body and is excreted in the urine.
- **Uric acid** is produced by the metabolism of certain plant and animal cells called purines and is excreted in the urine.

Gases are oxygen, carbon dioxide, and nitrogen.

- **Oxygen** is necessary to maintain life and is taken into the body by the process of breathing.
- **Carbon dioxide** is a waste product exhaled by the lungs.
- **Nitrogen** is necessary for the building of tissues.

Protective substances are antibodies, agglutinins, and bacteriolysins which help the body fight disease causing organisms and other harmful material.

Hormones are the products of the endocrine glands and are discussed in Chapter 15.

Blood Cells

Blood cells are 45% of the blood volume of an individual. The blood cells are erythrocytes (red cells), the leukocytes (white cells), and platelets.

Erythrocytes, red blood cells (RBCs), carry oxygen and carbon dioxide. They are shaped like disks with each side having a bowl-like depression which gives the cell a greater area for oxygen intake. Adult RBCs have no nucleus. Immature red cells are **reticulocytes.** RBCs are formed in the red bone marrow and live only an average of 120 days, resulting in a constant process of dying and disintegration.

- **Hemoglobin** (Hgb), the iron-containing pigment in RBCs, combines with oxygen from the lungs. The Hgb carries the oxygen to the tissues where it is exchanged for carbon dioxide.
- **Hematocrit** (Hct) is the percentage of total blood volume which consists of RBCs.

Leukocytes, white blood cells (WBCs), are classified as *granular* if granules are in their cytoplasm and *agranular* if no granules are in their cytoplasm. WBCs function as **phagocytes**—they ingest and destory bacteria and other harmful substances. Most WBCs have the ability to leave blood vessels and travel to an injured or infected area, earning them the name of scavengers. The life span of a WBC is very short, from two to twelve days. A differential count is the percentage of each kind of white cell in 100 white blood cells.

- **Granular** WBCs originate in the red bone marrow and are the **neutrophils, eosinophils,** and **basophils.**

- **Agranular** WBCs are **lymphocytes** and **monocytes** which mostly originate in the lymph glands although a few are formed in the red bone marrow. The lymphocytes aid in the production of antibodies.

Platelets are disk-like structures with no nucleus and are formed in red bone marrow. Platelets initiate **coagulation** (clotting). They stick to each other and to the edge of an injury to form a clot.

Blood Types

An **antigen** causes antibodies to form and may be produced in, or introduced into, the body. Blood types are named according to the antigen on membranes of red blood cells.

- **Type A** blood contains antigen A on red cell membranes; the plasma contains anti-B antibodies.
- **Type B** blood contains antigen B on red cell membranes; the plasma contains anti-A antibodies.
- **Type AB** blood contains both antigen A and antigen B on red cell membranes, and the plasma contains no antibodies. Type AB is the universal recipient; it is compatible with all other types.
- **Type O** blood contains neither antigen A nor antigen B on red cell membranes; the plasma contains both anti-A and anti-B antibodies. Type O is the universal donor, it can be given to all other types.

The **Rh factor** is an antigen. About 85% of the population is *Rh positive* (Rh +), that is, the antigen is present on the red cells. The other 15% have no antigen and are *Rh negative* (Rh −).

Blood must be typed and crossmatched before a transfusion can be given. A **crossmatch** means that the blood from a possible donor is mixed with the blood from the possible recipient and observed for **agglutination** (clumping) of red blood cells. If any clumping occurs, that donor cannot give to that recipient. Clumping is lethal.

| THE HEART

The heart is a cone shaped organ about the size of the two closed fists. The function of the heart is to pump blood to the body and receive the returning blood so that there is a constant circulation of blood.

The **apex** of the heart is the lower end of the cone, the point.

Mediastinum is the space between the lungs in which the heart lies. About two-thirds of the heart lies to the left side of the sternum.

The **atria** are the two top chambers of the heart. The *right atrium* and the *left atrium* are divided by the **interatrial septum**.

Ventricles, the lower and larger chambers, are divided by the **interventricular septum.**

The **pericardium** is a two-layered membrane that surrounds the heart. The *fibrous layer* supports the heart by attaching it to the sternum and the diaphragm. The *serous layer* on the inside consists of the **parietal** portion which lines the fibrous layer and the **visceral** portion which adheres to the heart. The pericardial space between the parietal and visceral portion contains a small amount of pericardial fluid, which acts as a lubricant and allows the two portions to move across each other easily.

Myocardium, the heart muscle, is an involuntary muscle that contracts in a special pattern giving the heart a pumping action.

Endocardium lines the myocardium. It is a serous membrane that is continuous with the lining of arteries.

Valves of the heart keep the blood flowing in the right direction.

- **Tricuspid valve** has three flaps and allows blood to flow from the right atrium to the right ventricle.
- **Pulmonary valve** opens from the right ventricle into the pulmonary artery.
- **Mitral valve,** or bicuspid valve, allows blood to flow from the left atrium to the left ventricle.
- **Aortic valve** leads from the left ventricle into the aorta, the largest artery of the body.

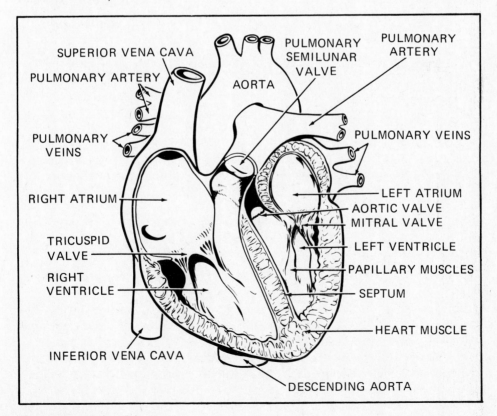

Figure 11-2. Interior of the Heart.

Blood Flow

Blood from the lower part of the body enters the right atrium from the **inferior vena cava;** blood from the upper body enters the right atrium from the **superior vena cava.** The vena cava is the largest vein of the body. The blood travels first from the right atrium through the tricuspid valve to the right ventricle then passes through the pulmonary valve to the pulmonary artery, which branches to the right and left lung. As the blood circulates through the lungs, it picks up oxygen and gives off carbon dioxide, which is carried away by the process of breathing. The oxygenated blood returns to the left atrium via the right and left pulmonary veins. This is the only time veins carry oxygenated blood. The blood then travels through the mitral valve into the left ventricle and through the aortic valve into the aorta, which delivers the blood to all areas of the body by way of smaller arteries.

Electrical Impulse

The walls of the heart chambers have a rhythmic contraction and relaxation pattern due to a special conduction system of nervous tissue which stimulates the muscle fibers by generating electrical impulses. A **node** is a tightly packed group of cells which conduct impulses.

- **Sinoatrial node** (SA node), the pacemaker, starts the activity and determines the rate of the heart beat. The SA node lies just below the opening in the right atrium where the superior vena cava enters. The impulse from the SA node causes both atria to contract.

- **Atrioventricular node** (AV node) lies in the lower right atrium near the interatrial septum. The AV node picks up the impulse and passes it down to the atrioventricular bundle **(bundle of His),** a band of specialized fibers originating at the AV node and dividing into two branches in the ventricular septum.

Purkinje fibers are branches of the bundle of His which run to all parts of the ventricles. Impulses from the Purkinje fibers cause the ventricles to contract.

Cardiac Cycle

One complete contraction and relaxation wave of the heart is a cardiac cycle. The period of contraction is called the **systole** and the period of relaxation is the **diastole.** When listening to the heart with a stethoscope, you hear the beat as a lubb, dupp, pause rhythm. The cardiac cycle can be recorded because the electrical impulses are detectable on the surface of the body. A record of this cycle is an **electrocardiogram** (EKG or ECG).

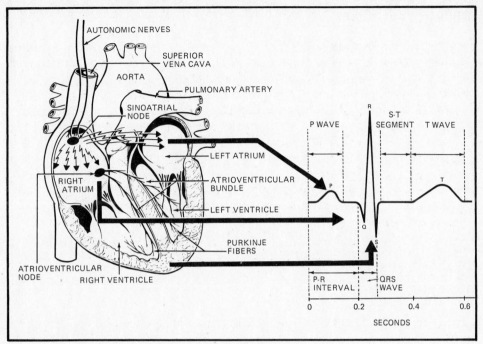

Figure 11-3. Heart Activity Correlated with EKG Pattern.

BLOOD VESSELS

Blood vessels are a network of tubes with elastic properties that can expand with an increase in internal pressure and can contract when the internal pressure decreases. The pressure of the heart on the blood and the pressure of surrounding tissues determines the amount of expansion of the vessels. The blood vessels are arteries, veins, and capillaries.

Arteries

Arteries carry blood from the heart to the body. Because arteries carry oxygenated blood (except the pulmonary artery), the color of blood in the arteries is bright red.

The **aorta,** the largest artery of the body, arches upward from the heart and branches into the innominate, the left common carotid, and the left subclavian, then each subdivides into smaller arteries.

Coronary arteries supply the heart muscle and enter the heart muscle from the base of the aorta, just above the mitral valve.

The **thoracic aorta** is the part of the aorta that turns down from the arch and supplies the chest area with blood.

The **abdominal aorta** is the part below the chest which supplies the organs of the abdominal cavity. It divides into the right and left iliac which subdivide first into the femoral and then into the popliteal arteries.

Arterioles are the very small branches of arteries which lead into **capillaries,** minute blood vessels that connect arterioles with small veins.

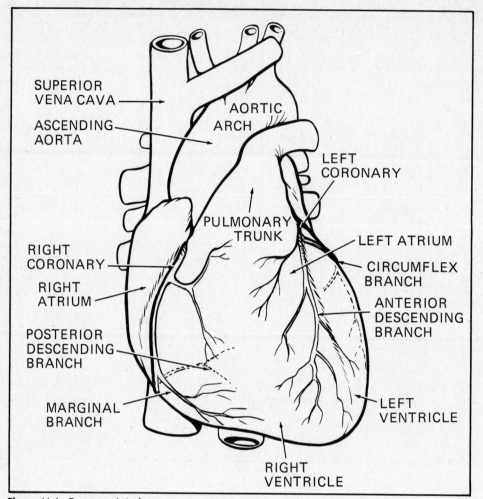

Figure 11-4. Coronary Arteries.

Veins

Veins carry blood from the body to the heart. Blood in veins contains more carbon dioxide than blood in arteries, so the venous blood is dark. Veins have thinner walls than do arteries, and many have valves that prevent a backflow of blood. Veins parallel the arterial tree.

Vena cava, the largest vein of the body, is divided into the inferior vena cava for the lower part of the body and the superior vena cava for the upper part of the body.

- **Inferior vena cava** divides into the common iliac, which branches to each side of the body. The iliac veins subdivide into the femoral and then into the popliteal veins, which return blood from the legs.
- **Superior vena cava** branches into the innominate, jugular, and subclavian veins, which further subdivide to return blood from the head, neck, and upper extremities.

Venules are the very small veins that lead into the capillaries.

THE LYMPHATIC SYSTEM

The lymphatic system consists of **lymphatic vessels, ducts, nodes** (masses of lymphoid tissue), and a fluid called **lymph.** The vessels branch over the entire body, similar to the blood vessel tree. The lymph resembles plasma except that its protein content is lower and it is 95% water. Lymph is sometimes referred to as tissue fluid. It is formed when plasma parts pass through the capillary wall into tissue spaces. Lymph acts as an exchange media connecting the blood and the cells.

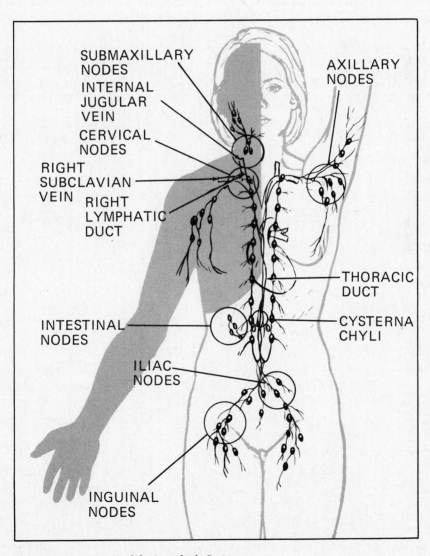

Figure 11-5. Structure of the Lymphatic System.

Lymph vessels are made of connective tissue. They begin as closed channels, **lymphatic capillaries,** in the tissue spaces. The capillaries lead into larger vessels, **lymphatics,** which empty into the great thoracic duct and the right lymphatic duct. These ducts empty into the jugular and subclavian veins.

Lymph nodes or glands are bodies of lymphatic tissue enclosed in a capsule of fibrous connective tissue. Blood vessels enter and leave through a slight depression, the **hilus.** Nodes occur in chains in the neck, armpit, and groin. Nodes produce lymphocytes and monocytes and have a filtering action to prevent bacteria and other harmful substances from entering the blood stream.

Spleen

The spleen is the largest mass of lymphatic tissue in the body. It is oval shaped and lies behind and below the stomach in the upper left quadrant of the abdomen. About 350 ccs of blood are stored in the spleen and can be released rapidly if hemmorhage occurs. Worn-out blood cells are removed from the blood and the iron is returned by the spleen's action. Microorganisms are also destroyed. Monocytes, lymphocytes, and plasma cells are formed in the spleen.

Thymus

The thymus gland is an **endocrine gland,** a gland that produces a secretion which is carried by the bloodstream. It is mentioned here because it is composed of lymphatic tissue. The thymus plays a role in immunity and seems to control the antigen-antibody responses from birth to several years of age.

TERMINOLOGY

Agglutination—clumping of blood cells when incompatible bloods are mixed

Anastomosis—an end to end union of two vessels and may refer to blood vessels, lymphatics or nerves. It can also refer to the joining of structures, such as the intestines

Aneurysm—occurs when a weak spot on a wall of a vessel develops into a saclike enlargement on the wall

Anoxemia—an inadequate supply of oxygen in the blood

Anoxia—a deficient supply of oxygen. It may be caused by an inadequate amount of oxygen carried by the blood or by an inadequate amount of oxygen in the air taken in by the lungs.

Antibody—a substance produced by a foreign material when it enters the body and makes the body immune to the effects of the material

Antigen—may be either within the body or introduced into the body; any substance that causes antibody formation

Apex—a point

Arrhythmia—an abnormal pattern of electrical activity of the heart; common ones are atrial fibrillation, atrial flutter, ventricular tachycardia, ventricular fibrillation, premature ventricular contractions, sinus tachycardia, and sinus bradycardia

Asphyxia—unconsciousness due to lack of oxygen and increased carbon dioxide

Blood pressure—the force that moves the blood through the vessels. The **systolic pressure** is the force in the arteries as the ventricles contract, the top reading of a blood pressure reading. The **diastolic** is the force in the arteries as the ventricles relax, the lower reading. Average adult blood pressure is about 120 systolic and 70 diastolic, recorded as 120/70. Blood pressures vary according to the size of a person.

Bradycardia—a slow heart rate

CPR—cardiopulmonary resuscitation

DNR—do not resuscitate, the patient is too ill to benefit from CPR

Fibrillation—a quivering action of either the atria or the ventricles instead of a forceful contraction

Hilus—the place in an organ where blood vessels enter

Ischemia—inadequate flow of blood to a part of the body

Leukocytosis—the condition of an increased number of white blood cells

Leukopenia—a condition of a decreased number of white blood cells

Normal sinus rhythm (NSR)—normal electrical activity of the heart with the impulse originating in the sinoatrial node

Paroxysm—the sudden attack of symptoms of a disease or disorder that occurs periodically

Peripheral—outermost surface; blood vessels close to the skin are peripheral vessels

Phlebotomy—the procedure of taking blood from a vein

Pulse—the striking force of the heart beat that is felt in peripheral arteries. The pulse can be felt in several places:

- Brachial artery on the inside of the elbow
- Carotid artery in the neck
- Pedis artery on the top of the foot
- Radial artery at the wrist
- Temporal artery above and to the side of the eye.

An **apical** pulse is taken with a stethoscope at the apex of the heart.

Shunt—shift from one pathway to another; this may be a condition or may be created surgically.

STO—support therapy only; no CPR.

Syndrome—a group of symptoms that appear together to give a certain picture of a disease process

Tamponade—a massive accumulation of fluid in the pericardial space

DISEASES AND DISORDERS

Blood

Anemia is an abnormally low number of RBCs. The Hgb is low due to hemorrhage, nutritional deficiencies, poisons, or unknown causes. There are several types of anemia.

- **Aplastic anemia** is a condition in which RBCs, WBCs, and the platelets are greatly decreased. The bone marrow is fatty with few cells. The cause may be toxins or may be unknown. **Tx:** Androgens, transfusion of RBCs, bone marrow transplant.
- **Iron deficiency anemia** may be due to poor nutrition or to bleeding somewhere in the body. **Tx:** Treatment of underlying cause, iron preparations, transfusions.
- **Pernicious anemia** is due to a lack of Vitamin B_{12}. The intrinsic factor in gastric secretions is absent, and Vitamin B_{12} is not absorbed from food. **Tx:** Vitamin B_{12} IM at various intervals the rest of life span.
- **Sickle cell anemia** is an hereditary disorder found more often in blacks than in other races. The RBC is shaped like a sickle, and the blood is more viscous causing the obstruction of blood flow. Patients have periods of pain in the arms, legs, and abdomen because of the obstruction. **Tx:** Analgesics during periods of pain, oxygen, transfusions. The life expectancy is diminished and many complications may result.

Hemophilia is an inherited disorder that is transmitted by females to male offspring. One of the blood components that aid in clotting is missing. Bleeding may occur spontaneously or after surgery, injury, or dental work. **Tx:** Absolutely no ASA, cryoprecipitate is given IV, ice applied to bleeding area, prednisone.

Infectious mononucleosis involves the lymph system, and there are abnormal lymphocytes in the blood. Symptoms resemble those of the flu with a sore throat. A virus is believed to be the cause. **Tx:** Bedrest, fluids, IV fluids if necessary, good nutrition, ASA or other antipyretic drugs, antibiotic in some cases.

Leukemia is sometimes called cancer of the blood. The blood-forming tissues produce an excess of white cells that are abnormal. Leukemia is classified as acute or chronic. Types are:

- **Acute lymphatic leukemia** (ALL) may involve any organ. The lymph nodes, liver, and spleen are enlarged. **Tx:** Antineoplastics, prednisone. Radiation of the cerebrospinal axis may provide remissions.
- **Acute myeloblastic leukemia** (AML) occurs most often in adults. Patients have severe bone pain; there may be involvement of the central nervous system. **Tx:** Antineoplastics and radiation provide remissions.
- **Chronic lymphatic leukemia** (CLL) occurs in persons over 30 years of age. The onset is slow. **Tx:** Started only after symptoms appear, which may be some time after diagnosis is made. Antineoplastics, radiation, steroids.

- **Chronic myeloblastic leukemia** (CML) is due to a chromosome abnormality. This occurs most often in young adults. **Tx:** Antineoplastics and radiation give remissions.

Polycythemia vera is most common in middle-aged men. The RBCs are increased, blood is more viscous, and bone marrow shows increased activity. **Tx:** Radiophosphorous, phlebotomy of 500 cc at a time, chemotherapy.

Congenital Defects of the Heart

These are defects that are present at birth. Surgery is the treatment for all the defects.

Aortic stenosis is a narrowing of the aortic valve, which limits the flow of blood and puts pressure on the ventricles. This problem may also be caused by rheumatic heart disease.

Atrial septal defect is an opening in the septum which allows blood to flow from atria to atria, resulting in a mixture of oxygenated and unoxygenated blood.

Coarctation of the aorta is a narrowing of the aorta in a localized area. There is increased pressure in the head and arms.

Patent ductus arteriosus is a connection between the pulmonary artery and the aorta. This connection usually closes spontaneously shortly after birth; prematurity or other causes may keep it open.

Tetrology of Fallot has four abnormalities. There is a ventricular septal defect, a hypertrophy of the right ventricle, an abnormal placement of the aorta to the right, and an obstruction of the pulmonary outflow.

Transposition of great vessels occurs when the pulmonary artery branches from the left ventricle and the aorta branches from the right ventricle and, therefore, the blood is not oxygenated.

Ventricular septal defect is a hole in the septum which lets oxygenated blood and unoxygenated blood mix. As a result, the blood to the body has less oxygen than normal. The defect sometimes closes spontaneously, so surgery is done late in childhood if necessary.

Heart

Aortic insufficiency is due to incomplete closure of the aortic valve, producing increased blood flow from the left ventricle and a back flow into the left ventricle **(regurgitation).** The left ventricle is **hypertrophied** (LVH). **Tx:** Digitalis preparations, diuretics, surgery to replace the valve.

Bacterial endocarditis is an infection of the lining of the heart. Streptococci are frequently the cause, but another organism may be responsible. The infection may be secondary to an infection in some other part of the body. The disease is **acute,** (ABE) or **subacute** (SBE) according to the severity of onset. The acute type causes sudden chills, fever, extreme weakness, and rapid changes in heart murmurs. The subacute has a slower onset. Blood cultures are taken in series, usually three at a time, and repeated in one or two hours in ABE. Antibiotics are started as soon as cultures have been collected. In SBE, blood cultures may be taken two or three times a day for several days before the antibiotic is started. Any person who has cardiac abnormalities should be given penicillin before dental surgery or other surgery to prevent the occurrence of endocarditis. **Tx:** Antibiotics are given IV for several weeks. Blood cultures following treatment are taken each week for several weeks to make sure the organism has been eradicated. Fungus infections may require excision of valve tissue. Convalescence is long and many complications may arise.

Congestive heart failure (CHF) develops when the work load of the heart is increased. Circulation through the lungs is impaired, causing fluid to accumulate in the lungs and in the tissues of the body. CHF is secondary to other heart diseases. **Tx:** Bedrest c̄ BRP, digitalis preparations, low sodium diet, diuretics, oxygen, water restriction, vasodilators, treatment of underlying cause.

Mitral insufficiency causes enlargement of the left atrium as a result of regurgitation and failure of the left ventricle. **Tx:** Digitalis preparations, diuretics, mitral valve replacement.

Mitral stenosis occurs most often in women. The narrowing of the valve is often due to rheumatic fever. The left atrium pressure is increased causing increased pressure in the pulmonary veins. **Tx:** Quinidine if atrial fibrillation present, diuretics, repair or replacement of valve.

Myocarditis is an inflammation of the muscle of the heart. The cause may be organisms, chemicals, electrical shock, or a systemic disease. **Tx:** Treatment of underlying cause, same medications as for CHF, corticosteroids.

Pericarditis is an inflammation of the pericardium. The process may be due to an organism, a systemic infection, a trauma, or a tumor. **Tx:** Antibiotics, corticosteroids, diuretics, digitalis preparations, analgesics, sedatives, pericardiocentesis.

Tricuspid stenosis and tricuspid insufficiency is usually associated with mitral valve disease. **Tx:** Valve replacement for stenosis. Mitral valve replacement may decrease tricuspid insufficiency.

Coronary Artery

Angina pectoris, also called **ischemic heart disease** (IHD), is a syndrome caused by decreased blood flow to the myocardium from the coronary artery. Pain occurs in the chest and radiates down the inside of the left arm. The patient becomes very apprehensive. Pain is usually caused by exertion. **Tx:** Nitrates, coronary bypass surgery if condition unstable and medications do not help, plaque compression by a balloon catheter.

Myocardial infarction (MI) is the death of tissue in the muscle of the heart due to obstruction of a coronary artery. MI is also called coronary occlusion and heart attack. The pain may resemble indigestion or pain associated with gallstones. Nausea, vomiting, dizziness, dyspnea, and anxiety follow onset of pain. **Tx:** Bedrest c̄ continuous monitoring of heart activity, pain medication, anticoagulants, oxygen. After recovery, an exercise program is established. Coronary bypass surgery may be necessary.

An unexpected cardiac arrest is a life-threatening emergency. Hospitals have routines for such emergencies. A name such as "Code Blue" or "Dr. Heart" is used for this type of emergency. Each nursing unit has an emergency cart with IV fluids, drugs, and equipment. All nursing personnel and respiratory therapy personnel are trained in **cardiopulmonary resuscitation** (CPR). The first person to find the patient calls the operator who pages three times, "Dr. Heart for (number) floor, room (number)." CPR is started as soon as the call is made to the operator. Key personnel respond to the page. Doctors respond and the first one to arrive takes charge. RT is quick to respond and brings the defibrillator. An anesthetist responds to insert an airway if needed. For small hospitals, you may be expected to help and will need to know the location of the emergency medications on the cart and which ones will be used first. Larger hospitals have enough personnel so you will not be involved in the actual care of the patient. Your responsibility is to see that the emergency cart gets to the room as soon as you hear the page. Help with the family if any are present. If you are asked to call the patient's family, tell them that a change in the patient's condition has occurred and that the nurse would like the family to come to the hospital. Questions should be answered by saying that is all the information you have and the nurse is busy with the patient. Watch for the family to arrive, and escort them to the conference room. Pastoral care personnel will help with the family. You will call the office of the doctor taking care of the patient and say, "This is (number) floor at (name) hospital, and we need to notify Dr. Smith that there is a Dr. Heart in progress on patient (name) in room (number)." Each hospital will explain their procedure and what your duties will be in this type of emergency.

Heart and Blood Vessels

Aneurysms of the aorta may occur in any area of the great vessel. **Thoracic aneurysms** result from trauma or fatty deposits in the artery. **Abdominal aneurysms** are usually due to fatty deposits. Rupture of thoracic or abdominal aorta is a life-threatening emergency requiring immediate surgery. **Femoral and popliteal aneurysms** impair circulation to the legs. **Tx:** Surgical repair with grafting if defect is large.

Buerger's disease is also called **thromboangiitis obliterans** (TAO). There is inflammation of the arteries and veins in the extremities, especially the legs, with clot formation. Males in the 20 to 40 age group who smoke are most often the ones with this disease. **Tx:** Absolutely no smoking; good nutrition; protection of extremities from heat, cold, and trauma; exercises to promote circulation in the limbs. Amputation of the leg may be needed in extreme cases. Sympathectomy helps some cases.

Hypertension is increased blood pressure. The upper limit of normal is considered to be 160/95. **Primary or essential hypertension** has no specific cause. **Secondary hypertension** may be due to renal disease, a tumor of the adrenal glands, coarctation of the aorta, restrained anger, or other systemic problems. **Malignant hypertension** is a sudden rise in BP with the diastole reading of 130 or more. **Tx:** Antihypertensive drugs, diuretics, low sodium diet, mild sedatives. Any underlying cause is treated.

Phlebitis is the inflammation of the wall of a vein. Standing in one position without shifting weight causes pooling of blood in the calf of the leg, which may lead to inflammation. If a clot forms, the condition is called **thrombophlebitis. Tx:** Elastic hose help prevent the condition. Bedrest with leg elevated, heat to area, anticoagulants for clot formation.

Raynaud's disease involves the arteries of the fingers and, sometimes, the toes. Exposure to cold causes the fingers to become pale or cyanotic. Warmth turns fingers bright red and causes swelling with throbbing. The sympathetic nervous system seems to be involved. The disease is progressive. **Tx:** Protection of the fingers and toes from cold, lotions to keep skin moist, vasodilators, no smoking, sympathectomy if attacks are severe.

Shock is a condition resulting from inadequate circulation to the tissues of the body so that there is not enough blood to sustain life. Shock may be caused by trauma, infections, hemorrhage, burns, surgery, or cardiovascular problems. **Tx:** General measures are oxygen, maintainance of blood volume by IV fluids and/or transfusions, vasodilators, plasma products, steroids, monitoring of urine flow, central venous pressure readings. Antibiotics are given if infection is present.

Varicose veins are the dilated veins that occur when the valves are not working correctly. The cause may be an inherited tendency, pressure from standing in one position, or a disease process. Blood is not pushed toward the heart but flows back through the valve causing the vein to be stretched in that area. **Tx:** Support hose, vein stripping and ligation.

Lymph System

Lymphadenitis is an inflammation in the lymph nodes, usually secondary to an infection elsewhere. It disappears when the primary infection is treated.

Lymphangitis is inflammation of the lymph vessels. The streptococcus and staphylococcus are the usual organisms that cause the condition. **Tx:** Analgesics, hot, moist compresses to area, the appropriate antibiotics.

Lymphomas are malignant tumors that originate in lymph nodes or lymphatic tissue. **Hodgkin's disease** usually begins in the lymph nodes of the neck and progresses to other nodes and tissues. A biopsy verifies the diagnosis. **Tx:** Radiation, chemotherapy. In other lymphomas, radiation is not effective. Chemotherapy, allopurinal, and prednisone are combined for treatment.

SURGERIES AND PROCEDURES

Aneurysmectomy is the resection of an aneurysm. Reinforcement with a mesh material may be necessary if the defect is large. A synthetic prosthesis may be used if a section of an artery has to be removed.

Arterial graft is done when an artery is occluded. A vein may be used to bypass the clogged section by anastomosing the vein to the artery above and below the occlusion. A synthetic prosthesis may be used. Permits will state which artery and the type of graft.

Central venous catheter (CVC) is inserted into the subclavian vein through the skin above the left clavicle and threaded into the superior vena cava. The catheter is sutured to the skin. The **central venous pressure** (CVP) is measured at the tip of the catheter by a gauge connected to the external catheter, which is also connected to tubing for IV fluids. The measurement of the right atrial filling pressure is a guide for ordering IV fluids. It helps determine the presence of right ventricular failure, and a sudden rise may indicate the beginning of an arrhythmia. The catheter is inserted by a doctor and may be done on the unit. A central supply tray is needed.

Coronary bypass surgery for severe angina or following a heart attack uses a vein from the leg to graft onto the occluded artery and bypass the obstruction. The number of grafts in one procedure will be specified on the permit. The patient is connected to the heart-lung machine during the operation. The incision is down the chest, through the sternum. The patient is connected to monitors following surgery until stability is achieved. Exercise begins in a few days.

Embolectomy is removal of a blood clot from a vessel. Permit will specify location.

Endarterectomy is performed to clean out the plaque build-up in an artery. The most common artery involved is the carotid. The patient has a history of **transient ischemic attacks** (TIA), and arteriograms, scans, and doppler studies show a blockage in the artery. Neurosigns are taken before OR as a base line. Orders post-op concern possible respiratory problems due to edema, ability to speak, chewing and swallowing ability, memory for recent events, balance and coordination.

A *Hickman catheter* is used when a patient is to receive IV fluids for a long period of time. It is also used for long-term chemotherapy. A catheter is placed in the right atrium of the heart via the superior vena cava and cepahalic vein. The other end of the catheter is guided through a pathway under the skin, which has been created surgically, into the area over the sternum to the outside of the chest. Tubing is attached at this point for IV fluids. The patient is taught how to care for the point of exit so infection does not occur.

Sympathectomy is cutting the central mass of nerve fibers to an area. Occlusive diseases of arteries benefit by lumbar sympathectomy. Thoracic and cervicothoracic sympathectomy relieve pain of angina pectoris that is uncontrolled otherwise.

Valve replacements are accomplished with a plastic prosthesis or homografts.

Vein stripping and ligation is performed for varicose veins that are large and are impairing circulation. The vein is tied off on one end and pulled out through an incision at the other end. The veins are peripheral ones and the other veins take over the circulation.

Cardiology Lab Procedures

Doppler studies involve the changes in frequency sound waves. The sounds are amplified. Blood vessel studies show the flow of circulation and the presence of any obstructions. Small doppler machines are used to count the pulse when it is so weak it can't be felt.

ECG or EKG is an electrocardiogram which records the electrical activity of the heart. Cardiac monitors in ICU and CCU are a continuous ECG recording. Electrodes are placed on the body and transmit the electrical impulses to a machine which records the waves. The oscilloscope for monitoring can print out the ECG when needed. Leads are the waves viewed between two points of the body. The routine ECG has 12 leads or 12 pairs of points. A rhythm strip is one lead. Many students take an additional course to become monitor technicians in the special units.

Echocardiogram is a picture produced by sending sound waves through the body and using the echo to create a picture. An Echo M-mode traces the activity and shows functioning of each chamber and the pericardium. Echo 2-D means two dimensional and is performed with deeper ultrasound to show the valves

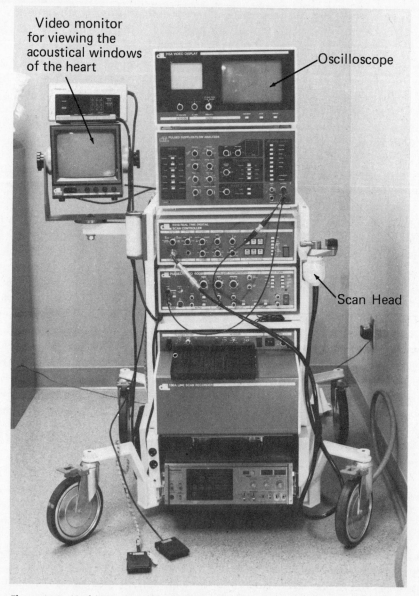

Video monitor for viewing the acoustical windows of the heart

Oscilloscope

Scan Head

Figure 11-6. Mark III System Echocardiograph *(Courtesy of ATL Ultrasound).*

and interior and to determine if any abnormalities exist. A routine echogram includes both the M-mode and the 2-D.

Heart catheterization is performed with the aid of the fluoroscope x-ray. A radiopaque catheter is introduced into the heart. For a right heart cath, the catheter is inserted into the right basilic or femoral vein, then into the vena cava, and finally into the right atrium. Blood samples are taken, and the catheter is passed on to the right ventricle where more samples are taken. The catheter is then pushed into the pulmonary artery where pressures are measured. For a left heart cath, the catheter is introduced into the right femoral artery, then into the abdominal aorta to the thoracic aorta, and finally into the left ventricle where samples of blood are taken. The catheter is then pushed into the left atrium for more samples and then into the coronary arteries. Dye may be injected into the arteries for visualization of obstruction. Heart caths show the condition of the valves, the oxygen content in each chamber, and the hematocrit values. Orders following heart caths will involve monitoring vital signs, administering IV fluids for a specified period, applying a sandbag to the area if an artery was used for entry, and specifying when the patient may eat and get out of bed.

Holter monitor is an ECG recording for 12 or 24 hours of the patient going about his/her usual activities. The small ECG recorder is enclosed in a small pack that has a shoulder strap for carrying. Only three leads are on the chest and wires are connected to the ECG in the pack. An hourly diary is kept by the patient so that abnormalities seen on the ECG can be correlated with activity at that time.

Intra-aortic balloon pump is used for left ventricular impairment. A catheter with an attached balloon at the end is inserted into the aorta via the femoral artery. The external portion is connected to a panel for control. The balloon inflates at the beginning of diastole to assist the left ventricle by forcing blood into the coronary arteries and the extremities of the body. Deflation occurs just before systole to decrease the resistance pressure for the left ventricle. The length of time the pump is used depends entirely on the patient's condition and response. The ECG is usually the control for inflation and deflation. A Swan-Ganz catheter is also in place for measurements of pressure. Orders following placement are for pulmonary artery pressure (PAP), pulmonary capillary wedge (PCW) pressure, cardiac output, urine output, CVP readings, pulse checks by doppler, suction for throat and trachea. These patients are in CCU.

Left heart assist device (LHAD) shunts some blood away from the left ventricle through the aorta. A cannula from the left atrium carries blood to an external ball-like pump which forces blood into another cannula placed in the ascending aorta. The cannulas are inserted in surgery. Cardiology lab places a Swan-Ganz catheter in place for measurements to assess heart function. Patients are gradually weaned from the device when the left ventricle is able to take over the work. The cannulas can be removed without further surgery. Orders will involve PA and PCW pressure readings.

Pacemaker implants are mechanical devices that trigger the heart just as the normal pacemaker of the heart would if it were working correctly. Temporary ones may be connected by wires to an external control box. Permanent ones are implanted under the muscle of the chest, and a catheter leads from the device to the right atrium where the tip stimulates the heart activity. A pacemaker lasts for a number of years. Patients who have one should have a card with them that states the type of pacemaker and where it was inserted so that if they are involved in an accident, the rescue squad will have that information.

Percutaneous translumenal coronary angioplasty (PTCA) is used in place of coronary bypass surgery in some cases. A catheter with a balloon tip is inserted through another catheter into the brachial artery to the heart and into a blocked coronary artery. Fluoroscopy visualizes the procedure to assure proper placement. The balloon is then inflated to compress the plaques in the artery against the wall. When dilatation is accomplished, the balloon is withdrawn and dye is injected to make sure the pathway is open. The patient will be in CCU for monitoring. This requires only two or three days hospitalization.

Swan-Ganz catheter is inserted into the subclavian vein into the vena cava through the heart to the pulmonary artery. The catheter usually has four lumen: one to inflate the balloon at the end of the catheter, one for wires to a machine to measure cardiac output, one to measure PA and PCW, and one to measure right atrium pressure or CVP. The readings show the function of the heart and help to maintain fluid balance. An x-ray following insertion is needed to check for proper placement. Orders will be in regard to the different measurements.

Treadmill exercise ECG records heart activity while the patient walks on an exercise walker. The angle of slant is increased and the rate of walk is increased to tolerance.

LABORATORY TESTS

- ABG
- ABG-VBG simultaneous (A-V gases)
- A-V difference
- Blood C&S
- Blood crossmatch
- Blood typing
- Bone marrow biopsy
- Cardiac enzymes and isoenzymes
    CPK
    LDH
    SGOT
    SGPT
- CBC
- Cholesterol
- Coagulation studies
    ACT
    PT
    PTT
- Coombs, direct and indirect
- Cryoglobulins
- Electrolytes
- ESR
- Hgb, Hct
- IBC
- Immunoglobulins
- Iron (Fe)
- Lipids
- Lipoprotein electrophoresis
- Lymph node cytology
- PCO_2
- pH, blood
- Platelet count
- Reticulocyte count
- Sickle cell test
- Triglycerides

RADIOLOGY AND NUCLEAR MEDICINE EXAMS

Angiograms visualize blood and lymph vessels after dye is injected. Studies involving dye require permits because invasive tests have a certain degree of danger. Orders will specify which vessel.

Arteriograms visualize arteries after dye is injected. Any time blood supply is insufficient to an area, arteriograms aid in the diagnosis. Orders will state which artery.

Lymphangiograms show the lymphatic system. A dye is injected into the lymph vessels between the toes. The blue color is very visible on the feet for some time.

Perfusion scans show the blood flow to an area or the flow of the lymph. Radioactive isotopes are used.

Venograms help determine blockage and extent of damage. Dye is used.

X-ray of chest shows size and configuration of the heart and large vessels. PA and Lat are the most common type of chest x-ray.

X-ray of thighs and legs show if any calcification of the superficial femoral and popliteal blood vessels is present in an occlusive disease.

MEDICATIONS

Antianginal or nitrates

Also called vasodilators, these drugs relax the smooth muscle of blood vessels.

- Cardilate—PO or sublingual—10 mg prior to expected attack and at HS, increase as needed.
- Iso-Bid—PO—40 mg cap q 12 hrs.
- Nitro-Bid ointment—2 inches q 8 hrs spread over a 6 × 6 area of the chest.
- Nitrostat—sublingual—tab ī at first sign of attack, repeat q 5 min. until pain relieved.
- Peritrate—PO—10 or 20 mg qid, increase as needed to 160 mg/d.

Antiarrhythmics

Antiarrhythmics return the heart to normal sinus rhythm (NSR).

- Bretylol (bretylium)—IM, IV—dosage individualized for ventricular arrhythmias that do not respond to other drugs.
- Inderal (propranolol)—PO, IV—individualized dosage.
- Lidocaine—IV—bolus of 200 mg over a 15 to 30 min period or may be mixed in 1000cc of solution for continuous drip.

- Procainamide HCl capsules—PO—dosage individualized.
- Quinidine gluconate—IM, IV—dosage individualized.
- Quinidine sulfate—PO—dosage according to arrhythmia.
- verapamil—IV—10 mg over 2 min, repeat in 30 min prn.

Anticoagulants

These drugs prolong the clotting time of blood.

- Coumadin (warfarin)—IM, IV, PO—dosage determined by prothrombin time. Doctor will order daily after the results of the Pro-T for that day have been reported.
- dicumarol—PO—dosage depends on prothrombin time.
- heparin—IV or intrafat injection—dosage is in units. An ACT or PTT test one hour before the time of a dose determines the amount given. Protamine sulfate IV or IM is used to counteract an overdose of heparin.

Antihypertensives

Antihypertensives reduce blood pressure. Dosages are individualized.

- Apresoline—IV, IM, PO
- Catapres—PO—available in 0.1 mg and 0.2 mg tabs.
- Inderal—IV, PO
- Minipress capsules—PO
- Serpasil (reserpine)—PO—tabs and elixir, IM.

Antihypertensives with diuretics reduce blood pressure and remove fluid from the body tissues.

- Aldactazide—PO—tabs i̅ to 8 daily according to response
- Dyazide—PO—cap i̅ or i̅i̅ bid
- Hydrodiuril—PO—50 to 100 mg/d
- Ser-Ap-Es—PO—tab i̅ or i̅i̅ tid

Antineoplastics

Antineoplastics are used to treat cancer. Dosages are individualized.

- adriamycin for leukemias, lymphomas
- BCNU (carmustine), CCNU (lomustine), and MeCCNU (semustine) for Hodgkin's and myelomas
- bleomycin and vinblastine for lymphomas
- Mechlorethamide (nitrogen mustard) for Hodgkin's, lymphomas
- methotrexate (MTX) for leukemia
- vincristine for ALL, Hodgkin's
- 6-mercaptopurine (6-MP) for ALL

Blood Products

- Antihemophilic factor

- Buminate 5%, normal human albumin
- Cryoprecipitate
- Fresh frozen plasma (FFP)
- Hespan, a plasma expander
- Packed red cells
- Platelets
- Proplex, factor 1X complex
- Salt poor albumin (SPA)
- Whole blood

Calcium Blockers

Calcium blockers are used in many cardiac conditions, but mainly for angina.

- nifedipine—sublingual—10 to 30 mg tid.
- verapamil—IV—individualized dosage for paroxsymal atrial tachycardia—PO—80 to 120 mg tid or qid to depress AV conduction or for control of angina.

Diuretics

Diuretics increase the flow of urine and decrease edema.

- Diuril—PO—500 mg to 1 Gm/d.
- Edecrin—PO, IV—individualized dosage.
- Hydrochlorthiazide—PO—50 to 100 mg/d.
- Lasix—PO, IV—40 to 120 mg/d.
- Renese—PO—1 to 4 mg/d.

Cholesterol and Lipid Reducers

- Atromid-S—PO—500 mg/d.
- Choloxin—PO—1 to 2 mg/d, may increase to 4 or 8 mg/d.
- Nicobid—PO—1.5 to 3 Gm/d with or after meals.
- Questran—PO—one packet mixed in fluid tid or qid.

Digitalis

These preparations increase the force of heart contractions.

- Cedilanid—PO, IM, IV—individualized dosage.
- Crystodigin (digitoxin)—PO, IV—individualized dosage.
- Lanoxin (digoxin)—PO, IM, IV—individualized dosage.

Vasodilators, peripheral

Peripheral vasodilators increase the blood supply to the extremities.

- Arlidin—PO—3 to 12 mg tid or qid.
- Cyclospasmol—PO—1200 to 1600 mg/d then decrease to between 400 and 800 mg/d for maintenance.

- Ethaquin—PO—tab ī tid.
- Nico-400 Plateau Caps (nicotinic acid)—PO—cap ī q 12 hrs.
- Vasospan—PO—cap ī q 12 hrs.

Vasopressors

Vasopressors increase blood pressure. Dosages are individualized.

- Aramine—SQ, IM, IV
- Intropin (dopamine)—IV
- Levophed—IV

EXAMPLES OF PHYSICIAN'S ORDERS

Dx: Angina, CHF

1. Bedrest c̄ BRP
2. Low sodium diet
3. EKG
4. Nitroglycerin 1/150 sublingual, tabs īī q 5 min. for anginal pain. If no relief, give Demerol 50 mg c̄ Vistaril 50 mg IM.
5. Tylenol gr × PO q 4 hrs prn for minor discomfort
6. Nitrobid 6.5 Plateau Cap ī bid
7. Lasix 40 mg PO @ 9 AM q Mon, Wed, Fri
8. Slow K ī PO qid pc and HS
9. Nifedipine 10 mg PO 30 min ac & HS
10. Colace 100 mg PO prn
11. Valium 5 mg PO HS prn
12. Call me if Demerol and Vistaril do not relieve pain.

Dx: Coronary insufficiency

1. CBC, SMA-20, UA
2. EKG
3. Up ad lib
4. DAT
5. Dalmane 30 mg HS MR × 1
6. Sign permit for left heart cath and coronary angiography.
7. Hold breakfast in AM.
8. 1000cc D5W in AM at 0600. Use left arm.
9. Demerol 50 mg c̄ Vistaril 25 mg IM on call to cath lab
10. Shave right groin.

Post Cath orders 0830:

1. Sandbag to right groin for 4 hrs. Observe for bleeding and VS check q 15 min × 4, q 30 min × 4, q hr × 4, then routine if stable.

2. Flat in bed until 1400
3. DC IV when completed if no N/V
4. Resume diet.
5. EKG in AM
6. Percodan tab ī PO q 6 hrs prn pain
7. Dalmane 30 mg HS
8. Notify Dr. if any bleeding or severe pain.

REVIEW QUESTIONS

1. Name the structures of the circulatory system.
   _____
   _____

2. List the functions of blood.
   _____
   _____

3. Arteries carry _____ from the _____ to the
   _____.

4. The function of the heart is _____.

5. The upper chambers of the heart are the _____, the
   lower chambers are the _____.

6. The aorta is the largest _____ of the body.

7. The vena cava is the largest _____ of the body.

8. Why is the spleen important?
   _____
   _____

9. Irregularities in the rhythm of the heart are called _____.

10. You receive a phone call from a patient's relative just minutes after a
    Dr. Heart has been called on the patient. How do you respond? _____
    _____
    _____

11. You are working in ICU and a doctor is inserting a Swan-Ganz catheter.
    What exam can you anticipate following completion of the procedure?
    _____

12. A heart attack is also called _____
    or a _____.

13. CPR means _____.

14. List the functions of the lymphatic system. _____
    _____
    _____

15. State whether the following diseases/disorders are of the blood, the heart, the blood vessels, or the lymphatic system:

Leukemia _____

Hodgkin's disease _____

Thrombophlebitis _____

Aortic stenosis _____

Anemia _____

16. Define:

heart catheterization _____

coronary bypass _____

embolectomy_____

EKG _____

echocardiogram _____

17. Classify the following medications:

Inderal _____

heparin _____

Nitrostat _____

verapamil _____

Lasix _____

Vasospan _____

Lanoxin _____

18. Name three laboratory coagulation tests. _____

_____

19. Name three cardiac enzyme studies ordered from the lab. _____

_____

20. A patient on the unit is a terminal cancer patient. She is only 47 years of age but the breast cancer has metastasized to the bones. Chemotherapy and radiation plus several surgeries have failed to control the disease. You know from the conversations between doctors and nurses that the patient is near death. Would you expect a Dr. Heart to be called on the patient? _____

_____

Chapter 12 | Respiratory System

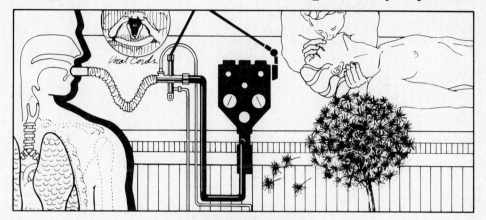

OBJECTIVES

Study of this chapter will enable you to:

1. List the structures of the respiratory system.
2. Describe the functions of the respiratory system.
3. List and define terms relating to the respiratory system.
4. List some diseases and disorders of the respiratory system.
5. List and classify medications that effect the respiratory system.
6. List some surgeries of the respiratory system.
7. List some laboratory exams that relate to the respiratory system.
8. List some radiology exams that aid in diagnosing diseases and disorders of the respiratory system.
9. Transcribe Physician's Orders for patients with respiratory problems.

The respiratory system works with the circulatory system to supply oxygen to the cells of the body and to eliminate the carbon dioxide produced by the cells' activities. This exchange of gases between an organism and its environment is called **respiration.** Inspiration is the phase of respiration during which air is taken into the body; expiration is the phase where air is exhaled. The structures of the respiratory system are the nose, pharynx, larynx, trachea, bronchi, and lungs.

RESPIRATORY SYSTEM STRUCTURES

Nose

The openings into the external nasal cavity are the **nares** or nostrils. The external and internal cavities are separated into two parts by a **septum** composed of bones of the skull (ethmoid and vomer) and cartilage. **Cartilage** forms the framework of the external nose and gives it flexibility. The internal nose is a cavity above the mouth that connects with the throat through another pair of nares. There are three bones, the **turbinates,** that extend from each lateral wall of this cavity. Four sinuses, the frontal, sphenoid, ethmoid, and maxillary, drain into the internal nose. Mucous membranes containing **cilia** line the nasal cavity and the entire respiratory tract to the bronchioles. The nose provides warmth and moisture to inspired air, filters particles from the air, receives stimuli for the sense of smell, and provides a resonating cavity for the voice.

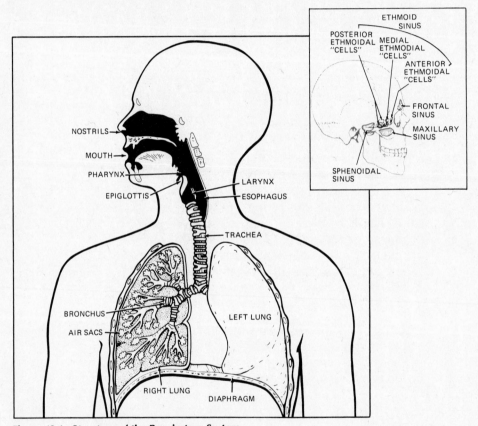

Figure 12-1. Structure of the Respiratory System.

Pharynx

The **pharynx** is usually called the throat. It is a muscular tube, lined with mucous membrane, that extends from the back of the nasal cavity and mouth to the larynx. The pharynx also functions as a resonating chamber for speech sounds. It serves as a passageway for air from the nose to the trachea and for food from the mouth to the **esophagus** (tube to the stomach). The top portion of the pharynx, the **nasopharynx,** contains openings to the tubes from the ears **(eustachian tubes).** The **adenoids** are masses of lymphatic tissue on the wall of the nasopharynx. The **oropharynx** is the portion at the back of the mouth which contains the tonsils. The **tonsils** are masses of lymphatic tissue, one on each side of the throat, that filter out bacteria.

Larynx

The **larynx,** or voice box, is composed of muscle and cartilage. The **thyroid cartilage,** the Adam's apple, gives the anterior wall a triangular shape that may be quite visible in the neck of some people. The **epiglottis** is the lid of the voice box which closes during swallowing. The mucous membrane lining of the walls folds over into two divided layers. The upper divided layer is called the false cords, and the lower divided layer is called the true vocal cords because sound is produced when they are vibrated. The space in the center, between the cords, is the **glottis.**

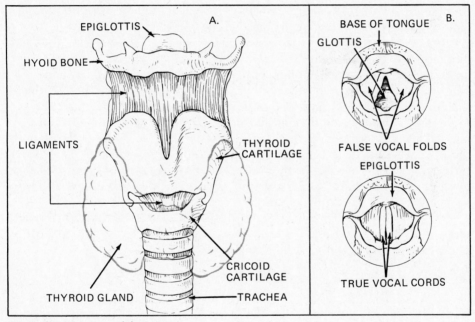

Figure 12-2. Structure of the Larynx.

Trachea

The **trachea** is a passageway for air and is usually called the windpipe. The tube leads from the voice box to the bronchi, a distance of about 4½ inches. The walls of the trachea have a partial circle of cartilage connected by a tough membrane on the posterior side. The open portion of the circle is next to the esophagus for flexibility during swallowing. The cilia in the mucous membrane lining move secretions upward to the throat.

Bronchi

Bronchi are tubes leading from the trachea to the lungs. The trachea divides into the right bronchus which leads to the right lung and left bronchus which lead to the left lung. The walls of the bronchi contain cartilage which gives support. As the branches get smaller, the cartilage gradually decreases and disappears. Each bronchus divides into smaller branches which subdivide into small **bronchioles.** The amount of smooth muscle increases; the lining contains no cilia in the ends of bronchioles. Microscopic bronchioles divide into **alveolar ducts** which terminate in several alveolar sacs that resemble bunches of grapes. The walls of the sacs contain many **alveoli,** air cells, composed of a single layer of cells. The alveoli are covered by capillaries, and gases are exchanged between the lung and the blood by diffusion. The branching of the bronchi into smaller and smaller tubes is referred to as the bronchial tree.

Lungs

The **lungs** are cone-shaped organs located in the thoracic cavity and sur-rounded by the ribs. The space between the two lungs is the **mediastinum.** The lung tissue is spongy and highly elastic. The right lung is shorter due to the diaphragm being higher on the right side to accommodate the liver. There are three lobes in the right lung: the upper lobe (RUL), the middle lobe (RML), and the lower lobe (RLL). The left lung has two lobes—upper lobe (LUL) and lower lobe (LLL)—and a tongue-like portion called **lingular segment.** The left lung is smaller and contains the cardiac notch in which the heart lies. Each lung is protected by a two-layered membrane called the **pleura.** The outer layer is the **parietal layer,** and the layer next to the lungs is the **visceral layer.** The **pleural space** between the layers contains a fluid secreted by the membrane for lubri-cating purposes. The **apex** of the lung is the narrow top portion. The **base** of the lung is the portion that fits over the diaphragm. The area of the lung lying against the ribs is the costal surface.

The lungs distribute air and exchange the gases, oxygen and carbon dioxide. The alveoli of the lungs and the capillaries of the circulatory system provide an enormous surface area for gas exchange.

| TERMINOLOGY

Acapnia—the condition of carbon dioxide depletion in blood and tissues
Airway—the path from the nose to the lungs
Allergy—the condition of unusual sensitivity to a substance which does not adversely affect others. The body reacts in a specific way such as a rash, itching, sneezing, vomiting, diarrhea
Apnea—a temporary cessation of breathing
Asphyxia—a lack of oxygen and an increase in carbon dioxide due to some interference with breathing
Auscultation—the process of listening with a stethoscope to sounds made by

body cavities, mainly the chest and abdomen

Bradypnea—a slow respiratory rate

Breath sounds—the noise made while breathing; described according to pitch, intensity, quality, and duration

Bronchospasm—an involuntary muscular movement that narrows the inner passageway of a bronchus

Cheyne-Stokes respiration—an irregular, repetitive breathing pattern that may occur in acute diseases of the lungs, heart, and nervous system. The breathing is first slow and shallow, then it becomes rapid and deep, then it becomes slow and shallow again until apnea occurs for a short time, maybe 20 seconds, and then the cycle is repeated.

Cilia—hairlike processes in epithelial tissue which help move dust, pus, and mucus up the bronchial tree.

Costal—pertaining to a rib

Costal breathing—term used when respirations move the rib cage.

Cough—a sudden and noisy expulsion of air from the lungs through the glottis. Lung disease patients are taught to cough effectively so that material in the lower bronchial tree may be forced upward and expectorated.

Cyanosis—a bluish color of lips, skin, and nail beds due to lack of oxygen.

Diaphragm—a dome-shaped muscular wall that separates the thoracic and abdominal cavities.

Diaphragmatic breathing—respirations that cause noticeable movement in the lower chest and abdomen instead of in the rib cage.

Dyspnea—difficult breathing; usually produces increased chest movement, flaring of the nostrils, restlessness, and anxiety.

Eupnea—normal respiration.

Expectorate—to cough up and spit.

Hering-Breuer reflex—pulmonary nerve impulses that control the normal depth and the rhythmic rate of respiration.

Hiccough, or hiccup—common term for singultus. The diaphragm is spasmodically lowered, causing the glottis to have periodic spasms that close it and produce an inspiratory noise. If prolonged, singultus can interfere with intake of oxygen and cause serious problems

Hypercapnia—above normal amount of carbon dioxide in the blood.

Hyperpnea—rapid breathing with unusually deep respirations.

Hyperventilation—excessive air exchange resulting in acapnia; characterized by very rapid breathing or very deep respirations

Intubation—insertion of a tube (endotracheal tube) into the trachea through the glottis to establish an airway

Laryngoscope—an instrument used to view the larynx

Lobe—part of an organ separted from other parts by definite edges

Orthopnea—an inability to breathe in the supine position

Palpate—to examine by feeling. Many organs can be palpated by applying the hands or fingers to the external surface of the body over the area of the organ.

Pectoral—refers to the chest.

Percussion—process of tapping the body lightly but sharply; may be done as a diagnostic aid or may be a procedure for the treatment of a condition.

Rales—abnormal sounds of the lungs heard via stethoscope. If the bronchi contain secretions, are constricted by spasm, or have thickened walls, there will be abnormal sounds as air passes through them.

Sigh—a deep inspiration, longer than normal, followed by a shorter expiration with a characteristic sound. Respirators can be set for a sigh cycle.

Sneeze—a strong expiratory blast through the nose and mouth produced by some irritating stimuli. Particles of material are expelled from the respiratory tract by sneezing.

SOB—an abbreviation for short of breath

Sputum—the material coughed up from the respiratory tract mixed with saliva

Stridor—the sound caused by an obstruction in the bronchi, trachea, or larynx. Breathing sounds are harsh with a high whistling noise

Suffocation—the state of being smothered by an obstruction of the air passages

Tachypnea—a rapid rate of respiration

Ventilation—the movement of air into and out of the lungs; it usually refers to the use of a machine to supply oxygen and artificial respiration

Yawn—a deep inspiration made with the mouth wide open. It occurs during times of fatigue, drowsiness, and boredom.

RESPIRATORY TREATMENTS

As you know, the RT department treats patients with breathing problems and conducts tests to see how the respiratory system is functioning. Many diseases of other systems cause respiratory problems.

Oxygen Therapy

The administration of oxygen is the most common treatment given by RT. Any time oxygen is being used, the door to the room is labeled, "Oxygen in use. No smoking." Oxygen is measured by percentage, by liters per minute (L/m), or both. Most hospitals have a central delivery system with wall outlets in each room or each patient unit. A metal connector with a gauge is inserted into the outlet. The gauge consists of a glass cylinder marked at intervals with lines and the numbers 0, 5, 10, and 15. A metal ball floats beside one of the numbers when the valve at the top of the gauge is opened. The bottom of the gauge has a fitting for a bottle of water (humidifier) to be attached. A tube leads from the humidifier to a device that fits on the patient. Several devices are used: catheter, nasal cannula, masks, T-pieces, croupettes, and tents.

Catheter

An oxygen catheter is inserted into the nose to a length corresponding to the distance from the tip of the nose to the lobe of the ear. The catheter is attached to the nose with adhesive tape. The oxygen flow rate for a catheter is usually from 4 to 7 L/m.

Nasal Cannula

A cannula is a plastic tube with small prongs that fit into the nostrils. The tubing crosses the cheek and loops over the ears and under the chin to keep it securely in the nose. Patients find cannulas comfortable, especially those who need oxygen for long periods. Oxygen may be ordered as low as 1 L/m or as high as 8 L/m. Average is 2 L/m to 4 L/m. Breathing through the mouth does not decrease the concentration of oxygen enough to be significant. Some patients prefer cannula prongs in their mouth instead of their nose; but the doctor's permission is required.

Masks

- *Rebreathing* masks cover the mouth and nose and have a reservoir bag. This mask is used for concentrations of 60–90% with a flow rate of 6 to 8 L/m.
- *Nonrebreathing* masks have a one way valve as well as a reservoir bag. Oxygen enters through the valve, and expired gases go through another opening. This type of mask can provide as much as a 100% concentration.
- *Partial rebreathing* masks deliver the oxygen from the reservoir bag, and exhaled gases go through openings on each side of the mask. Oxygen concentration is from 50–95%.
- *Venturi* masks are used for low oxygen concentrations. This mask needs an adapter for humidity.
- *Aerosol* masks are used for moderate concentrations with high humidity.
- *Tracheostomy* masks fit over the tube that has been surgically inserted into the trachea through an incision in the neck.

T-Pieces

All oxygen delivery systems need some way to add moisture to the oxygen so the mucous membranes do not dry out. T-Pieces are used with endotracheal tubes and tracheostomy tubes to supply humidity. Some have an opening for suctioning.

Croupettes

Croupettes are tents used in Pediatrics which supply oxygen and high humidity. This relieves the congestion of **croup** (laryngitis).

Tents

A plastic tent covers the head and thorax. The tent is securely tucked under the mattress and closed across the abdomen by a sheet. Humidity is supplied by filling an ice compartment. Zippers in the side allow insertion of arms for care of the patient. This method is very seldom ordered but may still be used in small communities that do not have RT departments.

IPPB Therapy

Intermittent positive pressure breathing acts as a mechanical bronchodilator because it makes the patient breathe deeper. Coughing is more effective. Medications may be administered as aerosols to liquify secretions so that they may be expectorated. IPPB may be ordered as a one-time treatment to obtain a sputum specimen.

Humidifiers

Room humidifiers are square containers of water with an enclosed motor that sits on top and rotates a wheel in the water. The water is converted to a mist and sprays out into the room. By keeping the door of the room closed, the humidity reaches a high level. Some types of surgeries require high humidity in the room post-operatively so that secretions will stay moist and not cause an obstruction to the airway.

Vaporizers

Vaporizers look like humidifiers but have a heating element so that steam is produced. The humidity is increased, and the room air is warmed.

Nebulizers (Nebs)

Nebulizers are devices that reduce liquids or solids to small droplets. Medications are given via the mouth by inhalation and go deep into the lungs to the bronchioles. This is often used in conjunction with IPPB therapy. **Ultrasonic nebulizers** (USN) convert liquids or solids into small particles by sound vibrations. These devices increase the humidity more and produce smaller particles than the ordinary nebulizer.

Ventilators

Ventilators are machines that carry on the process of breathing when a patient cannot breath adequately. Types commonly used are the MA–1, MA–2, BEAR–1, and Forreger.

The way in which the machine operates is called the mode. Intermittent mandatory ventilators (IMV) use positive pressure during inspiration at a slow rate to allow the patient to regain control. Control mode works independently of the patient and does all the work. Assist/control helps the patient and *can* take over control if the patient does not breathe regularly.

The settings on a ventilator are usually written as follows with a number after each setting:

- V_T or TV—tidal volume, volume of gas exchanged during a normal resting respiratory cycle
- f or RR—respiratory rate
- FIO_2—fractional inspired oxygen, oxygen percent
- PEEP—positive end expiratory pressure
- CPAP—continuous positive airway pressure
- Sigh or sigh rate—how often a sigh cycle is used

A typical order for ventilator:

$$V_T \ 1000$$
$$\text{f or RR}—12$$
$$FIO_2—30\% \text{ or } .30$$
$$\text{PEEP}—8$$

Orders are usually changed following an ABG report. So when ABG readings change, expect a change in ventilator orders.

Incentive Spirometer (IS)

Various devices are used; all encourage the patient to breathe deeply. Some devices have three compartments, and the depth of breathing is measured by how high the balls in the compartments move as inspiration occurs. Other devices have gauges. Incentive spirometers are used for the majority of surgical cases to help expel the anesthetic from the lungs. The RT department teaches the patient how to use the device the day before surgery. The RNs supervise the use following surgery.

Postural Draingage (P/D)

Patients with chronic lung disease or those with lung infections need to drain the affected side. Automatic beds may be placed in Trendelenburg position, and the patient lies on the non-affected side. If both sides are involved, the patient lies first on one side and then the other. Secretions move up the bronchial tree and are expectorated. If an automatic bed is not available, the patient lies on his stomach crosswise on the bed with chest and head over the side of the bed at a 90° angle.

Chest Physiotherapy (CPT)

This treatment is also called **percussion** and is usually done simultaneously with postural drainage. The patient is in Trendelenburg position with the lung to be drained superior to the other lung. The hands of the RT technician are cupped as the patient's chest (lateral, anterior, and posterior) is gently slapped. The resulting sound is like that made by a galloping horse. CPT loosens secretions.

Suctioning

RT technicians are skilled in tracheal suctioning for patients who have abundant secretions and are unable to cough effectively. RT assists the RNs in this procedure.

TERMINOLOGY FOR PULMONARY FUNCTION TESTS

ERV, expiratory reserve volume—maximum volume of gas that can be expired after a normal expiration.

FEV₁, forced expiratory volume—amount expired in a one-second time interval following a maximal inspiration.

FRC, functional residual capacity—amount of air in the lungs after a normal respiration.

IC, inspiratory capacity—maximum amount of air that can be taken in after a normal respiration.

IRV, inspiratory reserve volume—maximum amount of air that can be taken in after a normal inspiration.

RV, residual volume—amount of air in the lungs after the most forceful expiration.

TLC, total lung capacity—amount of air in the lungs following a maximal inspiration.

TV, tidal volume—amount of gas exchanged during a normal breathing cycle.

VC, vital capacity—maximum amount of gas that can be expelled from the lungs after a maximal inspiration. It measures a patient's ability to take a deep breath.

Types of Tests

Pulmonary Function Test (PFT) includes all of the measurements listed in above Terminology, taken with different machines. The type of disability and degree of disability can be determined by comparing all the components of the test results of a normal individual. PFTs may be done with or without ABGs.

Spirometry measures the vital capacity. This test is often ordered as a Pre and Post Bronchodilator. The patient takes the deepest breath possible, holds it a few seconds, and forcefully expels as much as possible. After a few minutes of rest, a medication in aerosol form is inhaled and the test is repeated. This shows whether or not the patient benefits from the use of bronchodilator medication. The test may be ordered as bedside spirometry.

Ear oximeter is a machine that attaches to the ear and measures the content of oxygen in the capillaries near the surface of the skin. This measurement is comparable to the oxygen in arterial blood, and this test is a much more comfortable test for patients than arterial blood gases. Numbers flash on the screen of the machine and are recorded. Ear oximetry is frequently used for patients with chronic lung diseases.

CO_2 analysis may be done by the Endotidal CO_2 Monitor-LB3. The machine is connected to an endotracheal tube and measures the amount of expired CO_2, which is comparable to the CO_2 content of arterial blood.

In the ICU, a respiratory technician is constantly checking equipment, changing ventilator settings, giving treatments, and doing tests. Therefore, when you have an RT order, you need only to tell the technician of the order and complete a requisition. You do not need to call the department.

On the regular units, call the department for treatment orders. The department may not have a secretary, which necessitates paging for new orders. The order is given over the phone so treatments may be started. Once the requistion is completed, it is either sent to the department or placed in a special box and collected by the department.

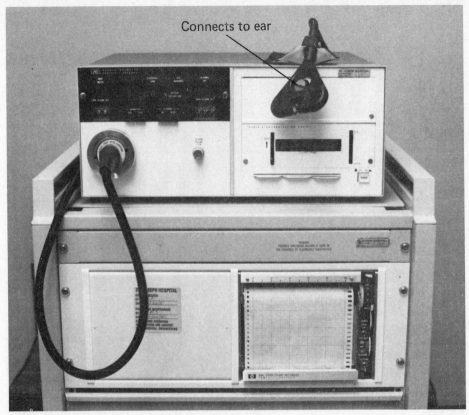

Figure 12-3. Ear Oximeter *(Courtesy of Hewlett Packard).*

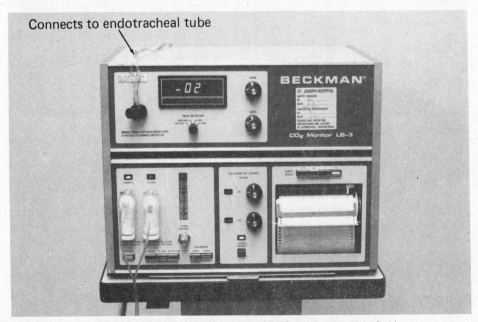

Figure 12-4. Endotidal CO$_2$ Monitor-LB-3 *(Courtesy of Beckman Instruments, Inc.).*

DISEASES AND DISORDERS

Nose

Deviated septum is an abnormal curve in the bony portion of the septum. This usually causes obstruction of air passages. **Tx:** Surgery.

Epistaxis (nosebleed) is caused by injury or diseases. **Tx:** Pressure on side of nose compressing it against the septum, local application of drugs to constrict blood vessels, use of cauterizing drugs to seal ends of ruptured vessels, electrocautery, packing of nasal cavity with gauze. The gauze may be saturated with medication or vaseline or may be inside a rubber finger cot. Any disease process that may be the cause is treated.

Fractures are caused by trauma. **Tx:** The cavity is packed to keep the septum straight, splints are applied to the exterior, cold compresses are applied to reduce swelling, and x-rays are taken to be sure realignment is correct.

Polyps, hypertrophied mucous membranes, cause obstruction and bleeding. **Tx:** Surgical removal.

Rhinitis is inflammation of the mucous membranes. The common cold is the usual cause; but it may be due to other viral infections or allergies. **Tx:** Treat the cause.

Sinusitis is an infection of one or more of the sinuses. The frontal sinus, above the eyebrows, causes a headache in the frontal area when an infection occurs. Infection of the ethmoid sinus (bone forming part of the septum and part of base of the cranium) causes pain around the eyes or in the eyes. Maxillary (upper jaw bone) sinusitis causes pain in the upper teeth. Sphenoidal (sphenoid bone forms anterior base of skull) sinusitis produces headaches in the back part of the head. **Tx:** Nasal swab cultures, antibiotics, antihistamines, vasoconstricting nose drops or sprays, moist heat. Frontal sinuses must be drained by surgery.

Pharynx

Adenoiditis (inflammation of the adenoids) obstructs the flow of air through the nostrils and obstructs the eustachian tubes. Serious complications may result if untreated. **Tx:** Antibiotics, surgical removal.

Peritonsillar abscess may develop after an infection of the tonsils. The tissues of the soft palate above the tonsils become inflamed and very swollen. **Tx:** Antibiotics, warm irrigations or gargles, incision and drainage if antibiotics are not given early enough to check the infection.

Pharyngitis (inflammation of the throat) may be caused by a virus or a bacteria. **Tx:** ASA for elevated temperature, ice collar for comfort, analgesics, throat culture to determine cause, antibiotics, force fluids, drugs to control cough, good oral hygiene.

Tonsillitis is a common source of some systemic infections. The infected tonsils give off toxins that are circulated throughout the body. **Tx:** Control infection with antibiotics and then surgical removal. Surgery is usually done in combination with adenoid surgery.

Upper respiratory infection (URI) refers to any of the numerous viral, bacterial, and chemical infections that cause a sore throat, husky speech, runny nose, and watery eyes. **Tx:** Try to find the cause, force fluids, prescribe antihistamines, provide humidity, provide proper diet.

Larynx

Cancer of the larynx carries a high cure rate if treated early. The cancer is found more often in men and has a tendency to run in families. Smoking is a predisposing factor. Hoarseness that does not go away should be investigated. **Tx:** Biopsy to verify diagnoses, radiation if one cord is involved, surgical removal.

Edema (swelling) of the larynx closes the glottis and cuts off the airway from the throat to the lungs. Allergic reactions or severe infections of the throat may cause edema. **Tx:** Provide airway by insertion of an endotracheal tube, treat cause.

Laryngitis, inflammation of the larynx, may be acute or chronic. Small children may develop an acute obstructive laryngitis called croup. **Tx:** Antibiotics if bacterial; vaporizers, corticosteroids for croup and croupette.

Polyps are growths of the mucous membranes usually caused by trauma from a strain. They may be due to overuse of voice during an attack of laryngitis. **Tx:** Surgical removal.

Trachea

Obstruction of the trachea interrupts air passage to the lungs and must be corrected. If a foreign object is lodged in the trachea and cannot be coughed up, a surgical opening in the neck with the insertion of a tube into the trachea may be necessary. The **Heimlich maneuver** helps prevent suffocation from choking on foreign particles, usually food. To perform this maneuver, position yourself behind the victim, wrap you arms around his waist, make a fist of one hand, and grab it with the other hand above the navel and below the rib cage. Press your fist into the victim's upper abdomen with a quick, upward thrust. This sudden, forceful compression of the lungs increases the air pressure within the trachea and ejects the object like popping a cork from a bottle.

Bronchi and Lungs

Asthma may be due to allergies or to infections. Either causes obstruction of air flow in small bronchi and bronchioles and results in periodic attacks of dyspnea with wheezing. Acute attacks of both types are treated with bronchodilator drugs, especially epinephrine and aminophyllin, Nebs with bronchodilator corticosteriods, fluids IV, and oxygen. Antibiotics are given if infection is present. **Status asthmaticus** is a state of acute respiratory distress due to a prolonged attack that does not respond to bronchodilators. These patients are given large doses of corticosteroids IV. Allergic asthma is treated by immunotherapy—skin testing is done to determine the allergens, and gradually increasing doses of the allergens are given by cutaneous injection at specific intervals for several years.

Atelectasis is a state of collapse; there is no air in the lung tissue. Pressure from disease or from obstruction may be the cause. Infection is usually present. **Tx:** Removal or treatment of cause, antibiotics, preventive measures following any anesthesia, surgical removal of affected portion.

Bronchiectasis may be congenital or acquired. Involved bronchi are dilated and inflamed. The alveoli of the affected bronchial branch are permanently dilated. Infection causes pus to collect in the alveolar sacs, and tissues are eroded. Hemorrhage may occur. The disease begins in the lower lobes and progresses gradually to other areas. Pulmonary function tests are of no diagnostic value; bronchoscopy and bronchogram are definitive diagnostic exams. **Tx:** Antibiotics, postural drainage, breathing exercises, bronchodilator drugs, surgical removal of affected area.

Bronchitis may be acute or chronic.

- **Acute bronchitis** usually follows a sore throat, and the tracheo-bronchial tree is infected. Cough is non-productive at first but progresses to production of mucopurulent sputum. **Tx:** Drugs to reduce fever and cough, humidifiers, force fluids, antibiotics according to sputum culture results, bronchodilator drugs.
- **Chronic bronchitis** can cause other lung diseases. Cough and sputum increase at frequent intervals, and the condition cannot be completely alleviated. **Tx:** Good nutrition, breathing exercises, prompt treatment of infections, humidifier, bronchodilator drugs.

Cancer of the lung is often metastatic. Primary lesions may be removed surgically if not of oat cell origin. Metastatic growths and primary lesions are treated with radiation and chemotherapy. The number of males with lung cancer used to be much greater than the number of females, but the female number is increasing as the number of female smokers increase. Primary lesions may cause the following complications: venous dilatations of the neck, face, and arms (superior vena caval syndrome); fluid in the pleural space; and central nervous system metastasis.

COPD or COLD, chronic obstructive pulmonary/lung disease, is a term referring to any of the long-term diseases of the lung that cause obstruction of the airway such as bronchitis, bronchiectasis, emphysema.

Cystic fibrosis is an inherited disease of the exocrine glands, the glands that produce secretions which are transported outside the gland directly, as in sweat, or indirectly through a tube or passageway. Pulmonary system involvement is the only part of the disease of concern to us at this time. The secretions of the respiratory tract become viscous (sticky) and fill the airway. The patient is unable to cough up and expectorate the sticky material. Abscesses may form. **Tx:** Antibiotics, ultrasonic nebulization to reduce viscosity, mist tent for sleeping, chest percussion, breathing exercises, mucokinetic drugs, suctioning to remove secretions, oxygen. The disease cannot be cured, and care must be constant. More males than females reach adulthood. Females are advised not to have children as the stress of pregnancy puts too many demands on an already "stressed" body.

Emphysema may be preceded by chronic bronchitis. The alveoli loose their elasticity and become enlarged, trapping air that the patient cannot exhale. The gas exchange is impaired, and CO_2 is increased. The lungs are constantly hyperexpanded causing a "barrel-chest." **Tx:** Breathing exercises using a flute-like instrument during expiration to increase positive pressure to exhale air in alveoli. If the instrument is not available, the patient may purse lips for the same effect. Regular exercise is important. Other treatments are Nebs or IPPB therapy with aerosol bronchodilators, prompt control of infections, chest physiotherapy, effective coughing techniques taught by RT, and oxygen at low liter flow.

Empyema is a secondary infection with pus in the pleural cavity. The infection may be from an infection of the surrounding area, from a chest wound, or from surgery. **Tx:** Aspiration of exudate with gram stains, aerobic and anaerobic cultures, antibiotics, surgical placement of a drainage tube kept in place until the cavity heals, breathing exercises. When infection resists treatment, surgical resection of the cavity may be necessary.

Hay fever, an allergic reaction, causes sneezing, runny nose, watery eyes, and wheezing respirations. Hay fever may lead to allergic asthma if not treated. **Tx:** Antihistamines, decongestants, skin testing so immunology injections may be given as explained under asthma. These are sometimes called desensitizing injections.

Influenza is an acute, contagious, viral disease. The muscles ache, the respiratory tract is inflamed causing sore throat and cough, and the intestinal tract may be involved with nausea, vomiting, and diarrhea. Pneumonia is a common complication. Persons with chronic lung diseases should be protected with influenza vaccines. **Tx:** Bedrest, force fluids, drugs to reduce fever, analgesics, humidity for respiratory symptoms, codeine cough medication, decongestants.

Pleurisy causes severe chest pain. The pleura is inflamed, and the layers rub together; this pleural rub is audible with the use of a stethoscope. Fluid may develop in the pleural space **(pleural effusion)** and is aspirated for cultures and cytology examinations. Pleurisy may be caused by pneumonia, other inflammatory lung diseases, tuberculosis, cancer, trauma. **Tx:** Treatment of the cause, analgesics and narcotics to control pain, x-rays to determine fluid level in effusion, aspiration of fluid with studies to determine causative agent.

Pneumonia has many causes. In pneumonia the alveoli are infected and become filled with fluid. Many types of bacteria cause pneumonia as well as viruses, fungi, and chemicals. Involvement of one lobe is referred to as **lobar pneumonia, bronchopneumonia** involves bronchi adjacent to the infected alveoli, **aspiration pneumonia** occurs when fluid is sucked into the lung during vomiting. **Pneumococcal pneumonia** is the most common bacterial type. **Nosocomial pneumonia** refers to infections acquired in the hospital. **Tx:** X-rays to show area of involvement, sputum cultures, antibiotics if bacterial, fungicides if fungus proven, blood cultures, force fluids, oxygen, analgesics, bedrest. Aspiration pneumonia requires suctioning of the bronchial tree. Patients with chronic lung disease should be given pneumococcal vaccine.

Pneumothorax means air in the pleural cavity. Traumas with a perforation of the chest wall or forceful trauma with rupture of the lung are common causes. Spontaneous pneumothorax indicates rupture of visceral pleura and is usually associated with pulmonary disease. However, it may also occur in healthy persons. **Tx:** Oxygen, insertion of a chest tube with suction expands the collapsed lung, surgical repair of wounds in trauma cases.

Pulmonary edema refers to an excess of fluid within the lung. Fluid accumulates in the alveoli and airways. If not controlled, a frothy fluid is forced from the mouth with each expiration. **Tx:** Oxygen, diuretics, IPPB therapy, alcohol by IPPB nebulizer if fluid obstructing airway. Treatment depends on cause. In cases due to congestive heart failure, treatment can include tourniquets rotated on all four limbs to reduce venous blood flow to the heart and morphine to decrease restlessness.

Pulmonary embolus means a blood clot traveling from some other site has lodged in a small artery of the lung. The deep veins of the legs may be the site of the original clot. Chest x-rays and scans aid in diagnosis. **Tx:** Oxygen, IV fluids, morphine or demerol for pain, anticoagulants. Patients who have repeated attacks of pulmonary emboli benefit from a vena caval filter which traps the clots before blood enters pulmonary circulation.

Respiratory distress syndrome (RDS) was formerly called hyaline membrane disease of infants. Prematurity is the most common cause. Breathing is labored, and lung volume is reduced. Etiology is unknown. RDS may be apparent at birth; if so, treatment starts immediately. **Tx:** Oxygen, IV glucose, electrolytes, and ABGs frequently as a guide to treatment. Intubation may be necessary in addition to the use of a ventilator. Infant should show signs of recovery in about three days. **Adult respiratory distress syndrome** (ARDS) is an unexpected, critical failure of the respiratory system. It may occur in an apparently healthy person. There are many causes, too many to discuss here, some of which are lung disease, shock, and drug overdose. Lung volume is reduced, breathing is difficult, and lungs cannot function well enough to oxygenate the body. Pulmonary edema may occur. **Tx:** Endotracheal intubation with ventilator, IV fluids, determination of cause, antibiotics if infection present. Complete recovery is possible.

Tuberculosis (TB) is infection of the lung by the tubercle bacillus. The disease spreads by sneezing and coughing, the droplets left in the air are inhaled. Saliva on dishes and silverware can also spread the infection. The Mantoux test is utilized to determine the presence of TB in the lungs. Tubercle bacillus extract is injected into the inner surface of the forearm, and within 48 to 72 hours, the reaction can be measured. If an inflamed area appears at the site of the injection, an x-ray should be taken. A positive result does not always mean active disease is present; a person may have been exposed to the tubercle bacillus, but the body destroyed the organism. The test is also called PPD (purified protein derivative of tuberculin) skin test. **Tx:** Specific drugs now control TB. The surgery that was previously done to resection the involved lung is no longer necessary.

Disease-Causing Organisms

- Actinomyces (fungus)
- Coccidioides (fungus)
- Hemophilus influenzae
- Histoplasma (fungus)
- Klebsiella
- Pneumoceptis carinii
- Pneumococci

- Proteus
- Pseudomonas
- Staphylococci
- Streptococci
- Tubercle bacillus
- Viruses

SURGERIES AND PROCEDURES

Nose

Caldwell-Luc surgery provides drainage of the maxillary sinus. An incision is made in the upper gum of the mouth above the canine and incisor teeth. This surgery is usually done in combination with a **submucous resection** (SMR) of the nasal cavity. The patient will have nasal packing with a sling of gauze placed under the nose and tied around the head. Orders will be for prn change of sling and ice across the nose to reduce swelling. The doctor will remove the packing in 48 hours and will need a suture set. You will need to know where these are kept on the unit.

Polypectomy is the removal of polyps. Nasal packing is used to control bleeding.

Rhinoplasty, the surgical repair of the nose, may be done for functional abnormalities or for cosmetic reasons. Nasal packing is used. All patients with nasal packing need humidity to keep the respiratory tract from drying out due to mouth breathing.

Septoplasty is the surgical repair of the nasal septum. Orders following Caldwell-Luc, SMR, rhinoplasty, and septoplasty are similar.

Pharynx

I and D, incision and drainage, may be necessary in peritonsillar abscess. A small incision is made in the center of the abscess and forceps are used to spread the opening and evacuate the pus.

T and A, tonsillectomy and adenoidectomy, are combined in one operation. Tonsils and adenoids are removed; no sutures are required. Ice collars prevent swelling. This is usually performed on children, so Pediatrics is probably the only unit caring for this type of surgical patient.

Larynx

Laryngectomy, removal of the larynx, is performed when cancer of the larnyx has spread to the area beyond the vocal cords. The entire larynx, the epiglottis, and some neck muscle with lymph nodes are removed. The extent of dissection depends on severity of involvement. When a laryngectomy is performed, a tracheostomy is necessary, and a permanent **stoma** (opening) is made in the neck to provide an airway. When healing is complete, the tracheostomy tube is removed. The patient must keep the stoma covered to prevent entry of dust, etc. The patient learns to talk again by esophageal speech—air is gulped and forced out of the esophagus to produce sound. Some patients become so proficient at esophageal speech that you may never realize they are speaking without a voice box. Mechanical devices held at the neck produce a harsh, grating sound. Progress is being made on development of an artificial larynx that could be implanted, eliminating the need for a stoma and giving a more natural speech.

A **laryngoscopy** is a visual examination of the larynx with a special instrument. A biopsy may be taken at the time of the exam.

Thyrotomy is performed when cancer involves only the vocal cords. The portion of the cord that contains the growth is removed. Temporary tracheotomy may be necessary.

Trachea

Tracheotomy provides an airway when an obstruction interferes with breathing or if surgery interrupts the continuity of passageways. An incision is made in the neck, the trachea is incised between cartilages, and a tube is inserted. Tubes are available in different sizes. The external portion of the tube has a shield around it with openings for ties which go around the neck to hold the tube in place. The tube has an inner cannula that may be removed for cleaning. Suctioning of secretions may be done through the tube. Patients cannot speak unless the tube is closed by use of a cork or by a finger being held over the opening. Before the tube is removed, it is corked for increasing time periods to make sure the patient has an adequate airway. Stitches may or may not be used to close the neck incision after tube removal. Usually, a small piece of tape will hold the edges together, and healing takes place quickly.

Tracheostomy is a permanent opening. When performed in radical cancer cases, a larger neck incision is made and the trachea is attached to the neck opening. There no longer is any connection from the mouth to the trachea. The tube is left in place until tissues are healed and then removed. The patient is taught how to protect the area and how to suction secretions through the opening.

Bronchi and Lungs

Bronchoscopy allows the doctor to view the bronchi and determine the condition of the mucous membrane, the degree of dilatation, and the amount of secretion in the lower tract. Exudate is usually removed by suction and sent to the lab for studies (bacterial, viral, and fungal) and to cytology for a cancer exam.

Bronchogram may be done with bronchoscopy. While the bronchoscope is in place, dye is introduced into the bronchial tree. X-ray films are taken and will show if any abnormality of the bronchial tree is present.

Lobectomy is removal of one or more lobes of the lung. The doctor will specify how to prepare the operative permit.

Pneumonectomy is the removal of an entire lung.

Segmental resection is the removal of a portion of a lobe.

Thoracentesis is a procedure done by the doctor in a patient's room. The patient sits on the side of the bed with arms on the overbed table. The doctor punctures the chest wall with a needle and aspirates fluid from the pleural cavity. Trays for this procedure are obtained from central supply. The doctor will also need sterile gloves, syringe, alcohol swabs, xylocaine or another local anesthetic agent, and an RN or LPN to assist and watch the patient. Fluid may be sent for bacterial and cytology studies.

Thoracotomy is the procedure of cutting into the chest. Operative permits may state, "thoracotomy with left lower lobe resection," for example. Chest tubes are used following chest surgery to equalize pressure and allow reexpansion of the lung and for drainage. The patient may have two tubes connected to water seal bottles, or a tube may be connected to an Emerson pump. The equipment is connected before the patient leaves the operating room, and orders will specify the operation and care of the equipment.

Cardiology Lab

Impedence phlebograph study (IPG) is done to show if any obstruction exists in the blood flow of the veins. It is useful in determining the cause of pulmonary embolus. The study is performed with a doppler machine.

LABORATORY TESTS

- ABG
- ACT
- AFB smear and culture of sputum, pleural fluid
- Blood cultures
- CBC
- Cultures of sputum, bronchial washings, pleural fluid
- Cytology of sputum, bronchial washings, pleural fluid
- Eosinophile count

- Electrolytes
- ESR
- PT
- PTT
- SMA-20
- Skin tests for:
  Coccidiodin (fungus infection of lung, also called Desert Fever, Valley Fever)
  Histoplasmin (fungus)
  Tuberculosis (tests such as Mantoux, PPD, and Tine)

RADIOLOGY AND NUCLEAR MEDICINE EXAMS

AP and L Chest show anterior, posterior and lateral views.

Bronchograms visualize the bronchial tree. Schedule the day before. NPO p̄ MN.

CT scan of the lungs shows all areas of the lungs. NPO for 3 hours prior.

Decubital views of the lung are taken when the patient is lying down.

Lung scans with ventilation and perfusion studies show defective circulation and gas exchange in alveoli. The order may be written "V/P Lung scan." Check with radiology for NPO orders.

Pleural ultrasound echogram shows the condition of the pleura.

Pulmonary arteriograms use dye to visualize the arteries of the lungs. Schedule the day before. Patient NPO p̄ MN.

Tomograms of sinuses and lungs give better views than flat x-rays.

Veinography of lower limbs utilize dye to show the veins of the legs; they are useful in determining the cause of pulmonary embolus. Schedule the day before. Patient NPO p̄ MN.

MEDICATIONS

Antibiotics

- ampicillin—PO—250 to 500 mg q 8 hrs
- Cefadyl—IM or IV—500 mg to 1 gm q 4–6 hrs
- erythromycin—PO—250 mg q 6 hrs or 500 mg q 12 hrs—give ac.
- Keflex—PO—250 mg q 6 hrs
- Keflin—IV, IM—500 mg to 1 gm q 4–6 hrs
- Kefzol—IV, IM—250 mg to 500 mg q 8–12 hrs
- tetracycline—PO—1 to 2 gm/d in 2 or 4 equal doses. Give 1 hr pc or 2 hrs ac. IM–250 mg q 24 hrs or 300 mg q 8–12 hrs. IV–250 to 500 mg q 12 hrs.

Anticoagulants

Anticoagulants prolong the clotting time of blood. Review those listed in Chapter 11.

Antifungal

These drugs inhibit the growth of or destroy fungi.

- Fungizone (amphotericin B)—IV—individualized dosage daily until fungus eradicated.

- Ketoconazole—PO—tabs ī daily until fungus destroyed.

Antihistamines

These drugs relieve the symptoms of an allergic reaction.

- Actifed—PO—tab ī or 10 cc tid.
- Benadryl—PO—25 to 50 mg tid or qid. IM or IV—10–50 mg.
- Chlor-Trimeton—PO—4 mg tid or qid.
- Dimetapp Extentabs—PO—tab ī AM & PM or q 8 hrs.
- Periactin—PO—4 mg tid.
- Triaminic—PO—tab ī tid. Syrup-2 tsps q 4 hrs.

Antitussives and Expectorants

Antitussives reduce cough. Expectorants increase cough efficiency by thinning secretions. All are given PO.

- Actifed c̄ Expectorant—2 tsps tid or qid. Not used for patients with asthma.
- Benylin Expectorant—1–2 tsps qid.
- Hycodan—tab 1–3 pc & hs. Syrup 1–3 tsps pc & hs.
- Phenergan VC Expectorant c̄ Codeine—tsp ī q 4–6 hrs.
- Tessalon-Perles—(10 mg) ī tid, up to 6/d.
- Tussionex—tsp, cap, or tab ī q 8–12 hrs.

Antineoplastics

Antineoplastics destroy or inhibit cancer growth.

- Adriamycin (antibiotics derivative)—IV only—individualized dosage q 21 days
- Cytoxan—IV—40/50 mg/kg given in divided doses over two to five days PO–1–5 mg/kg a day; maintenance individualized
- methotrexate—PO or IM—given for five days at intervals; dosage and schedule individualized

Decongestants

Decongestants shrink swollen membranes of the nose and relieve stuffiness.

- Afrinol Repetabs—PO—tab ī q 12 hrs
- Dimetapp-Extentabs—PO—BID. Elixir—PO—1 or 2 tsps tid or qid
- Neo-Synephrine—0.25% nose drops—2 or 3 drops each nostril q 4–8 hrs
- Novafed—PO—Cap ī q 12 hrs
- Otrivin nasal spray and drops 0.1%—2 or 3 sprays or drops each nostril q 8–10 hrs
- Sudafed (also bronchodilator)—PO—tab īī (30 mg each tab) q 4 hrs.

Bronchodilators

Bronchodilators open up the bronchial tree, reduce mucous membrane swelling in the respiratory tract.

- Alupent—PO—20 mg tid or qid. Aerosol Inhaler—1 or 2 whiffs tid or qid.
- Aerolone (isoproterenol hydrochloride)—by nebulization—dosage and frequency depend on severity of disease and patient's response.
- Aerolate (theophylline)—supplied in capsules. SR = 260 mg, JR = 130 mg, III = 65mg. PO—cap ī q 12 hrs. Type depends on severity of disease.
- Aminophyllin—PO—200 mg q 6 hrs. IV—250 to 500 mg in solution volume of 250 to 1000 cc.
- Bronkosol—nebulizer or IPPB—½ cc diluted 1:3—q 4 hrs or qid.
- Bronkotabs—PO—tab ī 4 to 5 × daily
- Isuprel—SL—10 to 20 mg tid. Nebulizer or IPPB—sol'n of 1:100 or 1:200, 0.5 cc diluted to 2 cc—4 or 5 × daily
- Metered aerosol inhalers are used as 1 to 4 whiffs tid or qid. Names- Duo-Haler, Medihaler, Metoprel, Nebair, Primatene, Proventil
- Slo-Phyllin—PO—tabs of 100, 200 mg. Gyrocaps of 60 mg, 125 mg, 250 mg; dosage of 60–250 mg bid, tid, qid per patient need
- Sus-Phrine—SQ—0.1 to 0.3 cc for severe asthma attacks
- Theo-Dur (theophyllin)—PO—200 mg q 12 h; dosage adjusted according to blood levels

Diuretics

Review those listed in Chapter 11.

Mucolytics

Mucolytics are drugs that thin secretions so that they can be expectorated.

- Alcohol—30%–50% as nebulization in treatment of pulmonary edema when fluid obstructs the airways
- Ammonium chloride—PO—0.3 gm qid with full glass of water
- Mucomyst—10% or 20% as nebulization—1–10 cc according to severity of disease
- Potassium Iodide (KI)—1 or 2 Enseals tid. Enseal = 300 mg
- Saline as nebulization—1 to 10 cc q 4 hrs
- Sodium Bicarbonate ($NaHCO_3$)—2.5 to 7.5%—1 to 10 cc tid or qid as nebulization.
- Tryptar nebulization—25,000 to 100,000 units in 3 cc NS 1–5 × daily

Steroids

Steroids reduce inflammation, swelling and allergic reactions.

- Prednisone—PO—given in large doses during periods of infection and then gradually decreased. Some patients may need a maintenance dose of 5 mg every other day for a long period.

- Solu-Cortef—IM or IV—supplied in 100 mg, 250 mg, 500 mg, 1000 mg doses, each patient considered individually for dosage. Used for bronchial asthma and pre-operatively for COPD patients who must have a general anesthetic.
- Vanceril Inhaler (beclomethasone depropionate)—2 inhalations tid or qid.

Other

Intol (cromolyn sodium) for inhalation only. The capsule (20 mg) is placed in a special spinhaler which punctures it, and the patient inhales the powder. Dosage is 4 caps a day to start, then reduce to 1 or 2 caps a day. If patient responds, steroids may be reduced or discontinued.

Specifics for TB

- Ethambutol—PO—15 to 25 mg/kg/d given with INH
- Isoniazid (INH)—PO—5 mg/kg/d up to 300 mg
- Rifadin (rifampin)—PO—Two 300 mg caps/d
- Seromycin (cycloserine)—PO—250 mg cap q 12 hrs

Vaccines

- Influenza vaccines are produced according to the formula established by the Public Health Service for that year. Protection lasts one year and only protects against specific types. Patients with chronic diseases should have the vaccine yearly; it is usually given in September.
- Pneumovax (Pneumococcal vaccine)—SQ or IM—0.5 cc—repeat every 5 years.

EXAMPLES OF PHYSICIAN'S ORDERS

Dx: COPD
Admission:

1. Lo salt diet
2. O_2 @ 1 L/m
3. ABGs before starting O_2
4. IV—½NS KVO
5. Aminophyllin 200 mg in 100 cc ½NS q 6°
6. Chest x-ray
7. CBC, UA, VDRL, SMAC, sputum culture

Next day:

1. Neb Bronkosol ¼cc in 3cc 0.45 NS tid between aminophyllin doses
2. Lanoxin 0.125 mg PO daily
3. Surfak 240 mg cap i̇ daily
4. Ambulate to tolerance
5. EKG

Next day:

1. Phenergan exp. ℥ii QID
2. Vibramycin 100 mg cap i̇ daily
3. Tranxene 3.75 mg TID
4. Dalmane 30 mg HS prn sleep
5. Old chart to floor please

Next day:

1. O_2 1 L/m at night, PRN for dyspnea only during waking hrs
2. Slow K tab ii Bid
2. DC phenergan
4. DC IV
5. DC aminophyllin
6. Slo-Phyllin 200 mg cap ii q 12 hrs

REVIEW QUESTIONS

1. Name the two gases that are exchanged during respiration.

   _____, _____.
2. An x-ray to visualize the sinuses would be _____.
3. What structure serves two systems? _____
4. Adenoids and tonsils are _____tissue.
5. The _____of the respiratory tract move secretions upward.
6. _____ is used to remove secretions when a patient is unable to cough effectively.
7. A _____is a machine that breathes for the patient.
8. The structures of the respiratory system are _____
   _____
9. The functions of the respiratory system are _____
   _____
10. List five diseases and disorders of the respiratory system.
    _____
    _____
    _____

11. Classify the following medications:

Benadryl _____

Sudafed _____

Aminophyllin _____

erythromycin _____

Mucomyst _____

Prednisone _____

INH _____

amphotericin-B _____

12. A lobectomy is _____.

13. A _____is often performed at the same time as a bronchoscopy.

14. _____ means cutting into the chest.

15. Laryngectomy is _____.

16. Explain the difference in a tracheotomy and a tracheostomy.

_____

_____

17. List five laboratory examinations relating to the diseases and disorders of the respiratory system. _____

_____

_____

18. An order reads "ABGs with patient on room air for 30 min." The patient is receiving O_2. How do you handle this order?

_____

_____

19. List four radiology and nuclear medicine examinations relating to the respiratory system. _____

_____

_____

_____

20. List three treatments performed by the RT department.

_____

_____

_____

Chapter 13 | The Digestive System

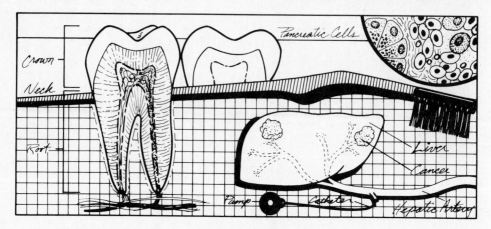

OBJECTIVES

Completion of study of this chapter will enable you to:

1. List the structures of the digestive system.
2. Describe the function of the digestive system.
3. List and define terms related to the digestive system.
4. List some diseases and disorders of the digestive system.
5. List some surgeries of the digestive system.
6. List and classify medications pertaining to the digestive system.
7. List some laboratory exams that aid in diagnosis and treatment of digestive system diseases and disorders.
8. List some radiology examinations that aid in diagnosis of diseases and disorders of the digestive system.
9. Transcribe Physician's Orders relating to the digestive system.

The digestive system organs form a long tube that extends through the body from the mouth to the anus. This system is sometimes called the **alimentary (nourishment) canal** or the **gastrointestinal (G.I.) tract**.

The organs of this system are the mouth, pharynx, esophagus, stomach, small intestines, and large intestines. Structures that assist the organs of digestion are the lips, teeth, gums, tongue, and salivary glands. The liver and pancreas are accessory glands with ducts leading into the main tract.

The digestive system breaks down food into nutrients that are carried by the bloodstream and the lymphatics to all the cells of the body. The food and digested food move along the tract as absorption takes place. The wastes are then eliminated as bowel movements.

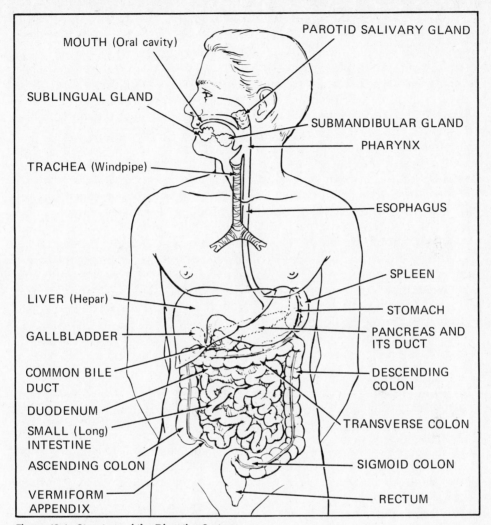

MOUTH (Oral cavity)

SUBLINGUAL GLAND

TRACHEA (Windpipe)

PAROTID SALIVARY GLAND

SUBMANDIBULAR GLAND

PHARYNX

ESOPHAGUS

SPLEEN

LIVER (Hepar)

GALLBLADDER

COMMON BILE DUCT

DUODENUM

SMALL (Long) INTESTINE

ASCENDING COLON

VERMIFORM APPENDIX

STOMACH

PANCREAS AND ITS DUCT

DESCENDING COLON

TRANSVERSE COLON

SIGMOID COLON

RECTUM

Figure 13-1. Structure of the Digestive System.

DIGESTIVE SYSTEM STRUCTURES

The **mouth** cavity contains the gums, teeth, tongue, hard palate, soft palate, and ducts from the salivary glands. The gums cover the bone that supports the teeth which grind up food by chewing (**mastication**). The tongue lies in the floor of the mouth and extends into the pharynx. The tongue is muscular, and its movements aid in chewing and swallowing. Taste buds are on some of the small projections (**papillae**) on the surface of the tongue. The lips form the opening of the mouth.

There are three **salivary glands** which secrete enzymes that aid in digestion.

- **Parotid glands**—anterior and inferior to the ears
- **Sublingual glands**—under the base of the tongue
- **Submandibular**—on the floor of the mouth anterior to the sublingual glands.

Digestion begins in the mouth as the enzymes are mixed with the food. **Saliva** (spit) is a combination of the salivary glands secretions and the fluid produced by the buccal glands of the mucous membrane lining of the mouth.

The action of the **pharynx** pushes food particles from the mouth to the esophagus. As the base of the tongue rises to activate swallowing, the epiglottis closes so that the food does not enter the larynx. The act of swallowing starts waves of contractions (**peristalsis**) in the esophagus that move the food into the stomach.

The **stomach** is an elastic organ with a mucosal lining that contains gastric glands. These glands secrete enzymes which act on food. Enzyme action plus peristalsis of the stomach converts the foods into a semi-liquid called **chyme**. Rennin, lipase, and hydrochloric acid (HCL) are enzymes produced in the stomach. The intrinsic factor, a secretion produced by stomach cells, is necessary for the utilization of vitamin B_{12} and certain proteins. Food leaves the stomach in about four hours. The upper portion is called the **fundus** and is guarded by the cardiac sphincter. The lower portion is called the **antrum** and ends in the pyloric sphincter. The greater curvature of the stomach is the **distal concave border**; the lesser curvature is the **proximal curve** on the border near the liver. The stomach is a reservoir for food and regulates the rate at which food empties into the duodenum.

The **small intestines** receive the chyme through the pylorus. There are three divisions of the small intestines:

- **Duodenum**—the first 10 inches
- **Jejunum**—the middle portion of about 7½ feet
- **Ileum**—last portion of approximately 31 to 35 feet and leads to the large intestines through the *ileocecal valve*.

There is a continuous flow of water and electrolytes between the blood and the intestines as food absorption occurs. The lining contains multiple projections called villi and microvilli which greatly increases the amount of surface area for absorption.

The **large intestines** are usually called the *colon*. The **colon** contains the bacteria necessary for the digestive process. The three sections of the colon are:

- **Ascending colon** extends upward on the right side of the body. The first part of the ascending colon is called the **cecum** which has an appendage called the **appendix**—a blind pouch.
- **Transverse colon** crosses the body from right to left.
- **Descending colon** extends downward along the left side of the body. The descending colon has an S-shaped section at the lower end called the **sigmoid**.

The **rectum** is approximately the last five inches of the colon. It is separated from the sigmoid by an internal sphincter. The **anus** is the external opening of the rectum and is guarded by the external sphincter.

The **pancreas**, an accessory organ to the digestive system, provides chemicals, enzymes, and hormones necessary for digestion. The pancreas is just behind the inferior edge of the stomach. The head is next to the curve of the duodenum, the middle section is called the body, and the tail section touches the spleen. The pancreatic juices flow into a duct in the center of the organ; the duct enters the duodenum from the head portion. The pancreas is also an endocrine gland and will be discussed further in Chapter 15.

The **liver** is important in digestion as well as in nearly 500 other activities. Located on the right side of the body under the diaphragm, it is the largest organ of the body and has a tremendous ability to regenerate. Some of the functions of the liver are:

- Forms, secretes, and stores bile
- Stores fats and sugars for release as the body needs them
- Removes wastes from the blood
- Aids in production of blood-clotting substances.

The bile goes into tiny ducts which lead to a main duct from the right side and main duct from the left side. These two join to form the **hepatic duct**.

The **gallbladder** lies on the underneath surface of the liver and is a storage bag for bile. Bile leaves the gallbladder via the cystic duct, which unites with the hepatic duct to form the **common bile duct**. The common bile duct enters the duodenum about three inches from the pyloric valve. The common bile duct is sometimes imbedded in the pancreas and joins the pancreatic duct.

Portal circulation refers to the flow of blood into and out of the liver. Blood from the stomach, spleen, pancreas, and intestines enters the liver through the portal vein, which branches all through the liver. Capillaries of the hepatic artery and the portal vein empty into the hepatic vein, which then empties into the inferior vena cava. Liver disease causes dysfunction of this system.

NUTRITION

Good nutrition is necessary for good health. There are four basic food groups you should have daily—**meat group**, the **milk group**, the **fruit and vegetable group**, and the **bread and cereal group**.

Foods in the meat group are meats, poultry, fish, eggs, nuts, dried beans, peas, and lentils. This group provides proteins, fats, minerals, and B vitamins. You need two servings each day from this group.

The milk group consists of all forms of milk, cheese, and ice cream. Adults need two servings a day; children and pregnant and nursing women need three to four. These foods provide calcium, phosphorus, protein, vitamin A, and riboflavin.

Fruits and vegetables provide vitamins, minerals, and roughage. Four servings a day are needed; this should include one dark green or deep yellow vegetable and one citrus fruit or fruit juice.

All breads and cereals that are whole grained, enriched, or restored and all pastas make up the bread and cereal group. You need three to four servings daily, which should include one cereal. All of these provide starch, bulk, proteins, vitamins, and minerals.

Calorie is the unit of measurement for the amount of energy produced by food in the process of digestion. Too many calories result in overweight or **obesity** (extreme fat on the body).

Proteins (Pro) supply the eight amino acids needed for growth and repair of body cells.

Fats (F) are a source of energy and essential fatty acids.

Carbohydrates (CHO) are starches and sugars, which provide energy.

Minerals aid in building blood, bones, and teeth and in the function of muscles and nerves.

Vitamins are necessary for proper use of food and for healthy functioning of the body. *Taber's Cyclopedic Medical Dictionary* contains a list of vitamins and their functions.

Dietitians utilize the above basic factors when assisting in patient care and in formulating daily menus. Many kinds of diets are needed to provide for all patients. Types of diets most commonly used are:

- **Regular**—a well-balanced diet, no restrictions, 2000 to 3200 calories
- **Mechanical regular**—same as regular except meats are ground, for patients with chewing difficulty
- **Soft**—restricted in fiber, composed of easily digested foods, 1100 to 2800 calories, for post-op patients, for patients with G.I. problems
- **Surgical soft**—same as soft with the elimination of milk, for post-op patients to prevent nausea and distention
- **Neuro diet**—ground meat, pureed vegetables, diced canned fruit, no clear liquids; for patients who are learning to swallow again
- **Surgical liquids**—clear liquids, no fruit juice; for post-op patients for a limited time only as it is nutritionally inadequate
- **Clear liquids**—consists only of coffee, tea, carbonated beverages, apple, grape, and cranberry juice, clear broth, bouillon, gelatin, sugar, and salt; for short time use for post-op patients and those with G.I. problems
- **Full liquids**—foods that are liquid at room temperature, strained soups, and strained cooked cereals; post-op patients progress from surgical liquids to full liquids
- **No added salt**—regular diet with no salt on tray, eliminates normally salty foods; for patients who require limited sodium, such as those with circulatory problems and some kidney conditions
- **2 gm Na (sodium)**—no salt in preparation of food, only three slices of bread a day, two glasses of milk, no salted crackers or normally salty food; for cases of edema and hypertension
- **Na restricted** (Dr. specifies amount of Na)—no salt in food preparation, for cases of edema and hypertension of varying degree
- **Progressive gastric diets**—Dr. writes number of diet he wants and when to progress (#1 for three days and #2 for four days, for example); for G.I. problem patients, especially those with gastric ulcer
- **Post-gastrectomy**—sugar limited, frequent small feedings; following surgery

- **Restricted gluten**—wheat, rye, oats, barley, buckwheat, and products of those grains are omitted; for celiac disease
- **Low residue**—elimination of foods that leave a lot of bulk after digestion, such as milk, whole grain products, some cheeses, nuts, seeds, coconut, and dried fruits; for patients who have irritation of G.I. tract
- **High residue**—regular diet with lots of fiber content food and vitamin B complex foods, used to stimulate peristalsis and improve muscle tone of G.I. tract
- **Restricted purine**—elimination or reduction of foods that produce uric acid, used for cases of renal calculi and gout
- **Low fat**—eliminates gas-producing foods, fried foods, and spicy foods; for gallbladder disease or patients who have trouble with abnormal amounts of flatus and for cardiovascular diseases
- **High protein, high carbohydrate (HiPro, HiCHO)**—used in diseases that cause loss of weight and chronic diseases
- **Low cholesterol**—elimination of milk and milk products, rich pastries, most cheeses, egg yolk, fatty foods, coconut and many meats; for heart disease patients and anyone with elevated blood cholesterol level
- **Giovannetti diet**—low protein, no salt, fluid restriction; for kidney disease patients
- **Hypoglycemic diet**—designed to maintain normal blood sugar level; specially for hypoglycemic patients (Hypoglycemia is discussed in Chapter 15.)
- **Diabetic diets**—five feedings, specific number of calories—American Diabetic Association (ADA) has diets for all diabetics; diabetes is discussed in Chapter 15.
- **Bland diet**—eliminates spicy and fried foods, for irritated G.I. tract

Remember that DAT means nothing to the dietary department; they need a specific diet. Be sure the entry on the kardex is DAT followed by a specific diet, which the RN can change as the patient's condition progresses.

- **Tube feedings** consist of blenderized foods, containing the nutrients of a well-balanced diet, or commercial preparations for use with patients who have a **feeding tube** (an NG tube of small caliber with a removable plug at the end) or **gastrostomy tube** (a tube leading directly into the stomach for feeding purposes). The doctor specifies the amount of calories per day. The RN and dietitian calculate the total amount of food needed, the amount of food for each feeding, and how often the patient is to be fed. Some commercial preparations are Ensure, Vital, and Vivonex.

TERMINOLOGY

Amylase—a pancreatic enzyme that acts on starches
Anabolism—the building up process of the body from food

Anorexia—loss of appetite

Ascites—an abnormal amount of fluid in the abdominal cavity

Bilirubin—reddish-orange or reddish-yellow pigment in bile

Biliverdin—the pigment that gives bile a green color

Calculus—a stone

Casein—a protein in milk

Catabolism—the breaking down of food into simple products for use by the body

Celiac—refers to the abdominal region

Chyme—the semi-liquid, partially digested food in the stomach and small intestines

Constipation—difficulty in having a bowel movement; the stool is hard and dry

Defecation—the elimination of wastes, a bowel movement

Diarrhea—frequent passage of watery stools

Distal—farthest away from the center of the body

Dysphagia—difficulty in swallowing

Emesis—to vomit

Feces—another name for stools

Fissure—a groove in tissue; this may be normal part of the structure or it may be due to injury or diseased tissue

Flaccid—a muscle has lost its tone and is flabby

Flatus—gas in the G.I. tract

Gastrin—a hormone secreted by the stomach, duodenum, and jejunum

Gastroenterologist—medical doctor who specializes in diagnosis and treatment of diseases and disorders of the G.I. tract and liver

Hematemesis–vomiting blood

Hepar—Greek for liver

Impaction—when stool cannot be evacuated; the rectum will be enlarged due to collection of stool

Ketones—acids produced during fat catabolism

Lipase—a pancreatic enzyme that acts on fats

Mastication—chewing

Melena—defecation of tarry stools

Mesentery—the part of the peritoneum that connects the intestines to the back portion of the abdominal wall

Paracentesis—the procedure in which a needle is inserted into the abdominal wall to withdraw fluid

Peristalsis—the wave-like movement of the esophagus, stomach, and intestines that keeps food moving

Peritoneum—the membrane that lines the abdominal cavity and covers the viscera of that cavity

Proximal—closest to the midline of the body

Ptyalin—an enzyme produced by the salivary glands and acts on starches

Pylorus—the area between the stomach and duodenum that acts as a gate-keeper because it ends in the pyloric-valve

Pyrosis—another name for heartburn

Sphincter—a circular muscle that opens and closes an orifice

Stoma—a surgical opening or mouth connecting a structure to the outside of the body

Trypsin—a pancreatic enzyme that acts on protein

Varices—dilated veins

Vomiting—the forceful ejection of the contents of the stomach through the mouth

DISEASES AND DISORDERS

Lips

Cancer occurs more often in persons who smoke, chew tobacco, or dip snuff. Sun exposure is also a predisposing factor. **Tx**: Surgery and radiation.

Herpes labialis, fever blister, is a viral infection. **Tx**: Drying agents such as Blistex.

Teeth

Cavities or caries are treated by a dentist. You may have consultations for dentists while a patient is hospitalized for the control of tooth pain or for tooth extractions.

Gums

Gingivitis is inflammation of the gums. This may be due to poor dental hygiene or a disease. **Tx**: Careful brushing, flossing, mouthwashes, saline rinses. A combination of table salt and soda for brushing is helpful.

Peridontitis is advanced gingivitis with loss of supporting bone. **Tx**: Surgery to clean out infection, antibiotics, intense dental hygiene.

Tongue

Fungus infections of the tongue and mouth may occur when antibiotics are used for a long period. A common one is thrush or moniliasis. **Tx**: Specific drugs.

Neoplasms are new, abnormal growths. The dentist is, many times, the person who notices neoplasms of the tongue and mucous membranes of the mouth. Regular dental check-ups are valuable for good health. **Tx**: Biopsy; if malignant, tx is surgery and radiation.

Salivary glands

Parotitis is inflammation of the parotid glands; it usually occurs in debilitated persons. **Tx**: Antibiotics, good nutirition. **Mumps** is an acute, generalized viral infection with parotitis. **Tx**; Bedrest, analgesics, sedatives, ice packs.

Stones may form after an infection. **Tx:** Extraction thru a duct in the mouth, removal of gland if frequent recurrences.

Tumors are usually of the parotid and usually malignant. **Tx:** Surgery and radiation.

Esophagus

Acholasia is a disorder involving the peristalsis of the lower esophagus causing a stricture. Complications are esophagitis, malnutrition, and predisposition to cancer. **Tx:** Bland diet, elevate head of bed, mechanical dilation, surgery.

Cancer of the esophagus spreads very quickly. The surrounding area is often invaded before the patient has any symptoms. **Tx:** Surgery if cancer in lower portion, radiation. Prognosis is poor.

Diverticulum is a ballooning out of the wall. Food then gets caught in the sac. **Tx:** Surgical removal.

Esophageal reflex occurs when changes in the lower esophagus result in dysfunction of the normal sphincter activity. This allows gastric contents to flow back into the esophagus. Inflammation of the esophagus (**esophagitis**) may or may not be present. **Tx:** Elevation of the head of the bed four to six inches; antacids; low fat diet with small meals; no tobacco, alcohol, chocolate, or citrus foods; no food or drink for four hours before bedtime; surgery if all else fails.

Esophageal varices are enlarged veins in the esophageal interior. They are due to a dysfunction of portal circulation which results in a reversal of blood flow and increased pressure in the veins. Portal hypertension may be great enough to cause rupture of the veins with massive hemorrhage. **Tx:** Use of a Blakemore-Sengstaken tube, which has a balloon to inflate and provides pressure on the wall of the esophagus to stop bleeding. Insertion of a nasogastric balloon with continuous irrigation of chilled, sterile solution may stop the bleeding. Surgery may be necessary. Recurrence is common.

Obstructive lesions may occur in iron deficiency anemia. Lesions are in the form of a web or a ring that interferes with swallowing. **Tx:** Mechanical dilatation.

Stomach

Cancer of the stomach may be felt by palpation before x-rays reveal the tumor. **Tx:** Surgical removal of involved portion and adjacent lymph nodes, chemotherapy.

Dyspepsia (indigestion) may be due to disease in the G.I. tract or be caused by disease of another system. **Tx:** Antinauseants, relaxants, bulk laxatives.

Gastritis is inflammation of the lining of the stomach. Acute gastritis is often due to food that is contaminated or to alcohol. **Tx:** Glucose IV until the vomiting ceases, antinauseants, bedrest. Chronic gastritis may occur in cases of uremia and portal hypertension. **Tx:** Easily digested food in several small meals, treatment of the underlying disease.

Hiatal hernia is an enlargement in the normal opening of the diaphragm through which the esophagus passes. The stomach protrudes into the thoracic cavity at times. Acid contents of the stomach are pushed into the esophagus causing damage to the lining. **Tx**: Elevation of the head of the bed eight inches, antacids, weight reduction, surgery if symptoms not controlled by other measures.

Mallory-Weiss syndrome usually is caused by excessive use of alcohol. Severe vomiting or retching for a prolonged period results in tears and bleeding of the gastric mucosa. **Tx**: Bedrest, antinauseants, sedatives, IV nutrition, ice lavage if bleeding is severe.

Peptic ulcer frequently occurs in the lesser curvature of the stomach but may occur in the duodenum. X-rays and gastroscopy exams aid in diagnosis. **Tx**: Specific drugs to control ulcers. Surgery is usually not necessary unless the ulcer perforates the wall of the area and causes a hemorrhage. Ulcers in the gastric area require surgery more often than those of the duodenum.

Small Intestines

Crohn's disease (also called regional enteritis or terminal ileitis) most often involves segments of the small intestines, although the inflammation can occur in any part of the intestinal tract. The inflammation is persistent and slowly involves adjacent structures. There are periods of quiet followed by periods of pain, nausea, and diarrhea. **Tx**: A low residue, high calorie diet, antinauseants, bedrest during acute episodes, IV nutrition if unable to eat, antibiotics if infection present, antacids, steroids, or surgery if no response to medical tx.

Enteritis, inflammation of small intestines, may arise from bacterial invasion. **Tx**: Antibiotics, IV fluids if severe diarrhea.

Gastroenteritis is an inflammatory process involving the stomach and intestines; it is usually acute when it involves food poisoning. Contaminates in food poisoning are most frequently salmonella and staphylococci. **Tx**: IV fluids, bedrest, antibiotics if infection proven. Isolation precautions (stool and tray) need to be taken for salmonella infections.

Gastroenteritis may or may not occur in **botulism**, a type of food poisoning in which toxins are produced. Home canned foods are the usual source. Neuromuscular involvement occurs quickly; there is dizziness, muscular incoordination, and difficulty in breathing. **Tx**: Antitoxins, ventilator, IV nutrition. Patient is in ICU and requires a long period of treatment. Fatalities are high.

Helminths are worms that infest the intestinal tract. **Trichinosis** is infestation by one of the round worms. Insufficiently cooked pork of diseased pigs contains egg cysts which develop when pork is eaten. The worms invade mucous membranes and embryos are carried by the bloodstream to all parts of the body. **Tx**: Specific drugs, steroids, analgesics for muscle pain. **Hookworm** is another roundworm. Eggs in dirt can be introduced into the G.I. system by dirty hands; embryos enter through the skin of bare feet. The worms that develop suck blood from the intestinal lining. **Tx**: Specific drugs, good nutrition, protein and iron supplements. **Pinworms** are common in children. Eggs are deposited around the anus by the female worm at night. The child scratches and hand-to-mouth contact causes reinfection. Contaminated food is the initial source. **Tx**: Specific drugs, daily washing of bed linen and pants, cleansing of the anal area each morning and apply an ointment to prevent itching.

Obstruction may be due to a hernia, a tumor growth, **intussusception** (a bowel pushing itself into an adjacent segment), adhesions, or damage to the nerve or blood supply. **Tx**: Nasogastric tube with suctioning, IV nutrition. Surgery is often necessary.

Paralytic ileus is a complication of abdominal surgery, kidney surgery, or back injuries and is a paralysis of the peristaltic movement. **Tx**: Enterotube with suction, Ilopan IM.

Colon

Appendicitis is an inflammation of the appendix. Pain may start in upper abdomen but localizes in RLQ. **Tx**: Surgical removal.

Cancer is usually not detected until late. Symptoms such as weight loss, weakness, and abdominal pain do not occur until the disease is advanced. Blood in the stool, detected only by laboratory exam, is probably the first clue. **Tx**: Surgery if involvement not extensive, chemotherapy, radiation.

Celiac disease (a childhood disease) is a chronic intestinal disorder with intolerance to gluten. This is thought to be an inborn metabolic error. Gluten is a protein found in most grains and some vegetables. **Tx**: Gluten-free diet. Rice, potatoes, corn, and cornmeal are allowed. This is a very difficult diet to prepare.

Diverticulosis refers to a condition in which sac-like protrusions appear along the bowel. These are blind pouches and become filled with food. If infection develops, the condition is called diverticulitis. **Tx**: High residue diet, bulk forming laxatives, antispasmodics ac and hs.

Ulcerative colitis is an inflammatory disease with ulcers in the colon. The patient has frequent stools that contain pus, blood, and mucus. **Tx**: Sulfa drugs for infection, bland diet with low residue and high proteins, vitamins, iron, sedatives, steroids, surgery.

Rectum and Anus

Abscess formation most often is located in the tissue around the anus. **Tx**: I & D.

Fissure is a tear in the anal canal or tissue surrounding the anus. **Tx**: Mineral oil or other stool softeners to regulate bowel habits, sitz baths, surgical excision.

Fistula is a sinus tract from the anal canal to the outside skin. Fecal material leaks through the tract. **Tx**: surgery.

Hemorrhoids, varicose veins, are internal if located in the rectum and external if located outside the external sphincter. **Tx**: Sitz baths, suppositories, bulk laxatives. Surgery if bleeding is a problem.

Peritoneum

Peritonitis is an inflammation of the peritoneum. The natural bacteria of the intestine cause infection if introduced into the peritoneal cavity. Most peritonitis cases occur following abdominal surgery, ruptured appendix, perforated peptic ulcer, or wounds to the abdomen. **Tx**: IV fluids, antibiotics, pain medication, oxygen.

Liver

Cancer usually originates in some other part of the body. Primary tumors have a rapid death rate and metastasize to the lungs quickly. **Tx**: Surgery if possible, chemotherapy.

Cirrhosis is a chronic disease caused by scarring of the liver. The function of the liver is impaired because of fibrous tissue and nodules. Causes include alcoholism, hepatitis, and chronic infection with bile obstruction. **Tx**: Diet high in calories with small meals frequently, vitamin supplements, antinauseants, diuretics if edema is present, withdrawal of fluid if ascites is present.

Hepatitis, inflammation of the liver, may be caused by drugs, chemicals, or viruses. **Tx**: Depends on cause.

Viral hepatitis is divided into three types:

- **Type A**—spread by feces contamination of clothing, toys, etc; this type does not leave lasting liver damage.
- **Type B**—spread by contaminated needles, blood transfusions, and other body fluids. Chronic hepatitis may result, and some persons become carriers of the disease.
- **Type Non-A, Non-B**—the A and B virus cannot be detected; this type can also lead to chronic hepatitis and is often spread by blood transfusion. **Tx**: Stool and tray isolation, good nutrition, antinauseants, rest. Gamma globulin gives protection to those exposed to Type A and sometimes to Type B.

Jaundice is a condition in which the bilirubin in the blood is increased, causing body tissues to have a bronze or yellow-orange color. The condition may be due to liver disease, hemolytic disorders, or obstruction of bile flow from the liver. **Tx**: Ascertain and treat the cause.

Gallbladder

Cholecystitis is inflammation of the gallbladder. Acute attacks may resemble the pain associated with heart attacks. **Tx**: Low fat diet, antispasmodics, analgesics, antibiotics. Surgery may be considered if attacks occur frequently.

Cholelithiasis is the presence of stone formation in the gallbladder. **Tx**: Surgery if the stones are producing problems.

Pancreas

Cancer usually occurs in the head of the organ and spreads rapidly. Prognosis is poor. **Tx**; Surgery, radiation, chemotherapy.

Pancreatitis is the result of autodigestion; the enzymes produced by pancreatic cells literally eat up the organ. Bacterial disease can cause infectious pancreatitis. Excessive use of alcohol may be a predisposing factor. **Tx**: IV fluids, nasogastric suction, drugs to reduce secretion of enzymes, pain medication. Antibiotics if infection present.

Disease-Causing Organisms

- Bacillus botulinus
- Escherichia coli (peritonitis)
- Salmonella
- Shigella
- Staphylococci
- Streptococci
- Vincent's bacillus

SURGERIES AND PROCEDURES

Gums

Full mouth gingivectomy (FMG) is done to clean out the infection of perio-
dontal disease. The gums are incised all the way around the mouth and infected
tissue is removed. The incision is filled with a paste-like material to allow healing
from the inside. Healing pushes the material out. Foil is placed over the teeth
and gums to prevent entrance of food particles. Liquids, full liquids, and soft
foods are eaten until the foil can be removed. The patient is in the hospital
overnight.

Tongue

Resection is performed for cancer treatment, usually in connection with a
laryngectomy. A feeding tube is inserted in the nose and into the stomach
before the patient leaves surgery. Good oral hygiene is important. Swallowing
and talking will be difficult and are not allowed the first few days. Frequent
suctioning is necessary.

Salivary glands

Parotidectomy is the removal of a tumor growth with the dissection of the
gland so that the facial nerve is not cut.

Esophagus

Biopsy is performed with the aid of an endoscope. The patient is observed
for bleeding following the exam.
Dilatation is a procedure to enlarge the area of constriction. The patient
swallows a thread, and a dilator is passed along the thread to the stomach. A
balloon attached to a dilator is placed in the stricture and inflated. This may

have to be repeated. Orders following will be to monitor the patient's vital signs and to report chest pain.

Esophageal resection is the removal of a portion of the esophagus. The stomach may be brought up into the thoracic cavity and sutured to the remaining esophagus. Plastic prosthetic devices may be implanted to replace the section removed.

Esophagomyotomy divides the muscle fibers at the area of stenosis and allows the passage of food into the stomach. This procedure provides good results for achalasia cases.

Stomach

Gastrectomy is removal of the entire stomach and duodenum. The esophagus is attached to the jejunum. Orders following may be CTDB q 2 hrs, oxygen prn, IPPB therapy, IV fluids. The patient will have to take Vitamin B_{12} the rest of his/her life.

Gastric reduction surgeries are performed for cases of **morbid obesity**, a condition in which a person has so much fat that it is life threatening. There are a number of surgeries: **stapling** is the process of reducing the size of the stomach by dividing off a portion of it with the use of staples; a **gastric wrap** uses a plastic mesh to encircle the stomach and reduce stretchability; a **balloon** may be inserted and inflated to give the stomach a feeling of fullness, thus reducing the appetite.

Gastric resection is removal of a part of the stomach, usually the lower three-fourths, with the attachment of the duodenum to the remaining stomach. IV fluids post-op and gradual return to diet are the usual orders. **Bilroth I** (gastroduodenostomy) is another name for the gastric resection of the lower stomach. **Bilroth II** (gastrojejunostomy) is removal of the lower portion of the stomach with the remainder sutured to the jejunum. The duodenum is left, and the end is sutured to form a stump.

Gastroscopy is the examination of the interior of the stomach with a scope. A biopsy may be performed at the same time.

Gastrostomy is a surgical opening into the stomach. It is usually performed for the insertion of a feeding tube when an intranasal feeding tube cannot be used for some reason.

Intubation of stomach and/or intestines is for the purpose of draining the contents of the G.I. tract or to decompress the tract. The tubes are connected to a portable machine called a **Gomco** or to a wall outlet suction. The common types of tubes are:

- **Levin tube** is a nasogastric tube of various sizes.
- **K-tube** is another type of nasogastric tube of various sizes.
- **Cantor tube** is an intestinal tube of about ten feet in length, size #18 French, and has a mercury filled bag at the end.
- **Harris tube** is an intestinal tube of about six feet in length with a metal tip next to the mercury filled bag at the end. This is used for suction and irrigation.
- **Miller-Abbott tube** has a lumen for inflation of the balloon at the end after insertion and another lumen for aspiration. It is an intestinal tube.

- **Salem nasogastric tube** is used for pyloric obstruction and has two lumen. This is sometimes referred to as a sump tube and has several holes along the tube instead of only one at the end.

Orders for tubes of this type specify the irrigating solution to be used, how often to irrigate, the kind of suction, and how much suction. Examples:

1. Irrigate NG tube with NS prn. Connect to low, intermittent Gomco suction.
2. Connect Miller-Abbott to constant suction. Irrigate with NS prn to keep open. Measure output q 8 hrs.
3. Clamp NG tube for one hr every three hours.
4. Clamp NG and give sips of clear liquids. Unclamp if pt becomes nauseated.

Pyloroplasty is the surgical repair of the pylorus to increase the size of the opening.

Vagotomy is the cutting of the vagus nerve which stimulates acid secretion. It is used for peptic ulcers in cases with excessive HCL.

Small Intestines

Ileostomy is a permanent opening in the abdominal wall to which the ileum is connected. The colon, rectum, and a small portion of the ileum are removed in ulcerative colitis cases. The stoma is then covered with an appliance. The

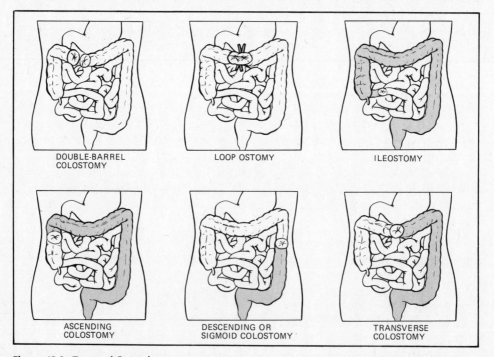

DOUBLE-BARREL COLOSTOMY   LOOP OSTOMY   ILEOSTOMY

ASCENDING COLOSTOMY   DESCENDING OR SIGMOID COLOSTOMY   TRANSVERSE COLOSTOMY

Figure 13-2. Types of Ostomies.

appliance may consist of a belt with a ring that fits around the stoma to hold a bag for discharges, or it may consist of a bag with an opening surrounded by adhesive material that sticks to the skin. Patients are taught by an RN Ostomy Specialist how to care for the stoma and appliance. The discharge of an ileostomy is semi-liquid and fairly constant in flow. Special care is needed so the skin around the stoma does not become raw and inflamed.

Resection of the ileum is a partial removal with the remaining sections sutured together. This may give some relief in Crohn's disease.

Large Intestines

Cecectomy is the removal of the cecum.

Colectomy is the removal of a part or all of the colon, usually a part, for ulcerative colitis.

Colostomy is incision into, sometimes removal of, a part of the colon with a stoma on the abdominal wall. Shaded areas in Figure 13-2 designate the part removed.

- **Descending** or sigmoid colostomy stoma will be on the left side. The stool is still formed in this type, and the patient may regulate evacuation time by an enema through the stoma if the doctor so orders. This allows a closed-pouch appliance and a little more freedom.
- **Transverse** colostomy stoma may be at any point along the transverse colon. Stools are usually semi-liquid and require full-time use of an appliance.
- **Ascending** colostomy stoma will be on the right side. The stool is semi-liquid, fairly constant, and irritating to the skin.
- **Double-barrel** colostomy is used to give the lower colon a rest in cases of inflammation or injury. There are two stomas. The one leading to the rectum is inactive. Post-op orders will refer to distal and proximal stomas. The colon can be rejoined and the abdominal wall closed after the colon is healed.
- **Loop-ostomy** is sometimes done as an emergency to relieve obstruction. Instead of making two stomas, the loop of the intestine is brought through the abdominal wall and cut for drainage. The loop is held in place by a plastic device. The colon can be sutured and replaced inside the abdominal cavity after the problem is corrected.

Sigmoidoscopy is the examination of the sigmoid colon with a scope. The patient is given enemas before the procedure. Trays are obtained from central supply. The medical unit usually has an examination room for such procedures.

Rectum and Anus

Fissurectomy is the excision of a fissure. Post-op orders pertain to dressing changes.

Fistulectomy is the dissection of a fistula. Post-op orders pertain to changing dressings or packing the wound.

Hemorrhoidectomy is cutting the hemorrhoid open and cleaning out the clotted material. No sutures are used; wounds heal from the inside out. Rectal packing is used. Post-op orders are for sitz baths and pain medication. Pack removal is usually done by the patient in a sitz bath.

Incision and drainage (I&D) is for the purpose of draining an abscess. The wound is packed, post-op orders are for packing removal.

Ligation of hemorrhoids consists of wrapping rubber bands around the hemorrhoid. This cuts off the circulation, the hemorrhoid shrinks, and the necrotic material sloughs off.

Proctoscopy is the examination of the rectum by using a scope. It helps determine any area of bleeding or any abnormality.

Liver

Biopsy is usually done in the patient's room. A tray is obtained from central supply. A special needle with retractable tongs is inserted into the liver, the tongs are released, and they grasp a portion of the tissue, which is withdrawn. The specimen is placed in a jar of preservative. The doctor will specify the examinations to be done. The jar with the specimen is labeled with the patient's ID and taken to the lab with a requisition. Orders will probably be for monitoring vital signs and applying a sand bag to the area for pressure to prevent bleeding.

Resection of the liver or lobectomy may be done to remove a diseased portion.

Transplants are the replacement of the liver with a liver from a donor.

Gallbladder

Cholecystectomy is the removal of the gallbladder. The operative permit may include exploration of the common bile duct. A T-tube may be placed in the common duct and connected to a drainage bottle. Post-op orders will specify how often to measure the drainage. Many patients ask for their gallstones, and the doctor will write an order to obtain them. You may also have a request sheet to be signed by the patient. The sheet is taken to the pathology lab where the stones, in a plastic bag with the patient's ID, will be given to you to take to the patient. Stones are various shapes, sizes, and colors. Some stones are different shades of green in a flat, square shape, and some patients make necklaces of this particular type.

Pancreas

Pancreatectomy is the removal of the entire pancreas, the lower stomach, and the duodenum. The common bile duct is connected to the end of the jejunum. The remaining stomach is connected to the side of the jejunum. This is usually performed in cancer cases.

Whipple procedure, or pancreatoduodenectomy, is removal of the head of the pancreas, the lower stomach, the duodenum, and part of the common bile duct. The jejunum end is connected to the remaining common bile duct, the body of the pancreas is connected to the side of the jejunum, and the remaining stomach is connected to the side of the jejunum below the pancreas connection. This procedure is used in cancer cases. Surgeries of the pancreas necessitate administration of insulin, a hormone produced by the pancreas and discussed in Chapter 15.

LABORATORY TESTS

- Calcium
- Carotene
- CBC
- CEA
- Cytology studies of tissues and fluids
- Electrolytes
- Enzymes:
  Alkaline phosphatase
  Amylase (blood and 2 hr urine)
  Gastrin
  LDH & Isoenzymes
  Lipase
  SGOT
  SGPT
- Feces:
  Cultures
  Fat, qualitative
  Fat, quantitative
  Occult blood (guaiac)
  Parasites and ova
  Pinworm exam
- Gastric:
  Diagnex Blue
  Gastric analysis
  Gastric analysis with Histolog
  Hollander test

- Glucose tolerance test
- Lactose tolerance test
- Liver function tests:
  A/G ratio
  Albumin
  Alkaline phosphatase
  Australian antigen (AuA, AA, HAA, HBAg)
  Blood ammonia
  BSP
  Bilirubin direct and total
  Cholesterol
  Lipoprotein electrophoresis
  Phospholipids
  Protein electrophoresis
  Total lipids
  Total proteins
  Triglycerides
- RAST
- Urine bilirubin
- Urine urobilinogen

RADIOLOGY AND NUCLEAR MEDICINE EXAMS

Some exams requiring dye or barium have to be in a specific sequence. Refer to your hospital's x-ray manual as this varies in different sections of the country.

Barium enema (BaE) visualizes the colon. The patient must be prepared so that the colon is free of fecal material. An Evac-U-Kit can be administered by the patient or by the RN if the patient is unable. The kit includes a laxative, directions for liquids, and a suppository for the next morning. You have to fill out medication cards for these. A special diet is required for the noon and evening meals the day before. The patient does not eat breakfast the morning of the test. The x-ray requisition is sent with the proper date for doing the exam. This routine is something you have to remember because the doctor writes only the x-ray order. If the doctor does not want the usual preparation, then orders must state that, the requisition states the same. Be sure the diet list and the kardex contain the diet information.

Barium swallow (Ba swallow) visualizes the activity of the tongue, pharynx, and esophagus during the swallowing process. The exam may be done without any preparation, NPO if doctor specifies. You complete the x-ray requisition and enter the information on the kardex. Take off NPO after the test, if that was ordered.

Barium burger swallow (may be written BB swallow or Ba Burger swallow) serves the same purpose as a barium swallow. The barium is placed in a hamburger patty instead of being a thick solution to allow the patient to swallow in a more normal manner. You may be responsible for ordering two hamburger patties from dietary when patient goes to the x-ray department or the x-ray personnel may do the ordering; this depends on hospital procedures.

CT scan of the abdomen shows any abnormality. The patient should be NPO for six hours. Schedule the exam with the scanning section, send the requisition, notify dietary and the RN responsible for that patient if the test is the same day, and enter the information on the kardex. Take the patient off NPO after the test. If the scan is scheduled for the following day, be sure to enter that information on the kardex.

Esophageal swallow is the same as Ba swallow and uses the same preparation.

G.B. series or cholecystogram uses dye to visualize the gallbladder. The patient is given tablets of dye with the special evening meal the day before the exam, NPO after midnight. You may have to make medication cards for the dye. If the unit does not have a file with directions for x-ray exams, the x-ray procedure manual on the unit explains the procedure. Be sure the x-ray requisition has the proper date. Inform the dietary department of the special evening meal and that breakfast should be held the next morning. Be sure the RN knows to give the dye and an entry is made in the kardex. The dye may be on the unit or may need to be ordered from the pharmacy. Following the test, take the patient off dietary hold.

G.B. and liver sonogram shows abnormality via an ultrasound visualization of the gallbladder and liver. You complete a requisition for the imaging section, call to schedule the exam (the department will tell you if there is any patient preparation), and enter the exam in the kardex.

Intravenous cholangiogram (IVC) uses IV dye to visualize the gallbladder and the bile duct. It is usually used when the patient is too nausated or too ill to tolerate oral dye. The patient is NPO after midnight; most patients are already NPO and have an NG tube so the exam may be done the same day it is ordered. You complete the requisition, enter on the kardex, and also enter on the diet sheet if necessary.

Papida scan visualizes gallbladder, common duct, and duodenum one hour after injection of a radioactive material. You probably will call to schedule the exam before sending the requisition. The department will give instructions for patient preparation. Enter the exam on the kardex and on the diet sheet if necessary.

Upper gastrointestinal series (UGI) visualizes the esophagus and the stomach. The patient is NPO after midnight. You complete the x-ray requisition with the proper date, enter on the kardex and on the diet sheet as a hold breakfast, and take the patient off dietary hold after the exam is completed.

UGI and small bowel series or stomach and small bowel series visualizes the stomach and the entire small bowel. The patient is NPO after midnight. Complete the x-ray requisition with the proper date, enter on the kardex and on the diet sheet as a hold breakfast. These patients will probably come back from x-ray with a note on the front of the chart stating, "Patient may eat, return to x-ray at (time)." You will notify dietary that the patient can eat, notify the RN in charge of that patient, and be sure the patient returns to x-ray.

Ultrasound of the pancreas shows abnormalities. You probably will schedule the test with the imaging section before sending a requisition. The department will tell you if any patient preparation is necessary.

MEDICATIONS

Amebicides

Ambecides kill amebae in the intestinal tract.

- Aralen—IM, PO—dosage calculated on body weight.
- Panaquin—PO—650 mg tid for 20 days.

Amino Acid preparations

Amino acid preparations supply the protein needed if patients cannot eat well or if food is not utilized because of a disease or disorder.

- Amigen—IV or central venous catheter—individualized dosage.
- Medamines—PO—tabs 10/d.
- Travasol—IV—individualized dosage.

Anorexics

Anorexics decrease the appetite for weight control.
- Dexatrim capsules—PO—cap ī mid-morning.
- Obestat long acting capsules—PO—cap ī mid-morning.
- Preludin—PO—25 mg tab ac tid.

Antacids

Antacids neutralize the acid in the gastrointestinal tract.

- Amphogel—PO—tsps ii or tabs of 0.3 Gm or 0.6 Gm between meals and hs.
- Delcid—PO—tsp i pc meals (½ to 1 hr) & hs.
- Gelusil—PO—tab ii or 10 cc 1 hr pc & hs.
- Maalox—PO—tsp ii to 4 or tabs ii to 4 one hour pc & hs.
- Mylanta—PO—tab i or ii or 5 to 10 cc between meals and hs.

Anthelminthics

Anthelminthics kill worms in the gastrointestinal tract.

- Antepar—PO—dosage per body weight—for roundworms and pinworms.
- Antiminth—PO suspension—per body weight—for roundworms and pinworms
- Povan—PO tabs—per body weight—for pinworms.
- Vermox—PO—tab i one time for pinworms. Tab i bid for 3 days for roundworm, whipworm, and hookworm.

Antibiotics

Antibiotics inhibit the growth of or destroy bacteria.

- Amikin—IV, IM—according to weight.
- Geopen—IV, IM—according to weight.
- Keflin—IV, IM—500 mg to 1 Gm q 4–6 hrs.
- Kefzol—IV, IM—250 to 500 mg q 8–12 hrs.
- Sulfa preparations are used before G.I. surgery. The type and length of the preparation depends on the doctor's order.

Antidiarrheals

Antidiarrheals reduce peristalsis and decrease the number of bowel movements.

- Cantil—PO—tab i or ii or tsp i or ii qid with meals and hs.
- Donnagel—PO—tbsp ii after each stool.
- Parapectolin—PO—tbsp i or ii after each loose stool up to 4 doses in 12 hrs.

Antiflatulents

Antiflatulents decrease the amount of gas in the gastrointestinal tract.

- Festal—PO—tab i or ii with each meal.

- Ilopan—IM—250 to 500 mg for treatment or prevention of post-operative distention. IV—500 mg mixed with glucose or LR and given slowly.
- Zypan—PO—tab ī or īī with meals.

Antinauseants

Antinauseants reduce or prevent nausea. Review those listed in Chapter 5 on page 105.

Antineoplastics

Antineoplastics are used for cancer therapy.

- BCNU (carmustine)—IV—individualized dosage.
- CCNU (lomustine)—PO—individualized dosage.
- 5-FU (5-Fluorouracil)—PO or IV—individualized dosage.

Antispasmodics

Antispasmodics reduce the painful contractions of the gastrointestinal tract.

- Combid spansules—PO—ī cap q 12 hrs.
- Donnatal—PO—tab ī or īī tid, qid.
- Enarax 5 and Enarax 10—PO—tab ī bid, tid.
- Pro-Banthine—PO—15 mg with meals. IM or IV—30 mg q 6 hrs.
- Valpin—PO—tab ī ac & hs.

Laxatives

Laxatives promote intestinal elimination.

- Metamucil—PO—tsp ī in 8 oz liquid daily to tid. Increases bulk.
- MOM (Milk of Magnesia)—PO—tbsp īī to 4 HS.
- Mineral Oil—PO—15 to 30 cc HS.
- Peri-Colace—PO—tab ī or īī or tbsp ī or īī of syrup HS—stimulates peristalsis and softens stool.
- Surfax—PO—cap ī daily as needed. Softens stool.

Specifics for Hemorrhoids

- Anusol ointment and suppositories—oint. has a tip for internal application as well as external use. Use q 3–4 hrs. Supp. bid or more often if necessary.
- Nupercainal ointment and suppositories-oint. into rectum bid and after bowel movements. Supp. ī p̄ each BM.
- Tucks pads—use as cleanser with toilet tissue, leave on area for 15 to 30 min. prn.
- Tucks Cream and Ointment—tid or qid locally or instilled in rectum.

Specifics for Peptic Ulcers

- Carafate (sucralfate)—PO—Gm i̇ qid.
- Tagamet (cimetadine)—PO—300 mg with meals and HS. IV or IM—300 mg q 6 hrs.

Steroids

Steroids are used to reduce inflammation.

- ACTH—IV—40 units over 8 hr period.
- prednisone—PO—40 to 60 mg/d.

EXAMPLES OF PHYSICIAN'S ORDERS

Dx: Small bowel obstruction
Admitted early AM:

1. CBC, SMA–20
2. UA
3. Flat plate of abd. STAT
4. IV fluids of D_5 ½ NS q 8 hrs
5. Miller-Abbott tube to constant suction (already done)
6. Phenergan IM 25 mg q 6 hrs for nausea
7. I & O
8. Irrigate MA tube with NS prn to keep draining

Same day:

1. Obtain permit for exploratory laparotomy with reduction of small bowel obstruction
2. Abdominal prep with Betadine scrub now
3. Anesthesia will write orders.

Anesthesia orders:

1. Demerol 75 mg ⎤ IM
   Atropine 0.5 mg ⎦ on call
2. Surgery scheduled for 5 PM.

Post-op Orders:

1. NPO
2. I & O
3. R/L at 80 cc/hr
4. Demerol 50 mg q 4 h prn pain
5. Compazine 10 mg q 4 h prn nausea

6. Kefzol 500 mg IVPB q 12 hrs
7. NG to intermittent suction
8. Cath q 8 hrs prn
9. TEDS

Next day:

1. Lytes this AM—call results to me.

Later same day:

1. Change IV to Isolyte M c̄ 30 mEq KCL/L. Add MVI amp i̇ to one liter per day.
2. Flat plate of abdomen, portable
3. Change Demerol to q 3 hrs prn.

REVIEW QUESTIONS

1. The function of the digestive system is _____
   _____
2. The digestive system consists of the _____, _____
   _____, _____, _____
   _____ and _____.
3. The large intestines are commonly called the _____.
4. The S-shaped portion of the colon is the _____.
5. The _____ and _____ are accessory glands of the digestive system.
6. The divisions of the small intestines are _____,
   _____ and _____.
7. Match the following terms with the definitions by placing the appropriate letter in the blank space.

a.	calculus	____	gas in the G.I. tract
b.	mastication	____	to vomit
c.	hepar	____	wave-like movement
d.	emesis	____	stone
e.	defecation	____	surgically created mouth
f.	dysphagia	____	Greek word for liver
g.	flatus	____	dilated veins
h.	stoma	____	chewing
i.	varices	____	bowel movement
j.	peristalsis	____	difficulty in swallowing

8. Define the following: (briefly)
   Esophageal varices _____.
   Gingivitis _____.

Hepatitis _____.
Crohn's disease _____.
Gastroenteritis _____.
Peritonitis _____.
Cirrhosis _____.
Cholelithiasis _____.

9. Classify the following medication:
Mylanta _____
Kefzol _____
Parapectolin _____
Antepar _____
Ilopan _____
Donnatal _____
Peri-Colace _____
Tigan _____
Tagamet _____

10. Fill in the blanks with the name of the department which performs the following examinations:
G.B. series _____
2 hr urine amylase _____
Occult blood, stool _____
Australian antigen _____
Papida scan _____
IVC _____
Ba swallow _____
CEA _____
BSP _____
U.G.I series _____

Chapter 14 | Urinary System

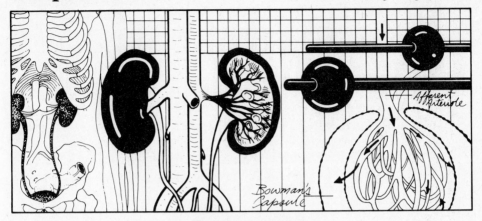

OBJECTIVES

Study of this chapter will enable you to:

1. List the structures of the urinary system.
2. Identify terms relating to the urinary system.
3. List diseases and disorders of the urinary system.
4. Define the types of dialysis.
5. List laboratory tests used in diagnosis and treatment of urinary diseases and disorders.
6. List radiology and nuclear medicine examinations that aid in diagnosis of urinary diseases and disorders.
7. List diagnostic procedures and surgeries of the urinary system.
8. Identify and classify medications used in treatment of diseases and disorders of the urinary system.
9. Explain how the location of the prostate gland effects the function of the urinary system.
10. List diseases and disorders of the prostate gland.
11. List laboratory tests used in diagnosis and treatment of diseases or disorders of the prostate gland.
12. List surgeries of the prostate gland.
13. Transcribe Physician's Orders relating to the urinary system.

URINARY SYSTEM STRUCTURES

The urinary system consists of two kidneys, two ureters, a bladder, a urethra, and a urinary meatus.

The **kidneys** are bean-shaped organs located in the retroperitoneal area of the abdomen at the level of the lower ribs. The right kidney is slightly lower than the left due to the space occupied by the liver. Each kidney is surrounded by a fibrous membrane, the **renal capsule**, that guards against trauma and infection. The outer portion of the kidney is called the **cortex**, the next portion is the **medulla**, both empty into a hollow space called the **pelvis**.

Nephrons are microscopic, structural units that fill the cortex and medulla. These units filter and help regulate the composition of the blood so that the chemical and physical properties remain the same. A nephron is composed of a long, tortuous tubule ending in a cup-like structure called **Bowman's Capsule** which is filled with a network of capillaries called the **glomerulus**. These capillaries branch into another network that surrounds the tubule. The process of filtering the waste products from the blood combined with tubular secretion results in the manufacture of urine. The urine travels down the tubules into

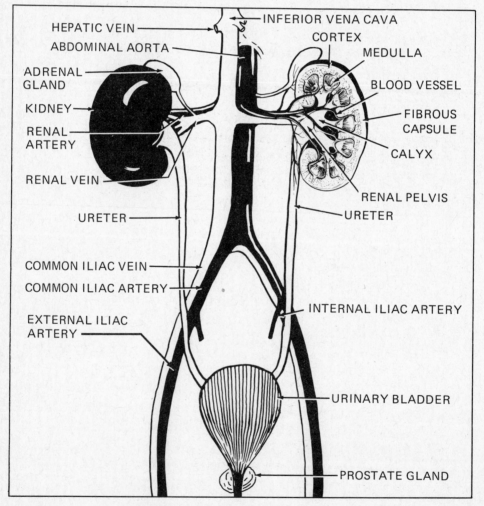

Figure 14-1. Structure of the Urinary System.

the kidney pelvis then down tubes (**ureters**) to the bladder.

The **bladder** is a hollow, muscular organ with great stretchability which serves as a reservoir for the urine. At the base of the bladder is a small triangular area, the **trigone**. The ureters enter the bladder at the base points of the triangle. The apex of the trigone contains the opening to the **urethra**, a canal that leads from the bladder to the exterior opening, the **urinary meatus**. The female urethra is approximately one and one-half inches in length. The male urethra is longer because it travels through the prostate gland and the penis to the meatus. Study these structures with the aid of Figure 14-1.

TERMINOLOGY

Anuria—absence of urine

Catheter—a tube for drainage of bladder, ureters, or kidneys. There are several different kinds of catheters.

Coude catheter—a firm, curved tip; used in urethral obstruction

Foley catheter—a balloon at the tip to be filled with water to keep the catheter in the bladder for continuous drainage. Types of Foley catheters are:

- **2-way Foley** has a lumen for the balloon and a lumen for drainage.
- **3-way Foley** has an extra lumen for irrigation.

French catheter is a straight rubber catheter for one-time catheterization.

Mushroom catheter has a preformed tip like a mushroom and is used for supra-pubic drainage.

Winged (Malecott) catheter has four parts at the tip, spread in wing fashion, for supra-pubic or kidney drainage.

UroSan is a soft external catheter for males; it resembles a condom.

UroSheath is a firm, pre-molded, external catheter for males.

Clean catch midstream (CCMS)—a specimen collected after the urinary meatus and surrounding area are cleansed with an antiseptic solution. The first part of the voiding is discarded, then the patient voids directly into the sterile container. Mark the requisition CCMS.

Closed drainage or dependent drainage (CD, DD) refers to one continuous line from the catheter to the drainage bag; the bag empties at the bottom.

Dysuria—painful or difficult urination

Glucosuria or glycosuria—an abnormal amount of sugar in the urine

Hematuria—blood in the urine; RBCs can be seen when urinalysis is performed

Hemoglobinuria—minute traces of hemoglobin in the urine; there are no red blood cells

Hemonephrosis—blood in the pelvis of the kidney

Incontinence—inablity to control the elimination of urine

Micturition—voluntary emptying of the bladder, voiding, urination

Oliguria—scanty urine

Polyuria—excessive secretion of urine
Pyuria—pus in the urine; WBCs found on urinalysis
Renal—refers to kidney; from the Latin word *renalis*
Retention—inability to expel urine from the bladder
Suppression—the complete failure of the natural production of urine
Toomey syringe—used to evacuate clots from the bladder.

DIALYSIS

Dialysis means a process for filtering wastes from the blood by some means other than the kidneys. It is used in kidney diseases or when another disease process causes dysfunction in the kidneys.

Peritoneal dialysis is used in non-emergency cases. A needle is placed in the peritoneal cavity, and fluid is introduced by a drip method similar to an IV drip. The specified amount of fluid remains in the cavity for 30 to 45 minutes and is then drained from the cavity. The instillation and drainage process is repeated until blood chemistries return to normal.

Hemodialysis requires uses of an artificial kidney machine. A vein and an artery in the forearm are connected to form a fistula. Needles are placed in the fistula and attached to tubing that carries all the blood from the body to the machine and circulates it so that the wastes are removed. The blood is then returned to the body. This is a continuous flow process and takes from four to seven hours. The frequency of the procedure depends on the severity of the disease; it could be every other day, twice weekly, or three times weekly. If a patient is scheduled for hemodialysis and laboratory blood work for the same day, the blood for the lab is drawn when the patient is connected to the machine. Lab requisitions go to the dialysis unit with the patient instead of to the laboratory.

Continuous ambulatory peritoneal dialysis, CAPD, can be used for some patients with chronic disease. Plastic containers for the fluid and collection are worn around the body so the patient may be active. Fluid bottles are easily changed. The biggest problem with this procedure is infection around the needle insertion site.

DISEASES AND DISORDERS

Glomerulonephritis, or Bright's disease, is the inflammation of the glomeruli and can be acute or chronic.

- In the *acute* disease, the glomeruli, tubules, blood vessels, and supporting tissue are seriously damaged and partially destroyed by an inflammatory process that usually originated in some other area of the body. Most cases are the result of streptococcus infections of the throat. **Tx**: Bedrest, antibiotics, diet low in protein and sodium, limited fluid intake, accurate I&O, and digitalis and oxygen if pulmonary edema and arterial hypertension develop.
- The *chronic* form may be present for a long time but show no symptoms and can occur without any apparent relation to an infection. An elevated blood pressure may be the first sign. **Tx**: Treatment of symptoms as they arise, antihypertensive drugs, antibiotics if infection present, and a high protein diet if BUN normal.

Acute renal failure is a sudden, severe reduction of renal function resulting from damage to the kidneys. Damage may be from physical injury, disease, poisoning, or the transfusion of mismatched blood. **Tx**: Dialysis; fluid restriction; diet low in Na, K, and protein; diuretics; daily weights; reverse isolation if needed to guard against infection.

Pyelitis is the inflammation of the kidney pelvis. **Tx**: Urine cultures to identify bacteria, antibiotics, and forced fluids.

Pyelonephritis is the inflammation of the pelvis and kidney tissue. **Tx**: Bedrest, identification of infection, antibiotics, kidney drainage, surgery in extreme cases.

Polycystic disease causes gradual degeneration of the kidneys with multiple cyst formation and is an inherited disease. **Tx**: According to symptoms. Dialysis keeps the patient alive for many years.

Nephroptosis, or floating kidney, is a downward displacement of the kidney due to an insufficient fat pad around the kidney. It may cause kinking or obstruction of the ureters. **Tx**: Surgery.

Nephrotic syndrome applies to renal disease, from any cause, that produces massive edema, excess protein in urine, and elevated cholesterol and lipids. **Tx**: Identify underlying cause and treat accordingly. Diuretics and low Na diet help reduce edema. KCL is needed to replace the potassium loss from diuretics.

Uremia is advanced renal insufficiency with wastes being retained in the blood. It can be produced by all types of kidney disease. **Tx**: Determination of specific cause, special diet, diuretics, antihypertensives, dialysis, and a kidney transplant if the disease cannot be controlled.

Stones or calculi may be in the kidney, the pelvis, the ureter, or the bladder. Stones are composed of either uric acid, calcium phosphate, or calcium oxalate. **Tx**: IVP to locate stone; forced fluids; straining of all urine; pain medication; x-ray refraction of stone, if it is recovered to identify cause; surgery if stone causes obstruction.

Cystitis is the inflammation of the bladder. The infection usually ascends through the urethra. Females are more prone to cystitis because of the short urethra. **Tx**: Forced fluids, identification of infection, antibiotics, antispasmodics, and analgesics.

Neurogenic bladder is a dysfunction of the bladder due to nerve injury caused by congenital abnormalities or injury or disease of the brain, spinal cord, or local nerves of bladder and urethra. **Tx**: Drainage of bladder by catheter or use of external catheter, bladder training exercises, urinary diversion surgery in some cases.

Neoplasms are new and abnormal tissue.

- **Wilm's tumor** is an adenosarcoma that occurs in the fetus but may not show symptoms for years. Usually a mass is discovered on physical examination, and IVP shows a mass. **Tx**: Surgery to remove kidney, chemotherapy with Dactinomycin, and radiation therapy.
- **Carcinoma of the kidney** occurs more often in males. IVP reveals the mass, and urinary cytology discloses the malignant cells. **Tx**: Radical nephrectomy with regional node dissection, chemotherapy, and radiation therapy.
- **Carcinoma of the bladder** is diagnosed by cystoscopy and biopsy. **Tx**: Surgical resection if tumor is superficial; cystectomy with urinary diversion if tumor is in the bladder wall; radiation therapy, and instillation of radium seeds.

Disease-Causing Organisms

- E. coli
- Klebsiella
- Proteus
- Pseudomonas
- Staph. aureus
- Strep. faecalis

SURGERIES AND PROCEDURES

Cystometrograms use a cystoscopic instrument to measure the capacity of the bladder and its reaction to pressure and then records the measurements on a graph.

Cystoscopy is the examination of the bladder interior with a scope while the patient is under anesthesia.

Cystoscopy with basket removal uses a cystoscopic instrument to introduce a wire basket beyond a stone. The basket opens and envelops the stone so it can be withdrawn.

Cystourethroscopic exams determine the degree of bladder outlet obstruction.

Ileal conduit (ureteroileostomy) is a surgical procedure in which the bladder is removed, and a pouch is made from a portion of the ileum. The ureters are attached to the pouch, and one end of the pouch is connected to an opening in the abdominal wall forming a stoma. A bag is worn over the stoma.

Kidney biopsy consists of removing a small piece of tissue for study in the pathology lab.

Kidney transplant is when a kidney is taken from one person and implanted into another person. The donor must have extensive tests for blood and tissue compatibility. A member of the immediate family is preferred as a donor.

Nephrectomy is the surgical removal of a kidney.

Nephrotomy is the surgical incision of the kidney for stone removal, drainage of an abscess, or other reason.

Urinary diversion or ureterosigmoidostomy may be done in cancer of the bladder. The bladder is removed and the ureters are connected to the sigmoid so that urine is eliminated via the rectum.

Urinary undiversion is used to correct congenital deformities or obstructions that cause a shortening of the ureters. A pouch is made from a portion of the ileum and connected to the bladder and the ureters are connected to the top of the pouch.

LABORATORY TESTS

- Albumin, blood and urine
- Blood urea nitrogen (BUN)
- Calcium (Ca), blood and urine
- CBC
- Cholesterol
- Creatinine
- Creatinine clearance, blood and 24 hr urine
- Magnesium, blood and urine
- Osmolality, urine
- pH, blood and urine
- Phenylsulfonphthalein (PSP)
- Potassium (K)
- Protein, urine
- Sodium (Na)
- Urea clearance, 24 hr urine
- Urine culture

RADIOLOGY AND NUCLEAR MEDICINE EXAMS

CT scan visualizes tumors and abnormalities.

Cystogram is a series of films which show the interior of the bladder and the voiding process after a catheter is inserted and dye is introduced into the bladder.

Intravenous pyelogram (IVP) or *intravenous cystogram* (IVC) uses an intravenous dye to visualize the kidneys, ureters, and bladder. The patient is usually given a laxative the evening before and liquids for breakfast. It can be done without any preparation.

KUB is a flat plate x-ray showing the kidneys, ureters, and bladder.

Renal arteriography outlines the circulation of the kidney.

Renogram uses radioactive iodine intravenously. The rate at which the iodine reaches the kidneys and is excreted is evaluated.

Renoscan uses radioactive mercury with the diuretic Neohydrin to visualize the kidneys; abnormalities such as tumors do not take up the dye so they show as solid spaces instead of the usual dots.

Retrograde pyelogram visualizes the drainage process during a cystoscopic exam by inserting catheters into the ureters and injecting dye into the ureters.

MEDICATIONS

Analgesics

- Pyridium—PO—200 mg tid c̄ meals. Urine turns reddish-orange.

Analgesic and antibacterials

- Azotrex—PO—Cap ī or īī qid. Given on empty stomach.
- Hiprex—PO—Tab ī (1.0 Gm) bid.
- Mandelamine—PO—1 Gm qid p̄ meals and HS.
- NegGram—PO—1 Gm qid for 1–2 weeks then 0.5 Gm qid.
- Urised—PO—Tab īī qid. Turns urine blue.

Antibiotics

- ampicillin—PO—500 mg q 6 hrs.
- Bactrim (co-trimoxazole)—PO—Tab īī q 12 hrs.
- Gantrisin (sulfisoxazole)—PO—2 to 4 Gm once then 1 to 2 Gm q 6 hrs.
- Garamycin (gentamicin)—IM, IV—1 mg|Kg q 8 hrs.
- Keflex—PO—250 mg q 6 hrs.
- Keflin—IM, IV—1 to 2 Gm q 6 hrs.
- Kefzol—IM, IV—250 to 500 mg q 8 or 12 hrs.
- Septra—PO—Tab īī q 12 hrs.
- Septra DS—PO—Tab ī q 12 hrs.

Antispasmodics

These relieve painful muscle contractions of the urinary tract.

- Cystospaz—PO—Tab īī qid.
- Cystospaz-M—PO Cap ī q 12 hrs.
- Cystospaz SR—PO—Cap ī q 12 hrs.
- Pyridium-Plus—Tab ī pc & HS. Turns urine reddish-orange.
- Pro-Banthine—PO—15 mg c̄ meals.
- Urispas—PO—Tab ī or īī tid or qid. Tab = 100 mg.

Others

- Prednisone—a corticosteroid used in individualized doses following kidney transplant

- Cyclosporin A—may be used after a transplant to help reduce the amount of prednisone required
- Imuran—an immunosuppressive given before and after a transplant to prevent rejection.

EXAMPLES OF PHYSICIAN'S ORDERS

Dx: Hematuria

1. NPO p MN
2. Shave and prep groin for cystoscopy and transurethral bladder biopsy.
3. Elastic hose pre and post op
4. Have patient sign permit for cystoscopy and transurethral biopsy of bladder tumor.

(Pre-op orders by anesthesiology)

Post-op orders:

1. VS q 15 min ×2, q 30 min ×2, qh ×2, then q 4h
2. Up ad lib this pm
3. Reg diet when over anesthesia
4. I & O
5. Tetracycline 250 mg IM now and 500 mg PO q 6h
6. IV fluids of $D_5/\frac{1}{4}NS$ at 125 cc/h first 4h then 100 cc/h
7. MOM 30 cc prn constipation
8. Dalmane 30 mg PO HS prn sleep
9. Tylenol #3 Tabs ī or īī prn q 3h for pain.
10. Foley to DD
11. Irrigate Foley q 1h and prn blood clots

Dx: Kidney stone

1. IVP ASAP
2. Demerol 50–75 mg IM q 3–4 prn pain
3. Up ad lib
4. DAT
5. Strain all urine
6. If stone recovered, send for x-ray refraction.
7. FF

Dx: Uremia

1. Restrict fluid to 600 cc/24h.
2. Low Na, K, protein diet
3. Daily Na, K, BUN, Cr
4. Daily weight

5. Accurate I & O
6. Send to dialysis Mon, Wed, Fri.
7. BR c̄ BRP

THE PROSTATE GLAND

The prostate gland is a part of the reproductive system but is discussed here, in part, because of the problems it causes the urinary system. The prostate gland is the size of a chestnut and fits around the urethra, just below the bladder neck, like a doughnut. The first inch or so of the urethra passes through the gland. If any swelling of the gland occurs, the gland protrudes into the urethra and blocks the flow of urine. The prostate gland is often called the "trouble-maker."

Diseases and Disorders

Prostatitis is an inflammation or infection of the prostate gland. An acute attack blocks the flow of urine. **Tx**: Catheterization, culture urine and prostatic secretions, antibiotics if infection proven, force fluids, bedrest. Surgery may be required after the swelling is reduced. **Chronic prostatitis** causes difficulty in voiding. **Tx**: Culture prostatic secretions, periodic prostatic massages, hot sitz baths, enzyme such as ananase.

Benign prostatic hypertrophy (BPH) occurs most often after the age of 50. The gland becomes enlarged and obstructs the flow of the urine. **Tx**: Surgery.

Cancer of the prostate is the most common malignant tumor of men over 65 years of age. **Tx**: Surgery if diagnosed early and the growth is localized. If inoperable, estrogen therapy, prednisone and radiation therapy are used.

Laboratory Exams

- Urine culture
- Prostatic secretion culture
- Acid phosphatase

Surgeries

Perineal prostatectomy is the removal of the prostate through an incision in the perineum.

Retropubic prostatectomy (RPP) is the removal of the prostate through a low abdominal incision between the pubic arch and the bladder so that the bladder is not entered.

Suprapubic prostatectomy (SPP) is the removal of the prostate via an abdominal incision for entry into the bladder. The patient will have a suprapubic catheter as well as a 2-way Foley.

Transurethral resection (TUR or TURP) is the removal of the prostate gland enlargement by cauterization with an instrument introduced through the urethra. The patient usually has a 3-way Foley with continuous bladder irrigation until the bleeding stops.

EXAMPLES OF PHYSICIAN'S ORDERS

Dx: BPH c̄ urinary retention

1. Insert Foley, connect to DD.
2. Demerol 75 mg IM q 4 hrs prn pain
3. Permit for cystoscopy and transurethral resection of the prostate
4. T&X for 2 U blood
(Anesthesia pre-op orders would follow)

Post-op: (next day)

1. Continuous irrigation c̄ NS at rate to keep urine clear
2. Hand irrigate for clots
3. I & O
4. DAT post anesthesia
5. Demerol 75 mg q 3–4 hrs prn pain
6. Pro-banthine 15 mg q 4–6h prn bladder spasms
7. D5/LR at 100 cc/h till taking fluids well
8. Colace 50 mg bid
9. Routine Foley care qid (This means that four times a day the meatal opening and the catheter at the opening is cleansed with an antiseptic and coated with a bacteriocidal ointment such as Neosporin. Each doctor usually has his own particular routine orders for this. When cath care is ordered be sure you order supplies if that is necessary.)
10. Dalmane 30 mg HS prn sleep.

1st post-op day:

1. Up in chair. Ambulate this PM

2nd post-op day: (if urine is clear and patient doing well)

1. DC irrigation. Hand irrigate if necessary.
2. Force fluids.

3rd post-op day:

1. Irrigate cath well and remove.
2. 3 bottle urine (This is not a lab test. The nurse gives the patient three bottles and instructs him to use the #1 bottle the first time he voids, #2 bottle the second time, #3 bottle the third time. By #3 the urine should be clear with little or no blood.)

3. Start Pyridium 100 mg tid if #3 urine clear.

4th post-op day: (if everything has gone well)

1. Home today
2. Appt. to see me in two weeks
3. Rx for Colace 50 mg bid for one week
4. Rx for Pyridium 100 mg tid for one week

REVIEW QUESTIONS

1. The purpose or function of the urinary system is _____
   _____
2. The structures of the urinary system are _____.
3. An IVP is an _____ exam that shows _____.
4. Dialysis is _____
   _____.
5. Name the types of dialysis. _____
6. Define the following:
   Anuria _____
   Pyuria _____
   Retention _____
   Suppression _____
   Uremia _____
   Calculi _____
   Wilm's tumor _____
   Cystoscopy _____
   Bright's disease _____
   _____
   Ileal conduit _____
   _____
7. Identify these abbreviations:
   BPH _____
   TUR _____
   SPP _____
8. List five medications and classify each according to their use in diseases
   and disorders of the urinary system.
   _____
   _____
9. List five diseases and disorders of the urinary system.
   _____
   _____

10. List six lab tests that relate to the urinary system or the prostate.

    _____

    _____

    _____

11. Name four kinds of catheters.

    _____

    _____

12. List four procedures or surgeries of the urinary system.

    _____

    _____

13. List four radiology and nuclear medicine exams relating to the urinary system. _____

    _____

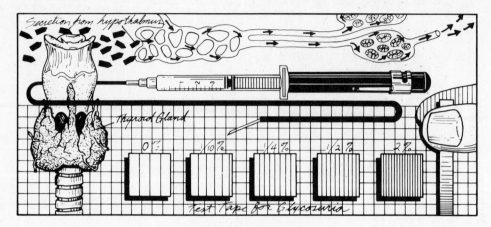

OBJECTIVES

Study of this chapter will enable you to:

1. List the endocrine organs.
2. Define hormone.
3. List some diseases and disorders of the endocrine system and the gland related to the disease or disorder.
4. List some laboratory examinations used in diagnosing and treating the diseases and disorders of the endocrine system.
5. List some radiology department tests relating to the endocrine system.
6. Classify some medications used in diagnosing and treating diseases and disorders of the endocrine system.
7. List some of the surgical procedures relating to the endocrine system.
8. Transcribe Physician's Orders relating to the endocrine system.

The word endocrine means to secrete. The endocrine system is composed of glands that secrete substances called **hormones.** The word hormone comes from the Greek word *hormon* which means to stimulate. The hormones are carried by the bloodstream to other organs, which they stimulate. We think of hormones as regulators. The hormones go from a gland to an organ, which is regulated by the action of the hormone on its cells. The receiving organs have a feedback action; this in turn helps regulate the amount of hormone produced by the endocrine gland.

The organs of the endocrine system are the pituitary, pineal, thyroid, parathyroids, thymus, adrenals, pancreas, and the sex glands—testes in male and ovaries in female. These glands do not have ducts that carry their hormones; the hormones are released into the bloodstream and carried throughout the body. All the glands except the sex glands will be discussed in this chapter. The testes and ovaries are discussed in Chapter 18.

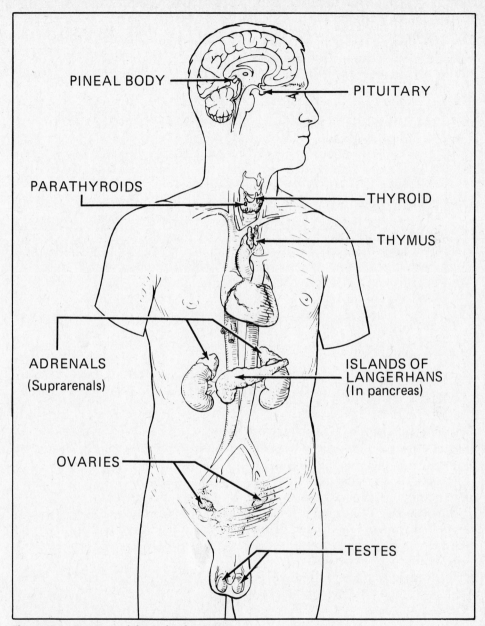

PINEAL BODY

PITUITARY

PARATHYROIDS

THYROID

THYMUS

ADRENALS
(Suprarenals)

ISLANDS OF
LANGERHANS
(In pancreas)

OVARIES

TESTES

Figure 15-1. Structure of the Endocrine System.

ORGANS OF THE ENDOCRINE SYSTEM

The **pituitary** gland lies in the skull like a cherry hanging by a stem. The stem penetrates the membrane covering the brain. The gland is protected by a fossa on the sphenoid bone called the sella turcica. This tiny gland has so many functions that it is often called the "master gland." There are two distinct parts of the gland, the anterior and the posterior.

The **anterior portion** secretes the following hormones:

- **TSH, thyroid stimulating hormone**, stimulates both thyroid growth and secretion of the thyroid hormone.
- **ACTH, adenocorticotrophic hormone**, urges the adrenal cortex to grow and secrete cortisol, usually called hydrocortisone.
- **FSH, follicle-stimulating hormone,** aids in the growth of the small egg sacs in the ovaries and in the manufacture of estrogen.
- **GH, growth hormone,** is also called **STH, somatotrophic hormone,** and is involved in the nourishment of the body. It speeds up the building of proteins in the body and the breakdown of fats and increases the rate at which glucose is released into the blood stream.
- **LH, luteinizing hormone,** in the female urges the ovum (egg) to mature and be expelled from the ovary. It also stimulates secretion of progesterone and estrogen.
- **ICSH, interstitial cell stimulating hormone,** in the male stimulates the growth and development of the testes and secretion of testosterone.
- **Prolactin** stimulates the changes in the breast during pregnancy and the production of milk after delivery.

The **posterior portion** of the pituitary releases two hormones:

- **ADH, antidiuretic hormone,** also called vasopressin, regulates the secretion of urine.
- **Oxytocin** is secreted in the female and stimulates contractions of the uterus during birth and contractions in the breast after birth to release milk for the infant.

The **pineal** gland is posterior to the pituitary. There is more calcification in the adult gland, but the activity of the pineal enzymes does not decrease. The hormone produced is **melatonin**, which acts on the ovaries; it is thought to regulate the menstrual cycle. Another hormone, **serotonin,** is not completely understood but is involved in the normal function of the brain.

The **thymus** is in the chest, behind the sternum. It has two lobes and is much larger in the infant. The gland becomes smaller and is atrophied by adulthood. The thymus is believed to be involved in immunity by enabling white blood cells to produce antibodies.

The **thyroid** gland is located below the larynx, with one lobe on each side of the trachea and a connecting piece that lies over the trachea. **Thyroxin** (T_4) is essential for growth and development. It increases the metabolic rate. Another hormone, **thyrocalcitonin,** regulates the amount of calcium in the blood.

The **parathyroids** are located on the posterior surface of the thyroid gland, two on each side. **Parathormone** (PTH) is excreted and acts on the kidneys and bones to maintain the calcium-phosphorous balance in the blood.

The **adrenal** glands are on the top of the kidneys, one on each kidney. The gland is divided into the cortex, the outer layer, and the medulla, the inner section. The **cortex** excretes glucocorticoids, the main one being **cortisol** or hydrocortisone. This group aids in metabolism, helps the body respond to stress, and has an anti-inflammatory action. Mineralocorticoids are also excreted by the cortex. The main one is **aldosterone** which is involved in the regulation of sodium and potassium in the blood. The **medulla** excretes **epinephrine** and **norepinephrine**, which aid in the response of the body to stress. They are often called the "fight-or-flight" drugs because of the increases in respiration, heart rate, blood pressure, and blood glucose level that accompanies anger and fear.

The **pancreas'** location you already know. The endocrine activity of the pancreas is performed by cells called **islets of Langerhans.** The hormone insulin is secreted by the beta cells, and glucagon is secreted by the alpha cells of the islets. **Insulin** decreases the amount of glucose in the blood and **glucagon** increases the amount of glucose in the blood, so they counterbalance each other.

TERMINOLOGY

Acetone—found in the blood and urine of patients who do not properly metabolize fats and glucose or who are malnourished. It has a distinctive sweet, fruity smell.

Acidosis—a condition that occurs when there is an accumulation of acid in the body. In uncontrolled diabetes mellitus, the urine has ketone bodies and breathing is disturbed. This may lead to coma if not treated soon enough.

Alpha—the first letter of the Greek alphabet and is used here to denote the larger cells of the islets of Langerhans.

Beta—the second letter of the Greek alphabet and is used here to denote the smaller cells of the islets of Langerhans.

Clinitest—a urine test which determines the amount of sugar excreted in the urine; it is performed in combination with acetest to determine presence of acetone in urine.

Coma—patient is in a deep sleep and can't be aroused; occurs if acidosis is not treated

Endocrinologist—a doctor who specializes in diagnosis and treatment of endocrine diseases and disorders

Feminizing—refers to the hormones that decrease body hair and increase breast size, give feminine characteristics.

Food exchange—in a diabetic diet means one food, with a certain calorie content and classification as a protein, fat, or carbohydrate, may be replaced by another one of equal value.

Glycosuria—urine contains glucose

Hyper—a prefix meaning more than normal

Hypo—a prefix meaning less than normal

Ketosis—results from improper metabolism of fatty acids; acetone present in the urine

Masculinizing—refers to hormone activity that gives masculine characteristics, such as body and facial hair, and undeveloped breasts

Polydipsia, polyphagia, and **polyuria**—all symptoms of diabetes mellitus. *Poly* means much, *dipsia* refers to thirst, *phagia* refers to food, and *uria* refers to urine. The diabetic has increased thirst, eats more than usual, and excretes a large amount of urine.

Post-prandial—after food; used in regard to tests

Provocative drugs—stimulate secretions or action of a gland or organ

Virilism—refers to hormone activity that causes facial hair and other secondary male characteristics in the female.

DISEASES AND DISORDERS

Endocrine diseases and disorders are mostly due to hyperfunction or hypofunction of a gland.

Pituitary

Acromegaly or gigantism results from excessive GH, usually due to an adenoma of the anterior pituitary. Bones of the face, hands, and feet are enlarged and the skin becomes thickened. **Tx:** Determine if oversecretion is due to a tumor of the pituitary and if other adenomas are present in the parathyroids, adrenals, or pancreas. Surgical removal of tumors, radiation therapy. Somatostatin, a synthetic hormone, inhibits the release of GH.

Diabetes insipidus is insufficient ADH hormone, resulting in production of a large amount of urine. **Tx:** Replacement therapy. The oral hypoglycemic drug, diabinese, is an effective antidiuretic in mild cases.

Dwarfism, which is due to a pituitary GH deficiency, causes the child not to grow at a normal rate. **Tx:** Replacement therapy must be before puberty.

Panhypopituitarism or Simmond's disease means that all the hormones of the pituitary are secreted in smaller than normal amounts due to stress factors or a tumor. Premature aging and the wasting process of tissues occurs. **Tx:** Replacement therapy, surgical removal of the tumor.

Pineal

Tumors occur more often in males and cause premature development of puberty. **Tx:** Surgery and radiation.

Thymus

Tumors are associated with other diseases and are discovered while testing in those diseases (myasthenia gravis, Cushing's syndrome). **Tx:** Surgical removal.

Thyroid

Cancer is either of a fast-growing type or a slow-growing type. **Tx:** Surgical removal in all cases, radiation therapy for areas of metastasis. For the slow-growing type, surgery and administration of radioiodine.

Cretinism is the result of a thyroid hormone deficiency in childhood. Dwarfism with mental retardation occurs. **Tx**: Thyroid hormone should be given early for results to be beneficial.

Goiter is the enlargement of the thyroid gland; and the usual cause is lack of iodine in the diet. **Tx**: Treatment of any underlying disease, increased iodine intake, surgery may be necessary.

Graves' disease (also called Basedow's disease and exophthalmic goiter) is hyperactivity of the thyroid gland. It occurs most often in women. The thyroid is enlarged, the eyes protrude, and the rate of metabolism is greatly increased. The condition may lead to a crisis situation if not controlled. **Tx**: Radioactive iodine, specific drugs, surgery after the condition is under control.

Myxedema is the condition resulting from hypothyroidism in an adult. Mental alertness is decreased, and metabolism is slowed. **Tx**: Replacement therapy; Synthroid is commonly used.

Parathyroids

Hyperfunction results in kidney stones, bone destruction, and bone tumors. **Tx**: Removal of enough tissue to restore the calcium-phosphate balance.

Hypofunction may cause **tetany**, a condition of increased nerve impulses. Muscle spasms and convulsions can occur. **Trousseau sign** means that the patient has a spasm of the hand when pressure is applied around the upper arm. **Chvostek sign** is a spasm of the facial muscle when the area over the facial nerve is tapped. Orders will contain instructions as to how often to observe the signs. **Tx**: Parathormone, calcium lactate, and Vitamin D.

Adrenals

Addison's disease results from decreased secretions of the cortex. The patient loses weight and is lethargic. Potassium blood levels are high, and sodium in the blood is low. **Tx**: Cortisol preparations.

Adrenogenital syndrome is the result of hypersecretion of sex hormones produced by the cortex. Premature sexual development occurs. **Tx**: Hydrocortisone.

Cushing's syndrome is caused by hypersecretion of the cortex. The patient presents a typical picture—the face is round and puffy, the abdominal tissue hangs freely, and the back develops a hump. **Tx**: Radiation therapy to the pituitary, surgical removal of benign adrenal tumors followed by replacement therapy, high protein diet.

Pheochromocytomas are tumors of the adrenals that cause hypertension. There is an oversecretion of hormones in the medulla. The increased epinephrine and norepinephrine keep the blood pressure elevated and the metabolic rate increased so that the patient feels worn out all the time. **Tx**: Antihypertensive drugs, surgical removal of the tumor.

Pancreas

Diabetes mellitus is a disorder where there is an inadequate production of insulin or the body cannot utilize the insulin that is produced and which has a variety of genetic causes. The National Institutes of Health classifies diabetes mellitus as:

- **Type I** *(formerly called juvenile diabetes) occurs when the pancreas produces little or no insulin and insulin must be given by injection. The cause may be genetic, viral, or an abnormal autoimmune reaction in which the body attacks and destroys its own insulin-producing cells. The majority of newly diagnosed Type I patients are very young.* **Tx**: Special diet, exercise program to establish a normal range of daily activity for the patient's age, testing of urine and/or blood, and insulin injections. It is extremely important that the patient understands that the treatment must be strictly controlled to prevent complications of the eyes, the circulatory, nervous, and urinary systems.

- **Type II** (formerly called maturity onset diabetes) is a disorder in which insulin is produced but the body cannot utilize it for some unknown reason. There is usually a strong familial tendency and the patient is usually obese. **Tx**: Special diet, monitoring of urine and blood sugar levels, oral hypoglycemic drugs, and insulin injections in some cases.

- **Diabetes mellitus associated with other conditions or syndromes** (formerly called secondary diabetes) is due to a glucose intolerance caused by poisons, trauma, or an illness. **Tx**: Same as Type II in most cases; if patient must have insulin, the treatment is the same as for Type I.

- **Impaired glucose tolerance** (formerly called latent diabetes) is a condition in which the blood sugar levels are between normal levels and diabetic levels. There is an increased susceptibility to atherosclerotic disease. **Tx**: Weight loss if obesity is a factor, regular blood sugar level checks.

- **Gestational diabetes** is the same name originally used and refers to patients whose diabetes begins or is first diagnosed during pregnancy. **Tx**: Maintain ideal weight following pregnancy, regular blood sugar level checks.

Diabetes monitoring may be testing the urine to ascertain how much sugar is spilled, evaluating the blood sugar level, or both. Blood sugar levels are more reliable and usually required for Type I. **Urine tests** are ordered as clinitest and acetest (C&A), fractional urines, or Ketodiastix. All are performed before meals and at bedtime. Insulin may be ordered on a sliding scale according to the results of the test and orders would be written:

> *(urine test name) ac and HS c̄ sliding scale:*
> trace give no insulin
> 1+ give regular insulin 5 U
> 2+ give regular insulin 10 U
> 3+ give regular insulin 15 U
> 4+ give regular insulin 20 U

If blood sugar levels are used, the order would state a number, such as 300 BS, in place of the urine values of 1+, 2+, 3+, 4+. The above order involves a treatment and a medication. The patient or the NA will do the test. The patient or the RN will give the insulin injection. The kardex entry will have the urine test under treatments or on the pre-printed page and the sliding scale will be entered under medications; both will be ac and HS.

Blood glucose monitoring may be accomplished by use of treated plastic strips or meter devices. Treated strips are Glucoscan test strips, Chemstrip bG, Dextrostix, and Visidex. The patient pricks the side of a fingertip and places a drop of blood onto the strip and waits a certain time span according to directions, and then compares the strip to the color code on the side of the container. The meter devices use one of the treated strips which is placed in the device and the read-out is automatic. Names of some meter devices are Dextrometer, Glucometer, Accu-Chek bG, Glucoscan-11, and Stat Tek.

Insulin delivery devices or pumps vary according to the company or institution that is trying to perfect the basic concept. The devices give a continuous flow of insulin at a very low dosage and give added insulin when food is eaten. One type consists of a needle inserted into the subcutaneous tissues of the anterior abdominal wall or thigh and connected to a radio-controlled pump. An implanted type consists of a pump, motor, battery, and insulin container enclosed in a capsule and implanted in the upper abdominal region. A catheter from the capsule is sutured to the peritoneum and tissue. There is an entry to the capsule from the skin so that the insulin supply may be replenished. The control has signals that can be seen and heard.

Functional hypoglycemia is a condition in which the pancreas releases too much insulin in response to sugar and causes a drop in blood sugar. The problem may lead to diabetes mellitus. **Tx:** A special diet of six small meals with high protein, low carbohydrate content.

SURGERIES AND PROCEDURES

Adrenalectomy is the removal of one or both adrenals. The permit will specify if bilateral or not. Solu-Cortef IM or IV in large doses is given the day of surgery, continued for a few days, and then gradually decreased. The patient is maintained on oral hydrocortisone.

Hypophysectomy is the removal of the pituitary gland. This may be performed by craniotomy (into the skull) or by transsphenoidal approach and use of microsurgery. Lasers are beginning to be used for this. Hormone replacement therapy depends on the amount of tissue remaining. Corticosteroids or thyroid and sex steroids may be administered.

Subtotal pancreatectomy is preferred to total pancreatectomy because patients survive longer. Insulin therapy is necessary after surgery.

Thyroidectomy is the removal of the thyroid. If surgery is not due to cancer, the total gland is not removed. Tetany is a threat after surgery, so orders may include that a tracheotomy set be kept at the bedside and Calcium Gluconate IV be ready for administration. Thyroid medication is ordered after surgery if the entire gland was removed or if tests show that thyroid production is inadequate.

Total parathyroidectomy is the removal of the parathyroid tissue. Part of one of the four glands is left to supply the hormone. The patient usually has an adenoma if this surgery is performed.

LABORATORY TESTS

- ACTH
- Aldosterone, blood or 24 hour urine
- Calcitonin
- Calcium, blood and urine
- Carotene
- CBC
- Electrolytes
- Glucose, blood
    Fasting
    Random
    2 hour PP or PC
- Glucose, urine
    Qualitative
    Quantitative
- GTT
- Insulin
- Ketones, urine
- Osmolality, blood and urine
- Parathyroid hormone
- Phosphorus (P), blood and urine
- Pregnanetriol, urine
- Sulkowitch test, urine

- Radioimmunoassay tests
    Cortisol
    FSH
    Growth hormone
    Growth hormone series
    LH
    Prolactin
    Testosterone
    T_3 (Triiodothyronine)
    T_4 (Thyroxine)
    Free T_4
    TSH
- 24 hour urine tests (Your lab requisitions will probably specify if a preservative is needed to add to the specimen bottle.)
    Catecholamines
    FSH
    Metanephrines
    VMA
    17-KS
    17-KGS
    17-OHCS (listed in Appendix II under K with other 17- tests)

SPECIAL TESTS

These are presented here instead of in the lab manual because you need to learn how orders for such tests are written.

ACTH Stimulation Test

Orders read:

Start 24 hr urine for 17-KS and 17-OHCS this AM. Tomorrow, after 24 hr urine collected, give ACTH 50 units IM and repeat daily for 4 days. Collect 24 hr urine daily for 17-KS and 17-OHCS; start test immediately after ACTH is given.

This test measures adrenal activity. Cushing's disease produces a marked rise in 17-KS and 17-OHCS values. Adrenal insufficiency causes a rise in 17-OHCS of less than 2 mg in 24 hrs. Inadequate pituitary function with normal adrenals causes a progressive rise over the five days.

Cortisol Test

(Other cortisone preparations may be used)

Orders read:

Draw plasma cortisol at 8AM tomorrow. Give Cortrosyn 0.25 mg IM after cortisol drawn; draw plasma cortisol 30 minutes after injection.

This test is indicative of Addison's disease if plasma cortisol does not rise by at least ten points after the injection.

Dexamethasone Suppression Test

Orders read:

Start 24 hr urine for 17-OHCS this AM. Tomorrow, after 24 hr urine collected, start Dexamethasone 0.5 mg PO q 6 hrs for two days. Repeat 24 hr urine for 17-OHCS each day.

Normally the steroid secretion would decrease. In Cushing's disease steroids do not decrease. If pituitary tumor is suspected, the test is repeated with dexamethasone 2 mg q 6 hrs for 8 doses. If a tumor is present, secretion of steroids is decreased with larger dose.

IV Corticotropin Test (other cortisone preparations may be used)

Orders read:

Start 24 hr urine for 17-OHCS this AM. Tomorrow give Cortrosyn 0.25 mg in 1000cc NS IV after urine collection. Repeat IV and urine daily for 3 days.

The urine values do not rise in Addison's disease. Pituitary insufficiency causing hypofunction of adrenals produces a rise in urine values slowly after several days of the IV medication.

Metopirone Stimulation Test

Orders read:

Start 24 hr urine for 17-OHCS this AM. Tomorrow start Metopirone 500 mg q 4 hrs for 24 hrs after urine collection completed. Repeat 24 hr urine tomorrow and next day.

Urine values are greatly increased if the pituitary function is normal.

Provocative Test

Orders read: (for patient with BP below 170/110)

Histamine 0.015 mg IV. Monitor BP q 5 minutes for 30 minutes. (This is usually given by MD. Order is written so you may obtain necessary items for MD.)

For patients with higher BP, Regitine is used in place of Histamine. Histamine causes quick rise in BP in cases of pheochromocytoma. Regitine reduces BP in pheochromocytoma.

Vasopressin Test (may be performed several ways, one example given)

Orders read:

Pitressin tannate in oil 5 units IM at 8PM today. Have patient empty bladder at bedtime. Urines for osmolality tomorrow at 7AM, 8AM, 9AM.

Urine values will show marked increase in diabetes insipidus.

RADIOLOGY AND NUCLEAR MEDICINE EXAMS

Ba swallow will visualize an enlarged thyroid that is low or intrathoracic.
CT scan of the body would show pituitary tumors and any delay in bone age.
Echoscan of pancreas visualizes tumors.
Echoscan of thyroid differentiates solid lesions from cystic lesions.
IVP is used in Cushing's syndrome to determine if any enlargement of the adrenal glands is present.
Radioactive scan and uptake of thyroid uses ^{131}I or ^{123}I. The ^{123}I has a lower radiation hazard. Scan outlines increased and decreased areas of activity.
Tomograms of sella turcica show size of pituitary.
X-ray of epiphyseal plates of long bones to show development. Delay in development process is seen in cretinism and hypothyroidism in young persons.

MEDICATIONS

The medications used for treatment or diagnosis in diseases and disorders of the endocrine system are regulated by the severity of the hypo or hyper function of the glands so no UAD is given.

Anterior Pituitary Hormones

- Pitressin (vasopressin)—SQ or IM
- Pitressin Tannate in oil—IM
- Pitressin nasal spray
- Oxytocin—discussed in Chapter 18.

Antithyroid Preparations

Antithyroid preparations reduce thyroid production or reduce the symptoms until the condition of hyperfunction can be controlled.

- Inderal—PO—reduces symptoms.
- Ismelin—PO—reduces symptoms.
- Lugol's solution—PO
- Propylthiouracil—PO
- Radioactive iodine—PO
- Sodium Iodide—IV drip
- SSKI (saturated solution potassium iodide)—PO
- Tapazole—PO

Calcium

Calcium preparations are used in hypocalcemic tetany.

- Calcium gluconate—PO, IV
- Calcium lactate—PO
- Parathyroid injectable—IM

Corticosteroids

Corticosteroids are used to replace hormones from the cortex of the adrenals.

- Alphadrol—PO
- Aristocort—PO, IV
- cortisone—PO
- Cortrosyn—IM, IV
- Decadron—PO, IM, IV
- dexamethasone—PO, IM, IV
- prednisone—PO
- prednisolone—PO, IM

Hyperglycemic Agents

Hyperglycemic agents are used to increase blood sugar levels.

- Glucagon—SC, IM, IV
- Proglycem capsules—PO

Hypoglycemic Agents

Hypoglycemic agents are used to decrease blood sugar levels.

- Diabinese—PO
- Dymelor—PO
- Humulin—first biosynthetic human insulin
- Orinase—PO

- Tolbutone—PO
- Tolinase—PO
- Insulins are given SC and are measured in units.
   Regular insulin is rapid acting, lasts 6 to 8 hours; given IV in insulin shock therapy
   Semi-lente is rapid acting, lasts 12 to 16 hours.
   Lente is intermediate in action, lasts 24 hours.
   NPH is intermediate in action, lasts 18 to 24 hours.
   PZI is long acting, lasts 36 hours.
   Ultra-lente is long acting, lasts 36 hours.

Somatotropin Hormone

The somatrotropin hormone replaces the growth hormone. Until recently, it was obtained from cadavers and was very expensive. It is now produced synthetically and is supplied to children who have undergone tests that show they would benefit by the hormone. The National Pituitary Agency of the federal government supplies the hormone, which is given by injection.

Thyroid

Thyroid preparations replace the hormone in hypofunction.

- Cytomel—PO
- Euthroid—PO
- Levothroid—POPo
- Proloid—PO
- Synthroid—PO, IM, IV.
- thyroid tablets—PO
- Thyrolar—PO

Vitamins

Vitamins that raise the blood calcium level are used to treat hypoparathyroidism.

Calciferol—PO—oil preparation for IM (Vit D)
Hytakerol—PO (Vit D)
Os-Cal—PO (calcium and Vit D)

EXAMPLES OF PHYSICIAN'S ORDERS

Dx: Juvenile diabetes (14 year old male) Type I diabetes

1. Random BS (blood sugar) stat. Call results to me.

2. SMA-20, UA
3. No routine chest

After BS results:

1. Give Reg. insulin 10 U with NPH 15 U now.
2. 2500 calorie ADA diet
3. FBS in AM

Next day:

1. Reg. insulin 10 U with NPH 15 U ac breakfast and supper
2. Random BS at 4PM, call results to me.
3. Have dietitian see patient to work out calorie need for activities of this patient.
4. Start diabetic teaching with RN Educator.
5. Have PT see and give exercises to correspond to patient's usual activities. (Recent studies show that regular insulin given with NPH before breakfast and before supper produce a more normal blood sugar level.)

Dx: Diabetic with neuropathy (involvement of nerves)

1. 1200 calorie ADA diet
2. BR, BRP
3. VS qid
4. SMA-20, CBC, UA with C & S
5. Tolinase 250 ī PO tid
6. Neurology evaluation c̄ EMG and NCV (nerve conduction velocities)
7. Zomax 100 mg PO q 4 to 6 hrs prn for pain

After NCV: (which showed a slow nerve reaction to stimuli)

1. Amitriptyline 25 mg PO tid (to relieve the pain in the feet and reduce the anxiety patient was experiencing)
2. FBS in AM

REVIEW QUESTIONS

1. Define hormone.

2. List the endocrine glands.

3. Write the name of the endocrine gland involved in these diseases:
   Diabetes insipidus _____
   Graves' disease _____
   Cushing's syndrome _____
   Diabetes mellitus _____
   Tetany _____

4. State which department performs the following exams:
   Tomograms of sella tursica _____
   24 hr urine for 17-OHCS _____
   Cortisol test _____
   Echoscan of thyroid _____
   Ketodiastix _____
5. Classify the following medications:
   Propylthiouracil _____
   Insulin _____
   Pitressin _____
   Decadron _____
   Diabinese _____
   Cytomel _____
   Os-Cal _____
6. List three surgeries of the endocrine system.

   _____

7. _____ is a threat after a thyroidectomy.
8. In transcribing orders for the special tests, what would be a major concern? _____
9. An order reads "2 hr PP tomorrow." What steps would you take to carry out the order? _____

   _____

10. At 8:30 AM you are checking charts for stat, ASAP, and now orders and read one that says, "Give Semi-lente 35 U this AM." How do you handle that order? _____

    _____

11. What would you check on the lab requisition if an order at 10 AM is for a BS today? _____
12. Orders for sliding scale insulin involve a _____ as well as the medication order.

Chapter 16

The Nervous System

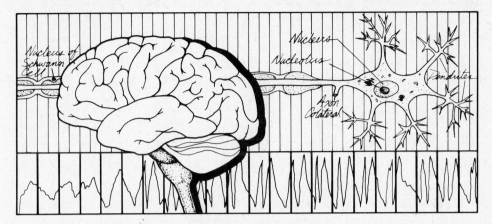

OBJECTIVES

Study of this chapter will enable you to:

1. List the structures that compose the nervous system.
2. List the functions of the nervous system.
3. List and define terms relating to the nervous system.
4. List the diseases and disorders of the nervous system.
5. List the laboratory tests relating to the nervous system.
6. List the radiology examinations relating to the nervous system.
7. List the surgeries of the nervous system.
8. List and classify the medications used in treating the diseases and disorders of the nervous system.
9. Transcribe Physician's Orders relating to the nervous system.

The nervous system controls and coordinates body activities by sending and receiving messages from all parts of the body. This coordination allows us to think, see, hear, smell, and taste. It also enables us to relate to our surroundings and to the natural habitants of those surroundings. In addition, it allows us to communicate with other people.

All nervous tissue is composed of gray matter, where impressions and impulses originate, and white matter, which conducts impulses.

The nervous system is divided into two parts:

The **central nervous system** (CNS) is composed of the brain and spinal cord. The CNS controls the body by receiving sensations and impulses, determining a course of action, and sending instructions to muscles and glands.

The **peripheral nervous system** (PNS) contains all the nerves which connect the CNS to the body. The PNS produces involuntary movement of muscles and glands to regulate body functions and produces the voluntary movement of the skeletal muscles.

CELLS OF THE NERVOUS SYSTEM

Neurons

Neurons, or nerve cells, are the structural and functional unit of the nervous system. They transmit impulses from one part of the body to another.

Structure
The **cell body** contains a nucleus and is vital to the life of the cell. Destruction of the cell body causes death to the entire neuron and regeneration is not possible.

Dendrites are thread-like projections which branch off one end of the cell body to receive impulses and relay them to the cell body.

The **axon**, or nerve fiber, extends from the other end of the cell body and carries impulses away from the cell body. Most axons are surrounded by a **myelin sheath** for protection and insulation. The sheath narrows at regular intervals to form nodes. The myelin sheath of axons that are located outside the brain and spinal cord is covered by another sheath called the **neurilemma.** Injured axons which have a neurilemma can be regenerated. This explains why injury to the brain and spinal cord is permanent, but injuries to peripheral nerves are not always permanent.

Nerve terminals are branches at the end of the axon which carry impulses from the axon to another neuron or an organ.

Types of Neurons
Sensory, or afferent, neurons carry impulses to the brain and spinal cord.

Motor, or efferent, neurons carry impulses from the brain and spinal cord to muscles or glands.

Association neurons, or interneurons, carry impulses from sensory neurons to motor neurons.

Neuroglia or Glia Cells

Neuroglia cells compose the connective tissue of the nervous system. They provide support for neurons and form the myelin sheath. In addition, they destroy bacteria and wastes caused by cellular activity.

THE CENTRAL NERVOUS SYSTEM

Brain

The brain consists of the cerebrum, the cerebellum and the brain stem.

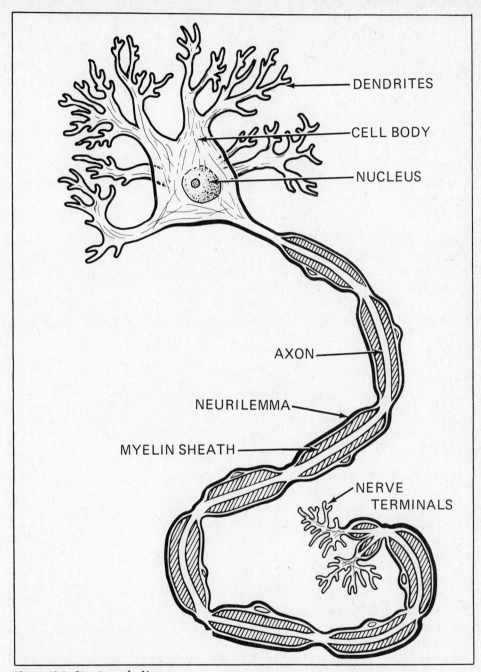

Figure 16-1. Structure of a Neuron.

Cerebrum

The cerebrum is the largest part of the brain. The outer layer, the **cerebral cortex**, is composed of gray matter; the central portion is white matter.

A long fissure divides the cerebrum into the right and left hemispheres. Other fissures divide each hemisphere into four lobes, each with the same name as the bone which covers the lobe—the **frontal, parietal, temporal,** and **occipital.**

The cerebrum controls all types of mental processes, such as controlling voluntary muscle movement, deciphering sensory impulses, and controlling emotional and intellectual performance.

Cerebellum

The cerebellum is the second largest part of the brain and lies under the posterior portion of the cerebrum. Like the cerebrum, the cerebellum is divided into hemispheres, and the cortex is gray matter. Below the cortex are tree-like branches of white matter with masses of gray matter deep within the branches.

The cerebellum coordinates and refines muscular movement to maintain the body's state of balance (equilibrium) and to maintain good posture.

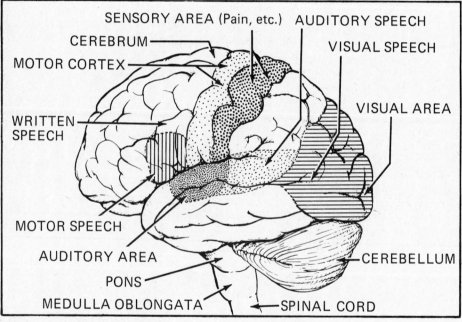

Figure 16-2. Structure of the Brain.

Brain Stem

The brain stem is a large bundle of nervous tissue divided into areas called the thalamus, hypothalamus, midbrain, pons, and medulla oblongata.

The **thalamus** is in the center of the base of the cerebrum and serves as a relay station by receiving stimula from the body and sending them to the cerebrum and by sending impulses from the cerebrum to other parts of the body.

The **hypothalamus** lies below the thalamus and controls body temperature, emotions, and sleep; regulates activities of internal organs and glands; and aids in memory regulation.

The **midbrain** is connected to the base of the cerebrum and joins the pons, cerebrum, and cerebellum. It is concerned with reflexes arising from auditory and visual stimuli.

The **pons** is just below the midbrain, in front of the cerebellum. The pons relays impulses and stimuli, connects the spinal cord to the brain, and connects the parts of the brain to one another.

The **medulla oblongata** connects the pons to the spinal cord. Most of the nerve fibers from the cerebrum to the spinal cord cross over where the medulla joins the cord. Therefore, the right side of the brain controls the left side of the body, and the left side of the brain controls the right side of the body. The medulla controls the heart beat, respiratory rate, and blood pressure. Injury to the medulla is critical and often fatal.

Spinal Cord

The spinal cord is a continuous column of nervous tissue that extends from the medulla to the second lumbar vertebra. The cord lies within the **spinal canal,** the hollow space of the vertebral column, and is protected by the vertebrae. Gray matter appears in the form of the letter "H" across the interior of the cord and is surrounded by white matter. Spinal nerves branch off the cord to travel to parts of the body.

The spinal cord serves as a pathway for conduction of impulses and responses between the brain and the other parts of the body and is the center of reflex action. A **reflex** is an automatic response to a stimulus. A reflex arc is the nerve pathway traveled by a stimulus to the cord and the response pathway from the cord to a muscle or organ. An example of a simple reflex arc is a pinprick (the stimulus) to a finger and the automatic withdrawal of the finger away from the pin (the response).

Meninges

The meninges are three layers of membranes that cover the brain and the spinal cord. The outer layer, next to the skull, is the **dura mater**. A cobweb-like

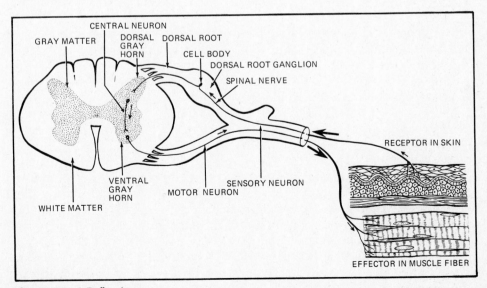

Figure 16-3. A Reflex Arc.

layer called the **arachnoid** is separated from the dura mater by the **subdural space**. The **subarachnoid space** is between the arachnoid and the innermost layer, the **pia mater**.

Cerebrospinal Fluid (CSF)

Cerebrospinal fluid can be found in the cavities of the brain, called **ventricles,** and in the subarachnoid spaces around the brain and the spinal cord. The circulating CSF acts as a shock absorber for the entire brain and cord, provides nourishment, and removes metabolic wastes. The CSF is formed in the ventricles, circulates through the CNS, and is reabsorbed into the blood via the veins of the brain. The process of formation, circulation, and reabsorption keeps the amount of CSF constant.

THE PERIPHERAL NERVOUS SYSTEM

Nerves are bundles of nerve fibers that connect the brain and the spinal cord to other parts of the body. Nerves have branches that communicate with branches of other nerves. There are 12 pairs of cranial nerves and 31 pairs of spinal nerves.

Cranial Nerves

The 12 pair of cranial nerves originate in the brain and emerge at the base of the brain, leading to the eyes, nose, face, ears, tongue, pharnyx, larynx, and thoracic and abdominal viscera. The names of the cranial nerves are often long so they are referred to by Roman numerals. Example: The glossopharyngeal nerve is commonly referred to as the IX (ninth) cranial nerve.

Spinal Nerves

The 31 pairs are divided into 8 cervical pairs, 12 thoracic pairs, 5 lumbar pairs, 5 sacral pairs, and one coccygeal pair. All spinal nerves originate on the spinal cord and are named according to the vertebral area from which they emerge. Each nerve has a dorsal or sensory root that conducts impulses to the cord and an anterior or motor root that conducts impulses away from the cord.

The roots of the spinal nerves below the first lumbar nerve do not leave the spine immediately; instead they go downward in the vertebral column and give the appearance of a "horse's tail," called **cauda equina**.

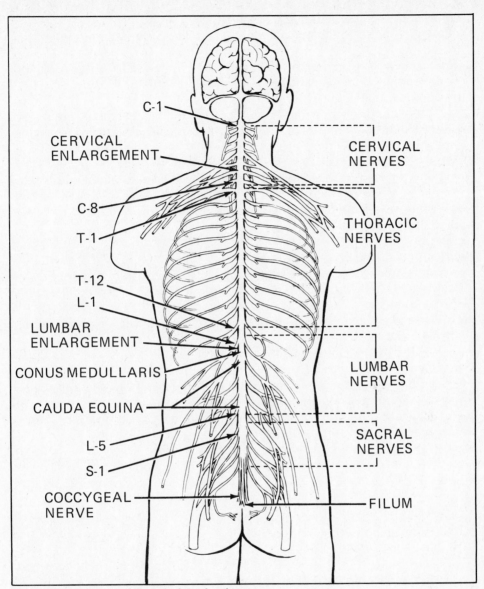

Figure 16-4. Structure of the Spinal Cord and Nerves.

TERMINOLOGY

Acetylcholine—a chemical that helps in the transmission of nerve impulses

Adrenergic—norepinephrine is released at the ending of the nerve fiber when the nerve is stimulated

Aphasia—loss of speech (either the ability to speak or to speak comprehensively or the ability to understand speech)

Ataxia—lack of or disorder of muscular coordination

Autonomic—spontaneous activities of the body, those that are not consciously controlled, such as breathing, heart beat, etc

Cholinergic—refers to the nerve endings that release acetylcholine when stimulated

Coma—a deep sleep, caused by illness or injury, from which the person cannot be aroused by external stimuli

Convolutions—the wrinkles on the cerebrum

Dyskinesia—abnormal or painful or difficult voluntary movement; often associated with the side effects of drugs classified as phenothiazines (Thorazine, Mellaril, Prolixin)

Fissure—a deep depression on the surface of the brain

Ganglion—a group of nerve cell bodies located outside the brain and spinal cord, such as the dorsal or sensory root of a spinal nerve

Glia—connective tissue cell of the CNS

Kinetic—refers to motion

Neuralgia—pain in a nerve

Neuritis—inflammation of a nerve

Parasympathetic—refers to the part of the autonomic nervous system that is controlled by neurons in the brain stem and the sacral portion of the spinal cord; produces involuntary functions that keep the body in homeostasis

Plexus—an interwoven network of nerves from which smaller nerves spread to cover an area

Seizure—a sudden attack of involuntary movement

Sympathetic—the branch of the autonomic system that dominates in emergency situations; impulses from this division prepare us for strenuous activity

Synapse—the space where dendrites of one neuron come close to the terminal ends of another neuron. An impulse passes from one neuron to another, in one direction only, at this space.

Tracts—groups of nerve fibers in the brain or spinal cord which form a pathway

Tremor—an involuntary quiver or continuous shaking of a part or parts of the body

| DISEASES AND DISORDERS

Amyotrophic lateral sclerosis (ALS) is a condition in which the motor neurons of the spinal cord, medulla, and cortex degenerate causing weakness of muscles with atrophy. The disease is progressive and incurable. **Tx**: Electromyogram (explained fully in the Special Tests section on page 335) aids in diagnosis. PT helps keep the muscles useful and gives the patient psychological support.

Cerebrovascular accident (CVA) or stroke occurs when the blood supply to the brain is deficient or cut off because of a hemorrhage or because of a thrombus or occlusion of the carotid artery. The location and extent of the brain damage depends on the cause. Prognosis is poor if a coma occurs and persists for days; full recovery is possible in cases where the brain tissue has not been destroyed. Paralysis occurs in severe cases, affecting the arm and leg on one side of the body. The leg paralysis may lessen with PT; the arm is less likely to return to functional use. Speech problems may vary from slight to complete loss of speech. **Tx**: Bedrest, IV fluids, tube feedings if patient is unconscious for a long period, surgery if a clot or narrowing of an artery is visible on CT scan or angiography; PT begins immediately to prevent atrophy of muscles. Any existing hypertension or arteriosclerosis is treated. Recovery may be slow and requires intensive care.

Encephalitis is the inflammation of the meninges around the brain and is caused by a virus more often than by bacteria. The disease may occur following influenza, measles, chickenpox, smallpox, or other illnesses. Children should be immunized against childhood diseases as a preventive measure. **Tx**: Mannitol to reduce intracranial pressure, oxygen, IV fluids, anticonvulsive medication.

Epilespy is a brain dysfunction in which episodes of uncontrollable muscular activity, called seizures, take place. This may be a congenital condition or may be acquired from trauma or disease, but there may be no discernible cause. The four main types of epilepsy are:

1. **Grand mal seizures** are major convulsions which may be preceded by a psychic or sensory warning called an aura. Unconsciousness may last from a few minutes to several, and return to consciousness is usually followed by a deep sleep.
2. **Petit mal seizures** are minor episodes with muscular jerks and a blank stare but no convulsions. Unconsciousness is only momentary.
3. **Jacksonian or focal seizures** begin in a muscle or group of muscles and may spread to adjacent muscles in a specific pattern.
4. **Psychomotor seizures** are seizures that do not fall into the other three classifications.

The types may appear separately or be mixed. The term **status epilepticus** refers to a series of attacks in rapid succession without consciousness being regained between the attacks and requires immediate care. **Tx**: Anticonvulsive medication, seizure precautions. Hospitals have routine procedures for seizure precautions which include placing a padded tongue-blade or an airway at the head of the bed and keeping padded siderails in the up position. If the patient has a seizure, the airway or tongue-blade inserted into the mouth prevents swallowing the tongue and the padded rail prevents injury during the thrashing around that a seizure produces. Examinations such as an EEG or CT scan aid in determining a cause for the epilepsy, if there is a discernible cause, and the portion of the brain where the dysfunction occurs.

Guillain-Barré syndrome is muscle weakness and polyneuritis with partial or complete paralysis following an infection, such as an URI or gastroenteritis, or following an immunization shot. **Tx**: Corticosteroids, PT when recovery begins. A respirator may be needed if respiratory paralysis occurs. Muscle weakness may persist for a long time or recovery may be complete. Respiratory failure or an infection may cause death.

Headaches (HA) may be a symptom of many diseases. The person with persistent headaches may undergo numerous tests to find the cause **Tx**: Analgesics, determination of cause.

Migraine headaches are thought to be caused by the constriction and then dilatation of blood vessels of the cerebrum and meninges. Visual disturbances may precede the pain. GI upsets often occur with the headache, which increases in intensity and lasts several days. **Tx**: Specific drugs are used at the onset. The patient should be in a dark room for several hours. Sedatives, tranquilizers, and antidepressants may help.

Head injuries are evaluated very carefully for signs of brain damage. X-rays and CT scans help determine the extent of the injury. A **contussion** is bruising of the brain. A *concussion* is loss of consciousness following injury and may last from a short period to 24 hours. **Tx**: Simple wounds of the scalp are cleaned and sutured, compound fractures are debrided and bone fragments removed, depressed fractures are elevated after the critical stage is over. Monitoring of intracranial pressure is done for all injuries. Other treatment includes frequent change of position and Foley catheter if the patient is unconscious. Neuro signs include vital signs, reaction of the eyes to light, the reaction to painful stimuli, strength of the hand grasp and the degree of orientation (awareness of date, time, and place).

A special bed is used for brain-damaged patients who are very restless and whose movements may be harmful to them. The bed is similar to a very large playpen—a larger than average mattress is placed on the floor and is surrounded by padded walls that may be opened to enter. The large size allows personnel to enter the area to care for the patient, the padded walls protect the patient. The bed is called a Craig bed.

Hemorrhages are named according to the location in the brain. **Extradural hemorrhages** occur on the outer side of the dura and usually follow a blow on the temporal area which ruptures the middle meningeal artery or vein. Intracranial pressure increases. **Tx**: Small disks are removed from the skull (trephining), and the blood is removed. The patient is monitored carefully. **Subarachnoid hemorrhage** is due to a ruptured aneurysm or a tumor of a blood vessel. The CSF contains blood. **Tx**: Bedrest, arteriography to determine cause, surgical removal of the blood, surgical repair of the aneurysm, and surgical removal of the tumor if at all possible. **Subdural hemorrhage,** commonly called subdural hematoma, is usually from a ruptured vein. **Tx**: Removal of the blood by trephining or craniotomy, careful monitoring.

Hydrocephalus is an excess of cerebrospinal fluid in the cranial cavity. The condition may be congenital or acquired. If congential, there is an enlargement of the head at birth or shortly thereafter. **Tx**: Shunting of the fluid by insertion of tubes into the ventricles and to the peritoneal cavity or to the heart. These are called ventriculoperitoneal shunts or atrioventricular shunts. Shunts may need revision at various intervals.

Meningitis is an inflammation of the meninges from a bacterial or viral infection and may be fatal if not treated quickly. **Tx**: An antibiotic is started immediately and changed if cultures of the spinal fluid indicate an organism not susceptible to the antibiotic. Other treatment includes IV fluids, respirator if necessary, and careful observation of neurosigns.

Multiple sclerosis occurs when the myelin sheath has areas of degeneration which cause a spastic paralysis, slurred speech, and inability to care for one's self. The condition occurs in early adult life and is slowly progressive. Periods of remission decrease as the disease progresses. **Tx**: PT and OT to keep the patient active as long as possible.

Myasthenia gravis is a disorder in which the skeletal muscles are very weak and tire easily. A defect in transmission of motor impulses caused by an antibody creates the disorder. Respiratory problems may be severe, requiring a respirator in cases where the patient is said to be "in crisis." **Tx**: Specific drugs control the symptoms.

Narcolepsy is characterized by attacks of muscular weakness that occur during emotional reactions and by frequently occurring periods of sleep that cannot be controlled. **Tx**: Specific drugs control the sleep problem but do not help with the muscular weakness attacks.

Neuralgia is pain in a nerve. The most painful type is **trigeminal neuralgia,** or Tic Douloureux, which affects the trigeminal nerve of the face that spreads out in three directions. **Tx** for trigeminal neuralgia: Anticonvulsants may control the pain, Vitamin B$_{12}$ helps in some cases, alcohol injections into the nerve may bring temporary relief. Surgery with radiofrequency can be performed to destroy the nerve.

Parkinson's disease is a degenerative nervous disorder characterized by muscle stiffness which produces a shuffling walk and a tremor of the hands that looks as if the person were rolling a pill between the thumb and the fingers. The disease may be **idiopathic** (no cause can be determined) or it may occur after encephalitis. **Tx**: Specific drugs relieve the symptoms.

Shingles or Herpes Zoster is a condition in which acute, inflammatory blisters caused by the herpes virus erupt on the body along a peripheral nerve. **Tx**: Bedrest, isolation until blistering and crusting are no longer present, medicated packs to the area for comfort and to prevent secondary infection.

Spinal injuries occur when trauma or disease cause damage to the spinal cord. When the spinal cord is permanently damaged, paralysis occurs from the level of injury down the rest of the spine. **Quadraplegia** is paralysis of all four limbs; **paraplegia** is paralysis of both legs. **Tx**: Keeping the spine straight, PT and OT after acute phase. Special beds are used to keep the spine straight. The Stryker frame is canvas stretched across a metal frame; the patient is turned by placing another frame on top of the patient, fastening the frames together, and rotating the frames. The circuloelectric bed has the frame in the center of an electrically operated circle. The Roto Rest Treatment Table, sometimes called the Kinetic bed, tilts at various angles while attachments keep the limbs in position. Rehabilitation is long-term.

Tumors may occur in the brain, in the spinal cord, or on the nerves. **Tx**: Surgical removal and radiation. The spinal cord tumors are most often benign encapsulated tumors. **Intrancranial tumors** may be present for a long time before any symptoms appear. Headaches that increase in severity, convulsions, and dizziness may be symptoms. Gliomas are the most common. Many tumors are metastatic. **Tx**: Surgical resection if possible, whether benign or malignant. Radiation therapy following surgery usually decreases symptoms. **Tumors of the nerves** are usually on peripheral nerves and cause subcutaneous nodules. The disease is benign. **Tx**: Removal if possible when the tumor is on a spinal nerve. Peripheral ones are removed only if they are bothersome.

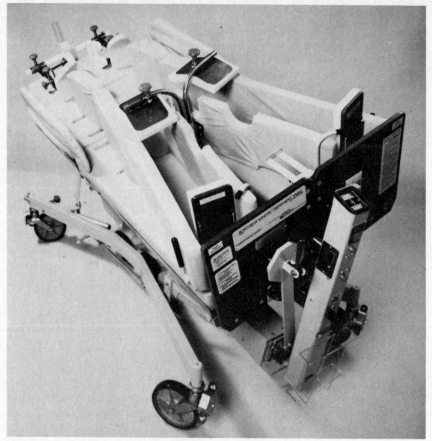

Figure 16-5. Roto Rest Treatment Table *(Courtesy of Kinetic Concepts).*

Disease-Causing Organisms

- Diplococcus pneumoniae
- Escherichia coli (E. Coli)
- Hemophilus influenzae
- Neisseria meningococcus
- Pseudomonas
- Staphylococcus

- Streptococcus
- Viruses
- Yeast and fungi
  Actinomyces
  Candida
  Coccidiodes
  Cryptococcus

| SURGERIES AND PROCEDURES

Biopsy of muscle differentiates between **neuropathy** (disease of nerves) and **myopathy** (disease of muscles). The symptoms of myopathies and neuropathic muscular disorders are so similar that it is difficult to make a correct diagnosis without an EMG and a biospy.

Blocks are injections of drugs into a nerve to relieve pain. Alcohol is frequently used. Marcaine hydrochloride, Novocain, and Xylocaine are all used for peripheral nerve blocks. Many times after surgery of the thoracic cage, the patient will have pain along the ribs, and a nerve block works when pain medications do not help. This procedure may be performed in the patient's room.

Cordotomy is a procedure in which the spinal pain fibers are severed in the cervical or thoracic region. These nerve fibers may be either cut or destroyed by radiofrequencies. To use radiofrequency, a needle is placed in the spinal cord with the aid of fluoroscopy, and the electrode is inserted through the needle. Cordotomy relieves the pain of terminal cancer.

Craniotomy is a procedure in which an incision is made in the scalp and the skull is opened. Operative permits will state the reason, such as "craniotomy with removal of tumor of (location)" or "craniotomy with debridement of fracture (location)." The head is shaved before surgery. The family should be consulted as to the disposal of the hair; certain cultures have specific rituals.

Lobectomy is the removal of the anterior portion of the temporal lobe. This may be performed in cases of temporal lobe involvement in epilepsy with psychiatric disturbances.

Peripheral nerve repair is a procedure in which severed nerves are rejoined. Techniques of surgery with a microscope have been successful in repairing deep, severed nerves when the extremities have been accidently amputated.

Radiofrequency neurectomy is the destruction of a nerve, usually the trigeminal nerve, by use of the radiofrequency electrode. The procedure is performed in the X-ray Department. The patient receives a local anesthetic in the area used for needle insertion. When the electrode touches the nerve to be destroyed, the patient is put to sleep while the radiofrequency is applied. The patient will have a numb feeling, in place of the pain, after the procedure.

Spinal puncture or spinal tap is a procedure in which a needle is inserted between two vertebra, usually the third and fourth lumbar, into the subarachnoid space and fluid is removed for laboratory examination. A gauge called a manometer is connected to the needle during the procedure to measure CSF pressure. The procedure is performed by the physician and may be done in the patient's room, in which case you will obtain a tray from Central Supply. The CSF to be sent to the lab may be in vials marked #1, #2, #3, and the doctor will specify what exam he wants for each vial. Spinal punctures are performed in surgery to administer spinal anesthesia. Patients should remain flat in bed for 8–12 hours after any spinal tap to prevent headache.

SPECIAL TESTS

Echoencephalograms (EchoEG) determine the position of the midline of the brain. By beaming pulses of ultrasonic waves through the head, from both sides, the echoes can be recorded on a graph. These can determine if a blood clot or tumor is pushing the midline and on which side the abnormality lies. The exam can be done at the bedside and is a quick diagnostic tool when the patient is unconscious and there could be several reasons for the condition.

Electroencephalogram (EEG) is a recording of the electrical activity of the brain. Electrodes are placed in various positions on the scalp and impulses from different areas are recorded. A sleep pattern may be needed for diagnosis, and the patient will be kept awake the night before so sleep will occur during the exam. Flashing lights may be used to determine if any abnormal activity occurs. The doctor will state if sleep studies are needed. Each hospital will have routine orders for EEG preparation. These are usually to wash the hair and be sure no spray or hair dressing is used. The patient is to eat a good meal before the exam so he/she will not be restless. An EEG may be done at the bedside for comatose or extremely ill patients. The EEG is used to determine if there is brain death when a patient has been on a respirator with no signs of recovery. EEGs aid in diagnosis of epilepsy, tumors, and brain damage.

Electromyogram (EMG) is a recording of the electrical activity produced by a muscle at rest and during contraction. Needle electrodes are inserted into the muscle and the electrical activity is seen on a screen and heard on a loud-speaker. The normal voluntary muscle is silent at rest; contraction gives a continuous smooth tracing on the screen and a low-pitched rumble sound. A muscle that has lost its nerve supply produces a series of small spikes on the screen during the resting stage with a ticking noise audible. Primary diseases of the muscle have distinct patterns for each disease. The EMG aids in determining if the disease is muscular or is from nerve damage. A neurologist must perform the EMG.

Evoked response tests are performed by the EEG department. Unlike the continuous response in an EEG, the response in an evoked response test is intermittent, caused by a stimulus, and recorded with a precise time control and a computerized signal averaging. Evoked response testing shows the functioning of a specific end organ (such as an ear) and the continuity of specific nerve pathways (for the ear it would be peripheral nerves leading to the auditory branch of the VIII [eighth] cranial nerve onto the point of origin in the brain). The brainstem evoked response (BSER) uses sound as the stimulus. The visual evoked response (VER) uses sight as the stimulus. The sensory evoked response (SER) involves touching the body as the stimulus.

LABORATORY TESTS

- Blood sugar
- CBC
- CSF exams
    Cell count
    Chloride

  Collodial gold
  Glucose
  Protein
  VDRL
  Cultures of CSF
- SMA-20

RADIOLOGY AND NUCLEAR MEDICINE EXAMS

Carotid angiography visualizes the carotid artery to determine if there is any obstruction of blood flow to the brain.

Cerebral angiography traces the blood vessels in the cerebrum to determine if any abnormality exists, such as a growth or an obstruction.

CT scan of the brain outlines tumors and abscesses and shows the extent of injury due to trauma.

Myelogram (explained in Chapter 10) visualizes any abnormality of the spinal cord.

Pneumography or pneumoencephalography shows the ventricles and the subarachnoid system by performing a spinal puncture with the patient in a sitting position and replacing withdrawn CSF with air or a gas. This exam is performed only when a CT scan does not give adequate information.

Positron emission tomography (PET) produces a picture of the metabolic activity of the brain. Glucose tagged with radioisotope is given to the patient in the nuclear medicine department. PET hopes to detect cancers before any symptoms arise and will aid in explaining how cancers spread to surrounding areas. It also aids in diagnosing mental disorders.

Radioisotope encephalography uses radioactive material injected via spinal tap prior to a brain scan. The pathway of the radioactivity demonstrates abnormalities in the circulation process of the CSF in the brain, such as obstructions or fistulas caused by injury.

Skull series x-rays visualize fractures and bone abnormalities. Head injury cases will probably have skull series ordered first and other tests, such as CT scan, later according to patient's condition.

Ventriculography involves a great deal of hazard because a needle is passed through brain tissue into the ventricles after burr-holes are made in the skull. CSF is replaced by air and films visualize the ventricles. CT scan and radioisotope encephalography are performed first; ventriculography is used only if other tests fail to give information needed.

MEDICATIONS

Antibiotics

- ampicillin—IV—500 mg q 6 hrs, up to 8 or 12 Gm a day for very severe infections. Drug of choice for meningitis caused by Neisseria meningococcus. PO—250 mg q 6 hrs for minor infections.
- erythromycin—IV—in dosage by body weight for severe infections when the patient is allergic to penicillin.
- Chloromycetin—IV—dosage per body weight, used in influenzal meningitis.
- gentamicin—IV—dosage per body weight, used for serious bacterial infections caused by E. coli, pseudomonas, and staphylococcus.

Anticonvulsants

- Dilantin—PO—100 mg tid and adjusted to needs. IV for cases of status epilepticus. Also used to relieve pain in trigeminal neuralgia.
- Depakene—PO—individualized dosage for epilepsy of mixed types.
- Mebaral—PO—400 to 600 mg daily, adjust to needs, used for grand mal and petit mal seizures.
- Milontin—PO—500 mg to 1 Gm daily, adjust to needs, used for petit mal seizures.
- Mysoline—PO—250 mg to start and increase as needed, used for grand mal seizures, psychomotor, and Jacksonian types of epilepsy.
- Peganone—PO—start with 1 Gm daily and increase as needed, used for grand mal and psychomotor types.
- Tegretol—PO—start with 200 mg bid and adjust, used for grand mal, psychomotor, and mixed type seizures that do not respond to other drugs. Also used in trigeminal neuralgia.
- Zarontin—PO—250 mg bid, used for petit mal seizures.

Antineoplastics

BCNU, CCNU, and methy CCNU—all individualized dosage.

Fungicides

- amphotericin-B—IV—individualized dose, used for meningitis caused by cryptococcus and coccidiodes.

Specifics for Cerebral Edema

- Decadron (dexamethasone) is a steroid—IV—4 to 6 mg q 6 hrs. Initial dose may be as high as 10 mg, then reduced. Inoperable brain tumors may be given 2 mg bid or tid. Orders for decadron may be gradual dosage decreases, but the doctor will write a series at one time. Example:
  Decadron 4 mg qid for 2 days then

Decadron 4 mg tid for 2 days then
Decadron 4 mg bid for 2 days then
Decadron 4 mg daily.

When orders are written in that fashion, be sure the dates on medication cards are correct for starting and stopping each dose. Kardex cards must contain correct information as to dosage, stop, and start dates.

- mannitol—IV—available in 15% and 20% solution, dosage is calculated by weight and given over a period of 30 to 60 minutes. May be repeated in 12 hours. Urine output is checked and the patient usually has a Foley catheter.

Specifics for Migraine Headache, Adrenergic Blockers

- Cafergot (ergotamine)—PO—tabs ii at start of attack and tab i every half hour till pain ceases or until 6 tablets have been taken. Supp i at beginning of attack, repeat in one hour.
- Gynergen (ergotamine)—IM—0.25 to 0.5 mg usually effective if given at start of attack. PO or sublingual—4 to 5 mg at start of attack then 2 mg q hr up to 11 mg a day.
- Sansert—PO—2 mg bid, tid with meals, up to 8 mg a day. After six months use, the drug must be stopped for several weeks to avoid pulmonary or cardiovascular problems.

Specifics for Myasthenia Gravis, Cholinergics

- Mestinon—PO—dosage individualized—available as a syrup, as tablets, and as timespan tablets.
- Mytelase Chloride caplets—PO—5 to 25 mg qid.
- Prostigmin (neostigmin)—SC or IM—0.5 mg. PO—tabs of 15 mg, 10 tabs over 24 hr period with patient adjusting schedule according to symptoms. Is sometimes used as a diagnostic test for myasthenia gravis since it causes symptoms to disappear.
- Tensilon—IV,IM—used as diagnostic test as it relieves the weakness quickly, used to test if patient is in myasthenic crisis or has been overtreated. This is not used for treatment on a continuing basis.

Specifics for Narcolepsy, Cerebral Stimulants

- Benzedrine—PO—10 to 20 mg tid, increase as needed.
- Dexedrine—PO—start with 5 mg each morning and increase prn.
- Ritalin—PO—5 to 10 mg tid or qid, increase prn.

Specifics for Parkinson's Syndrome

- Artane—PO—1 to 5 mg tid.
- Cogentin—PO—0.5 to 5 mg daily
- Larodopa—PO—250 mg tid, increase to tolerance.
- Sinemet 25/250—PO—tablets 3 to 6 a day.
- Symmetrel—PO—100 mg bid.

Valium

Valium may be used to control severe recurrent convulsive seizures, but it is not exclusively an anticonvulsant. It may be used to help in treating spasticity disorders of CNS seen in cerebral palsy and paraplegia. It is also used in short-term therapy of anxiety states.

EXAMPLES OF PHYSICIAN'S ORDERS

Dx: Myasthenia gravis

1. CBC, SMAC-20, UA
2. EKG
3. Bedside spirometry q 12 hrs
4. Notify me if any respiratory problems.
5. DAT
6. VS q 4 hrs
7. Up c̄ assistance
8. Mestinon ī PO q 3 hrs
9. Prednisone 25 mg qod—ask patient if she had any today.
10. Vit D 50,000 U PO once a wk
11. OsCal 500 ī PO bid c̄ meals
12. Mestinon timespan at 2200 daily
13. Eggcrate mattress (a foam mattress to prevent decubiti)

Dx: Organic brain syndrome, patient is aphasic.

1. O_2 @ 4 L/m
2. EKG today
3. Chest x-ray
4. VS, NS q ½ hr till stable
5. CBC, UA
6. D_5W TKO
7. Cardiac enzymes

Next day:

1. CT brain scan
2. Repeat EKG
3. DAT

Next day:

1. May sedate with Valium 10 mg PO prior to CT scan
2. Valium 5 mg PO q 6 hrs prn agitation
3. Serentil 30 mg PO HS
4. EEG tomorrow—no sleep deprivation studies
5. Ca, P, Alk phos, CBC in AM
6. Encourage oral fluids.

REVIEW QUESTIONS

1. The nervous system is composed of the _____,
_____, and _____.
2. The function of the nervous system is _____
_____
3. The inability to speak or speak comprehensively or to understand is
_____.
4. _____ is the supporting tissue of the CNS.
5. _____ refers to motion.
6. Inflammation of a nerve is _____.
7. _____ is a sudden attack of involuntary movement.
8. List five diseases and disorders of the nervous system.
_____
_____
_____
_____

9. Name the department that performs the following:
Evoked response tests _____
Carotid angiography _____
Craniotomy _____
CSF exams _____
Myelogram _____
PET _____
10. Classify the following medications:
Dilantin _____
amphotericin-B _____
mannitol _____
Sansert _____
Mestinon _____
Ritalin _____
Larodopa _____
11. An electromyogram is performed by a _____ for the purpose of _____.
12. EEG is the abbreviation for _____.
13. The structural unit of the nervous system is the _____.
14. The membranes that cover the brain and the spinal cord are _____
_____.
15. A refex arc is _____
_____
16. What medication may be ordered in decreasing dosages with the order
for several days written at one time? _____
17. What examination may be done on the unit that requires a tray from
central supply? _____
18. Name four special beds that may be used on the neurology unit.
_____

Chapter 17 | Eye and Ear

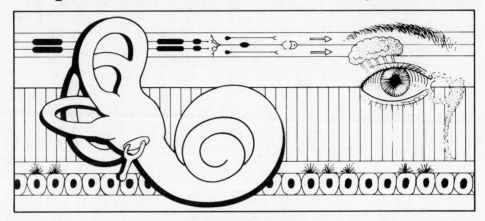

OBJECTIVES

Study of this chapter will enable you to:

1. List the structures of the eye.
2. List the disorders of vision.
3. Define glaucoma.
4. Define cataract.
5. List surgeries of the eye.
6. List and classify eye medications.
7. List the structures of the ear.
8. Define otitis media.
9. Define Meniere's Syndrome.
10. List common surgeries of the ear.
11. List and classify some ear medications.
12. Transcribe Physician's Orders for diseases of eye and ear.

The eye and the ear are organs of sensation. Both are very intricate organs that allow us to enjoy the beauty of the world in which we live.

STRUCTURE OF THE EYE

The eye is the organ of vision. The eyeball is composed of three layers. The outer layer, **sclera,** is composed of tough, fibrous tissue which provides protection. The very center of the front of the sclera is the **cornea,** which is transparent to permit the passage of light rays.

The middle layer is the uvea or vascular coat. The parts of this layer are the

choroid, the **ciliary body,** and the **iris.** The choroid is pigmented and contains blood vessels which nourish the eye. The ciliary muscle makes up most of the ciliary body at the front of the eye. The iris is behind the cornea, and the hole in the center is the **pupil.** These structures give the eye color. The muscles of the iris react to light. The pupil constricts in bright light and dilates in dim light. The crystalline **lens** lies just behind the iris, attached to the ciliary body by a ligament.

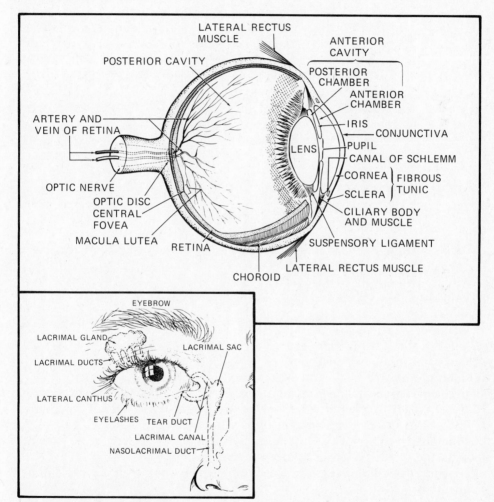

Figure 17-1. Structure of the Eye.

The **retina,** the innermost layer, covers the back two-thirds of the choroid. It leads into the optic nerve which leads into the brain. The retina contains rods, receptors for dim light, and cones, receptors for color and bright light. The **blind spot** is the area where the optic nerve enters and there are no rods or cones. This area is also called the **optic disk.** The lens refracts the light entering the eye so that the light focuses on the retina, which transfers the message to the brain and enables us to see.

The anterior cavity in front of the lens is filled with a watery fluid called the **aqueous humor.** This fluid flows into the bloodstream through the Canal of Schlemm.

The posterior cavity is filled with a jelly-like substance called the **vitreous humor.**

The **conjunctiva** is a mucous membrane that covers the front of the eyeball and lines the eyelids.

The **lacrimal glands** secrete tears, which are spread over the eye by blinking. This process cleans and lubricates the external surface of the eye. Tears enter the lacrimal ducts at the inner corner of the eye, and the ducts empty into the lacrimal sac. The nasolacrimal duct carries tears to the nose where the hairs move the tears to the nasopharynx where they are swallowed.

Study the structures of the eye with the aid of Figure 17-1.

| TERMINOLOGY

Accommodation—the ability of the ciliary muscles to change the curvature of the lens for seeing at different distances

Canthus—any corner of the eye

Gonioscope—an instrument for viewing the angle of the interior chamber where the cornea and iris are joined

Nystagmus—a constant, rapid, involuntary eyeball movement

Oculus dexter (O.D.)—right eye

Oculus sinister (O.S.)—left eye

Oculus uterque (O.U.)—both eyes

Ophthalmoscope—an instrument for viewing the interior of the eye

Ophthamologist—a medical doctor who specializes in eye care; examines eyes for glasses and diseases and performs surgery

Optometrist—a Doctor of Optometry (OD), trained and licensed to examine eyes and prescribe lenses to correct vision

Refraction—bending of light rays as they pass from one medium into another medium

Tonometer—an instrument that measures intraocular pressure

20/20 vision—a person can see at a distance of 20 feet the size letter on the examination chart that he should see at 20 feet.

Viscosurgery—microsurgery with the use of a viscous jelly called Healon that fills the eye cavity during surgery

Visual acuity—sharpness of vision

Visual fields—the area seen when looking straight at an object. A person should see for some distance on each side. Visual fields are reduced in glaucoma. An extremely narrow field is referred to as tunnel vision.

DISORDERS OF VISION

Astigmatism is a distorted focus rather than a sharp, point focus which results when the rays of light are not all focused on the retina. There are many types of astigmatism. **Tx:** Corrective lenses.

Diplopia is double vision due to muscular dysfunction or to a disease process. **Tx:** Determine and treat cause.

Hyperopia is farsightedness. Things at a distance are seen more clearly than things that are near. **Tx:** Corrective lenses to wear for near tasks.

Myopia is nearsightedness. Objects nearby are seen more clearly. **Tx:** Corrective lenses.

Poor eye coordination means that both eyes do not work as a team and vision is distorted. **Tx:** Eye exercises for vision training, corrective lenses with prism component, surgical resection of a muscle in extreme cases.

Presbyopia means that the focusing ability has decreased to a point where vision at a reading distance is blurry and difficult. This usually occurs between ages 40 and 45. **Tx:** Corrective lenses, bifocals, or trifocals.

Strabismus is crosseye. One eye or both eyes turn in or out. **Tx:** Corrective lenses, muscle training, surgery if necessary.

DISEASES AND DISORDERS

Achromatopsia is color blindness. This is an inherited condition that is due to the mutation of a gene in an X-chromosome. It is more common in men since they have only one X-chromosone. It causes an inability to fully see either red or green colors. There is no treatment.

Cataracts are a clouding of the lens, and light cannot get past the lens to the retina; they may be caused by age, disease, or injury. **Tx:** Surgery with implanted lens and/or corrective eyeglasses.

Choroiditis is an inflammation of the choroid. **Tx:** Atropine gtts, corticosteroids.

Conjunctivitis is an inflammation of the conjunctiva. **Tx:** Atropine eye gtts, corticosteroids.

Dacryocystitis is an inflammation of the lacrimal sac. **Tx:** Hot compresses to the area, antibiotics orally, and eye gtts. The condition may need surgery for drainage.

Detached retina means that the retina has separated from the choroid. **Tx:** Surgery.

Glaucoma is increased pressure within the eye due to an obstruction of the Canal of Schlemm. The acute type is sudden blockage of the canal and requires immediate medical attention. The chronic type may show no symptoms for a long time, but side vision is destroyed. **Tx:** Medications to reduce pressure, surgery if medication not helpful.

Iritis is an inflammation of the iris. **Tx:** Atropine gtts, corticosteroids.

Keratitis is an inflammation of the cornea. It is usually caused by the herpes simplex virus for which Stoxil eye gtts are specific.

Papilledema (choked disk) is swelling of the head of the optic nerve due to an increased intracranial pressure or due to interference with venous return from the eyes. **Tx:** Determine cause of intracranial pressure or blockage and treat cause.

Pterygium is a thickening of the conjunctiva, and it grows from the inner canthus to the border of the cornea. **Tx:** Surgical removal.

Retinoblastoma is a fairly common tumor arising from retinal cells. It accounts for 2% of childhood malignancies. **Tx:** Removal of eyeball or radiation therapy or both.

Sty is an infection of a sebaceous gland of the eyelid. **Tx:** Warm soaks, antibiotic ointment to area.

Disease-Causing Organisms of Eye

- H. Influenzae
- Herpes Simplex virus
- Staphylococci
- Streptococci

SURGERIES

Blepharoplasty is plastic surgery on the eyelid for cosmetic purposes or because the weight of the lid interferes with vision.

Cataract removal can be done several ways. **Cryosurgery** is extraction of the lens by a cryoprobe; the lens sticks to the cold probe and is easily withdrawn. The lens may be removed by suction. **Phacoemulsification** uses ultrasonic vibrations to liquify the lens, which is withdrawn through a very small needle. Post-op glasses or contact lenses are used in all types of surgery if intraocular lenses were not implanted at the time of surgery.

Enucleation is removal of the entire eyeball.

Evisceration leaves the sclera, but the rest of the eyeball is removed. This provides better motion for an artificial eye.

Iridectomy is surgical removal of a portion of the iris.

Iritomy or irotomy is the formation of an artificial pupil.

Keratoplasty is a corneal transplant.

Keratotomy is an incision of the cornea.

Kerectomy is surgical excision of a portion of the cornea.

Pterygium removal is surgical excision of the extra growth of the conjunctival tissue.

Retinal reattachment surgeries involve some method of exudate formation so that the retina adheres to the choroid. **Electrodiathermy** is the process of withdrawing the fluid below the detached retina by passing an electrode needle through the sclera. This causes an exudate to form on the choroid, and the retina adheres to it. **Retinal cryopexy** is the process of applying a cryoprobe to the sclera to cause very small damage. The choroid and retina adhere to the sclera as a result of scarring. **Photocoagulation** by laser beam (laser means light amplification by stimulated emission of radiation) is the process of directing a strong beam of light from a carbon arc source through the dilated pupil. This produces a small burn which causes exudate to form and seal the retina onto the choroid.

| MEDICATIONS

Eye gtts, solutions, and ointments are given in varying amounts individualized for each patient. No UAD will be given.

Miotics

Miotics are drugs that produce contractions of the iris and lower the intra-ocular pressure of glaucoma.

- pilocarpine 1% and 2% eye gtts
- Timoptic eye gtts
- Diamox tablets 250 mg, parenteral vials of 500 mg

Mydriatics and Cycloplegics

Mydriatic, drugs that cause the smooth muscle of the iris to relax, and cycloplegic drugs that cause paralysis or relaxation of the ciliary muscle are combined in the following medications:

- atropine 1% gtts
- Cyclogyl 1% and 0.5% gtts
- homatropine 5% gtts

Antiviral

- Vira-A Ophth Oint
- Stoxil (idoxuridine) Ophth Sol'n and Oint for herpes simplex keratitis

Antibiotics

- Chloromycetin Ophth Oint 1%
- Neosporin Ophth Oint and Sol'n
- Opthocort Ophth Oint

Steroids

Steroids are used to treat allergic reactions, nonpyrogenic inflammation, and severe injury.

- Hydeltrasol Ophth Oint and Sol'n
- Neodecadron Ophth Oint and Sol'n

EXAMPLES OF PHYSICIAN'S ORDERS

Dx: Cataract O.S.
  Pre-op orders:

1. Reg diet
2. Up ad lib
3. Sign operative permit for cataract extraction of left eye.
4. Cleanse face with phisohex tonight, repeat in early AM.
5. Cyclogyl Ophth Sol'n 1% gtts ̄ii O.S. 30 minutes before surgery time
6. Neosynephrine Ophth Sol'n 10% gtts ̄ii O.S. 25 minutes before surgery time
7. Send hearing aid to surgery with patient (Pre-op orders by anesthesiology)

  Post-op orders:

1. Have Neodecadron Ophth oint at bedside
2. Complete bedrest
3. Lie on unoperated side or back only
4. May elevate head of bed as desired
5. Soft diet, advance as tol
6. LOC prn
7. ASA gr × q 4h prn discomfort
8. Tylenol #2 tab ̄i if ASA not effective
9. Mouthwash prn but do not brush teeth
10. Instruct patient not to bend head forward or downward, not to sneeze, cough or move rapidly
11. Dalmane 30 mg HS prn sleep

STRUCTURE OF THE EAR

The ear is the organ of hearing. The fleshy external ear (the **auricle or pinna**) collects sound waves and directs them into the **auditory canal.** The **tympanic membrane** (eardrum) separates the auditory canal from the middle ear. The middle ear contains the three smallest bones of the body, the ossicles. The eardrum is attached to the handle of the **malleus** (hammer) which fits into the **incus** (anvil). Sound waves hit the eardrum and move the malleus and incus as one unit. Articulation of the incus with the **stapes** (stirrup) causes the stapes to move back and forth in the oval window. The oval window and the round window are small structures in the thin, bony partition that separates the middle ear from the inner ear. The **eustachian tube** leads from the middle ear to the pharynx and helps equalize air pressure.

The inner ear is referred to as the **labyrinth,** a complicated structure composed of bone and a membrane within the bone. The central portion is the **vestibule,** which leads to the **semi-circular canals.** The canals are three half circles filled with fluid. The **cochlea** in front of the vestibule looks like a snail's shell. It contains hair cells in a gelatinous membrane. As the stapes moves in the oval window, the movement causes waves in the fluid of the canals. A complex process of compression and decompression of air involving the oval window and the round window move the hair cells in the cochlea. This stimulates nerve endings which lead to the auditory nerve and into the brain where sound is interpreted.

The **mastoid** is a portion of the temporal bone behind the ear. The mastoid cells resemble a honeycomb. The middle ear has an opening into the mastoid.

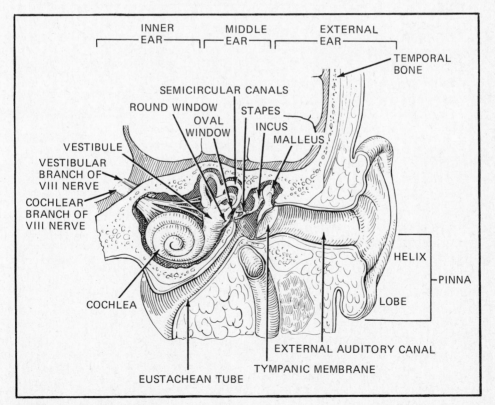

Figure 17-2. Structure of the Ear.

TERMINOLOGY

Otalgia—an earache

Otolaryngologist—a medical doctor who specializes in diagnosis and treatment of diseases of the ear and the larynx

Otologist—a medical doctor who specializes in the diagnosis and treatment of diseases of the ear

Otorhinolaryngologist—a medical doctor who specializes in diagnosis and treatment of diseases of the ear, nose, and throat; usually referred to as an ENT specialist

Otoscope—an instrument to examine the ear

Tinnitus—ringing in the ears

Valsalva maneuver—the act of forcing air into the middle ear when the mouth and nose are closed

DISEASES AND DISORDERS

Eustachitis is an inflammation or infection of the eustachian tube. **Tx:** Decongestants, antihistamines, antibiotics.

External otitis is an infection in the external canal. **Tx:** Keeping ear dry, antibiotic or antifungal ear gtts.

Labyrinthitis is an inflammation and infection of the inner ear. **Tx:** Antibiotics.

Mastoiditis is an infection in the mastoid bone. **Tx:** Antibiotics, surgical removal of mastoid cells.

Meniere's syndrome is a dysfunction of the labyrinth causing attacks of vertigo, vomiting, headache, incoordination. **Tx:** Anti-vertigo medications, vitamin therapy, testing for allergies, surgical use of ultrasound waves to labyrinth.

Myringitis or tympanitis is an inflammation of the eardrum. **Tx:** Decongestants, antibiotic ear gtts.

Otitis media is an infection of the middle ear. The **serous** type is when the eustachian tube becomes swollen and blocks air equalization. This allows fluid to enter the middle ear. **Tx:** Decongestants to open the tube. **Acute otitis media** occurs when a bacteria or virus enters the middle ear from the throat. Pus forms causing pressure on the eardrum, which may rupture. **Tx:** Antibiotics, surgery in some cases.

Otosclerosis is an hereditary condition in which spongy vascular bone fixes the footplate of the stapes and makes it immobile. **Tx:** Surgery.

Disease-Causing Organisms of Ear

- H. Influenzae
- Pseudomonas aeruginosa
- Staphylococci
- Streptococci

SURGERIES

Most surgeries of the ear are done with use of the otologic binocular microscope.

Mastoidectomy is the removal of the mastoid cells.

Myringotomy is the surgical perforation of the eardrum for drainage. Tubes are usually inserted to keep the hole open until healing occurs. The tubes will come out when tissues heal.

Otectomy is the surgical excision of the contents of the middle ear.

Stapedectomy is the removal of the stapes with an insertion of a prosthesis; it restores hearing in most cases of otosclerosis.

Tympanoplasty is the surgical repair of the eardrum. If the hole is small, the edges are cauterized and the hole is patched with a piece of cigarette paper. For large holes, an incision is made behind the ear and tissue is grafted onto the eardrum.

TESTS

Audiogram measures air conduction and nerve conduction by the tone of different pitches; it helps determine the type of hearing loss.

C&S (lab) of eye or ear drainage determines which antibiotic the infecting organism is affected by.

Audiogram measures air conduction and nerve conduction by the tone of different pitches; it helps determine the type of hearing loss.

Caloric test consists of instilling a fluid either colder or warmer than normal body temperature into the auditory canal. The normal response is dizziness; Meniere's Syndrome patients respond with severe vertigo.

Tuning fork tests use the vibrations of the prongs of the instrument to produce hearing. Where hearing occurs, in relation to where the fork is held, is an indication as to the cause of hearing loss.

MEDICATIONS

Decongestants

These drugs were listed in Chapter 12. Review them.

Analgesics

- Auralgan Otic Sol'n—fill canal and plug with cotton q 1–2 hrs.
- Tympagesic gtts—fill canal and plug with cotton q 4h.

Antibiotics

- ampicillin—PO—250 mg q 6 h. Children—50 mg/kg/day.
- Chloromycetin Otic Sol'n—gtts ii tid in canal.
- Orlex Otic Sol'n—gtts ii in canal tid or qid.
- Otic Domeboro Sol'n—gtts 4–6 in canal q 2–3 h.

Antivertigo

- Antivert—PO—25-100 mg/d in divided doses. Not for children.
- Niac Caps (nicotinic acid)—PO—300 mg Cap q 12 h.

EXAMPLE OF PHYSICIAN'S ORDERS

Dx: Meniere's Syndrome

1. Complete bedrest with siderails up at all times.
2. IV D5W c̄ 1 amp MVI at 100 cc/h
3. Keep room in dim light.
4. Disturb patient as little as possible.
5. Phenergan 25 mg IM q 4–6 h prn nausea
6. Low Na soft diet if tolerated. Assist patient.

Two days later:

1. DC IV
2. BRP c̄ assistance. Patient is not to get out of bed alone.
3. Antivert 25 mg q 6h

REVIEW QUESTIONS

1. The _____provides protection for the eye.
2. The structures that compose the vascular layer of the eyeball are _____, _____ and _____.
3. The _____layer of the eyeball gives color to the eye.

4. The _____contains receptors for light sensation that are called _____and _____.

5. The cornea is located _____.

6. The other name for the blind spot is _____.

7. The fluid in the cavity in front of the lens is _____.

8. The fluid in the cavity behind the lens is the _____.

9. Tears are produced by the _____.

10. A cataract is _____.

11. Increased pressure in the eyeball is _____.

12. The laser is used in what type surgery? _____

13. Name three disorders of vision. _____, _____,

_____

14. List three surgeries of the eye. _____

_____

15. The three tiny bones (ossicles) of the ear are the _____

_____

16. Name and define three classifications of eye medications.

_____

_____

_____

17. List three ear medications and classify each.

_____

_____

_____

18. The three divisions of the ear are _____, _____ and _____.

19. The structures of the labyrinth are _____, _____ and _____.

20. Define:
Otitis Media _____
Meniere's Syndrome _____
Mastoiditis _____

_____

21. Three tests for ear function are _____, _____ and _____.

22. Three surgeries of the ear are _____, _____ and _____.

Chapter 18

The Reproductive System

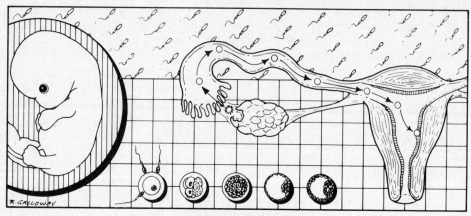

R. GALLOWAY

OBJECTIVES

Study of this chapter will enable you to:

1. List the structures of the male and female reproductive systems.
2. List diseases and disorders of the reproductive system.
3. List and define terms relating to the reproductive system.
4. List surgeries of the reproductive system.
5. List radiology examinations of the reproductive system.
6. List laboratory exams related to the reproductive system.
7. List medications used in diseases and disorders of the reproductive system.
8. Transcribe Physician's Orders relating to the reproductive system.

Reproduction in the human race occurs when a female egg (ovum) is fertilized by the male reproductive cell (spermatozoa or sperm). You remember from Chapter 15 that the endocrine system hormones greatly influence the function of the reproductive system. The hormones produced by the reproductive system will be discussed in this chapter.

MALE REPRODUCTIVE SYSTEM

The structures of the male reproductive system include the penis, scrotum, testes, prostate gland, Cowper's glands, vas deferens, and the seminal vesicles. The **scrotum** is a loose pouch that hangs from the inferior abdominal wall to hold the testes. It is composed of muscle and aerolar tissue covered by a wrinkled layer of skin. The internal part is divided by a septum so each testicle has its own compartment. The scrotum protects the testes and gives them a lower temperature housing since normal body temperature interferes with sperm production.

The **testes** are oval-shaped glands hanging from the spermatic cords. They develop in the abdominal cavity and descend into the scrotum about two months before birth. The left testicle is lower than the right one and has a longer spermatic cord. The testes are composed of lobules consisting of seminiferous tubules separated by interstitial cells. The tubules unite to form ducts which fold across each other to create a mass on top of the testis called the **epididymis.** The **vas deferens** is the duct from the epididymis to the urethra. The spermatic cord contains the vas deferens, blood vessels, and nerves. The tubules produce **sperm.** Sperm cells have a head that contains chemicals which help the sperm penetrate the ova. The middle section provides energy for movement. The tail movement enables the sperm to swim. The interstitial cells secrete **testosterone,** which produces male characteristics, controls growth and development of the male sex organs, aids in bone growth and protein build up, and controls normal sexual conduct.

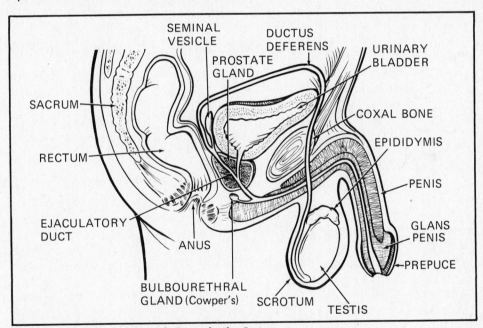

Figure 18-1. Structure of the Male Reproductive System.

The **prostate gland** secretes an alkaline fluid. The **seminal vesicles** are pouches, one on each posterior side of the bladder, which secrete a sticky fluid. **Cowper's glands** lie beneath the prostate, one on each side, and secrete an alkaline fluid. The fluid from the prostate gland, seminal vesicles, Cowper's glands, and sperm make up the semen which enters the ejaculatory duct on each side of the posterior bladder. The ejaculatory ducts open into the urethra. During sexual activity the ejaculatory ducts eject semen into the urethra.

The **penis** is the external sex organ which encloses the urethra. Urine is passed to the outside through the penis, and it also introduces semen into the vaginal canal of the female. The penis is usually flaccid but must become erect or firm to enter the vagina. Therefore, it contains erectile tissue in three columns. The erectile tissue contains large venous sinuses which fill with blood during erection. One layer of tissue is enlarged to form the glans at the end of the penis. The glans penis is covered by loose skin called the prepuce or foreskin.

FEMALE REPRODUCTIVE SYSTEM

The external organs are the labia majora, labia minora, hymen, clitoris, and vulvo-vaginal glands. The **vulva** is the term for all the external organs.

The **labia majora** are folds of skin from the mons pubis, a fatty pad of tissue over the symphysis pubis, to the perineum. The perineum is the area between the anus and vagina. The **labia minora** are smaller folds of skin inside the labia majora. The **hymen** is a thin membrane over the opening to the vagina and is easily perforated. The **clitoris** is similar to the male penis in that it contains sensory nerve endings and becomes erect during sexual excitement. It lies behind the point where the labia minora join anteriorly and is covered by a layer of skin called the prepuce; the exposed end of the clitoris is the glans. The urinary meatus is below the clitoris.

The internal organs are the vagina, uterus, fallopian tubes, and ovaries.

The **vagina** is a muscular organ lined with mucous membrane, which lies in folds called rugae. The opening to the vagina is below the urinary meatus. The vaginal walls lie against each other, but the vagina becomes tubular when something is inserted into it. The stretchability of the vagina is necessary for the passage of the baby during birth. Vaginal secretions are acid, which is destructive to sperm, so the alkaline secretions in semen counteract the acid. **Bartholin's glands,** one on each side near the vaginal opening, secrete a lubricating fluid.

The **uterus** is a pear-shaped organ connected to the vagina by the **cervix.** The cervix extends into the vagina and has an opening called the os. The cervical canal leads to the body of the uterus which contains the openings for the fallopian tubes. Above the tubal openings is the fundus. The uterus is held in place over the bladder by the broad ligaments. The muscle of the uterus is the myometrium. The lining of the uterus is the endometrium. The uterus receives the fertilized ovum and houses the fetus until time for birth, then the strong contractions move the baby through the cervix and vagina to the outside.

The **fallopian tubes** lead from the uterus and end near the ovary in fingerlike projections called fimbriae. The fimbriae catch the ova as it is released from the ovary and carry it to the uterus by peristaltic waves. If the egg is not fertilized, it is discarded through the vagina.

The **ovary** is an almond-shaped gland, and there is one on each side of the uterus. They are held in place by ligaments. The ovaries produce and release mature ova and secrete estrogen and progesterone. **Estrogen** controls the development of the female reproductive organs and is responsible for female characteristics such as the development of the breasts, aids in protein building, and keeps the fluid and electrolyte balance. **Progesterone** helps estrogen prepare the endometrium for pregnancy and the breasts for milk production. The ovarian cycle governs menstruation. Menstruation is the periodic discharge of blood, mucus, and fluid from tissue and cells from the endometrium. The lining of the uterus sloughs off, a little at a time, and new cells develop. An easy way to remember how the cycle occurs is to associate the changes with the letters *F-O-L-D.*

- *Folliculation* is the process by which an ova matures. Each ovary has about 200,000 follicles, eggs surrounded by a layer of cells, at birth. At the beginning of a cycle, a follicle begins producing estrogen. FSH from the anterior pituitary stimulates the follicle. The follicle enlarges and moves to the outer edge of the ovary. As it enlarges, more estrogen and some progesterone are produced. LH secretion increases and FSH decreases. The endometrium becomes thick.
- *Ovulation* occurs about day 14 in the average 28 day cycle. The follicle ruptures and an ova is released into the pelvic cavity.

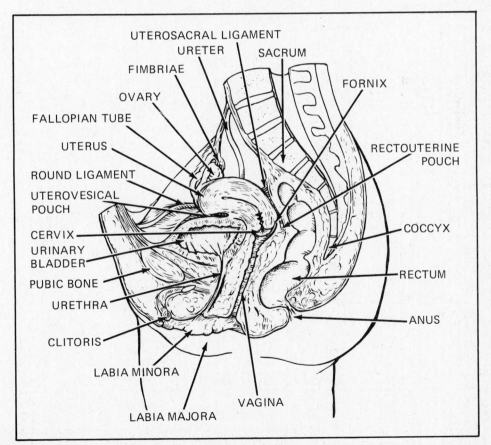

Figure 18-2. Structure of the Female Reproductive System.

- *Leutinization* refers to the changes in the follicle after rupture. The follicle absorbs the blood clot that results, and the cells enlarge to form the corpus luteum. Estrogen levels drop after rupture of the follicle and increase again as the corpus luteum develops. The corpus luteum secretes estrogen and progesterone. Progesterone levels are high in this phase.
- *Destruction* is the period of menstrual flow. If the ova is not fertilized, the follicle degenerates with decreased estrogen and progesterone, which causes the endometrium to slough off, and bleeding occurs. The drop in estrogen and progesterone causes FSH production again and another cycle starts.

The breasts are a part of the female reproductive system and are called the **mammary glands.** The breasts are affixed to the muscles of the chest by connective tissue. Each breast has compartments called lobes which divide into lobules containing the alveoli that secrete milk. Mammary ducts carry the milk to the nipple. The darker area of skin around the nipple is the areola.

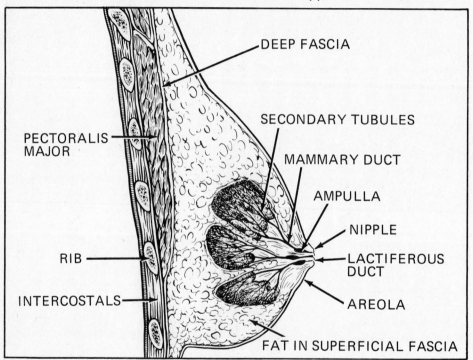

Figure 18-3. Structure of the Female Breast.

PREGNANCY AND CHILDBIRTH

Pregnancy occurs when the ova is fertilized and then becomes embedded in the endometrium. Fertilization takes place in the fallopian tube most of the time, but it can take place in the uterus. The concentration of sperm needed to liquefy the ova membrane for penetration is estimated to be 60,000,000.

Sperm counts below that probably produce sterility.

The menstrual cycle is absent during pregnancy. Any bleeding should be investigated. The corpus luteum remains functional six to eight months, secreting mainly progesterone.

The **placenta** is the growth in the uterine wall to which the embryo is attached at the navel by the umbilical cord. The placenta provides nourishment and produces the hormones estrogen and progesterone. The umbilical cord contains two arteries and a vein and provides for the exchange of nourishment and waste via the placenta.

The **amniotic sac** surrounds the embryo and secretes amniotic fluid. The fluid protects the embryo and provides warmth and moisture.

Identical twins result from the union of one sperm and one ovum. The fertilized egg divides into two embryo; there is one placenta and two amniotic sacs. The twins are the same sex.

Fraternal twins result from fertilization of two ova. There are two placentas and two amniotic sacs. The sex may or may not be the same.

A lunar month is 28 days. The growth of an embryo is spoken of in terms of lunar months. By the end of the first month all organs become differentiated. The embryo is about 9 millimeters long. The second month, the brain develops and the head enlarges, external genitalia appear, and the length is about 3 centimeters. Fingers and toes develop the third month, and nails are beginning. The fetus weighs about ½ ounce and is about 9 centimeters long. During the fourth month, sex can be determined, and hair appears on the head. Length is about 16 centimeters. The fifth month is the time movement is usually felt by the mother, heart sounds can be heard, and downy hair appears over the entire body. Eyebrows and eyelashes appear the sixth month. Length is now 34 centimeters and weight about 1¼ pounds. During the seventh month, a cheesy, greasy substance called the vernix caseosa covers the skin. The bowels contain a thick, green, sticky substance called meconium. The fetus is fully developed in the eighth month and weighs nearly three pounds. Iron, calcium, phosphorus, and nitrogen are being stored for use after birth. In the ninth month, fat deposits under the skin fill out the body and weight is about 5½ pounds, length between 40 and 46 centimeters. The end of the tenth month is time for birth. Average weight is 6 to 8 pounds and average length is 18 to 20 inches (48 to 52 centimeters).

Fetal circulation is different because the lungs do not function until birth. The ductus arteriosus closes after birth and circulation through the lungs begins with the baby's first breath.

LABOR AND DELIVERY

The onset of labor is one or more of the following: a bloody "show," a rupture of the membranes of the amniotic sac, or regular contractions of the uterus. A bloody "show" is expulsion of the thick plug of mucus that has filled the cervix during pregnancy.

Contractions of the uterus shorten and widen the cervix. Dilatation of the cervix is determined by rectal or vaginal examination. Full dilatation is 10 centimeters. The length of labor varies with each woman.

The baby moves through the cervix and vagina head first in the majority of cases. As soon as the baby is born, it cries or is made to cry. The mucus is cleared from the mouth. The cord is clamped in two places and then cut. The Apgar score is used to evaluate the heart rate, respiratory effort, muscle tone, reflex irritability, and color. An ID bracelet is placed on the baby before it is taken to the nursery.

The placenta detaches from the wall of the uterus and is expelled. The doctor examines the placenta to make sure a section did not tear off and remain in the uterus.

Some hospitals utilize birthing rooms for labor, delivery, and recovery. Others have separate rooms for each stage. The usual hospital stay is only 24 hours.

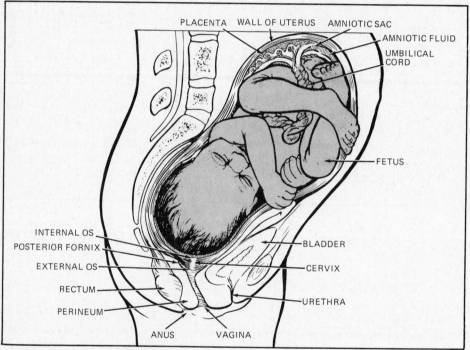

Figure 18-4. Fetus Inside the Uterus.

TERMINOLOGY

Abortion—the expulsion from the uterus of the products of conception if the weight is less than 500 grams. Types are:
- *Complete*—all products of conception are expelled
- *Incomplete*—part of placenta remains in the uterus
- *Induced*—a pregnancy is interrupted by an instrument or medication

- *Missed*—the fetus is dead but remains in the uterus
- *Spontaneous*—a pregnancy is interrupted by natural causes, a miscarriage

Antepartum—before birth; prenatal

Coitus—sexual intercourse

Cul-de-sac—a blind pouch in the peritoneal cavity between the vagina and the rectum

Embryo—a fertilized egg the first eight weeks

Fetus—the developing unborn from eight weeks to birth

Genitalia—the organs of reproduction; usually used in reference to external organs

Gestation—the period of pregnancy

Gravida—a woman that is pregnant

Induction—starting labor by mechanical or chemical means; usually means that pitocin is given to start contractions

Infertility—the inability to conceive and produce a living child.

Lactation—the secretion of milk by the breasts

Menarche—the first menstrual cycle

Menopause—the permanent cessation of menstruation, the change of life.

Neonatal—a newborn up to four weeks

Orgasm—the climax of the sexual act. In the male, the ejaculation of semen is the orgasm. In the female, orgasm consists of rhythmical contractions of the vaginal muscles combined with a diffuse pleasurable sensation.

Parturition—the labor of childbirth

Postpartum—after delivery

Premature labor—labor before the actual calculated due date.

Presentation—the part of the baby that will enter the outside first; the crown of the head is the most common and is called vertex presentation.

Primipara—a woman is giving birth for the first time or has only one child. Para refers to the number of pregnancies that have been carried past 20 weeks.

Puberty—the state of development at which a person is capable of reproduction.

DISEASES AND DISORDERS

Male

(You remember the prostate was discussed previously.)

Cancer of the penis usually occurs in males who have not been circumcised. The usual lesion is under the foreskin. **Tx:** Surgery.

Cancer of the testes most often occurs in men under 30. Seminomas are treatable by radiation. Chemotherapy is used for choriocarcinomas and metastatic tumors.

Cryptorchidism is incomplete or improper descent of the testes (one or both) before birth. **Tx:** Chorionic gonadotropin, surgery before age five or six if necessary.

Epididymitis is inflammation of the epididymis. **Tx:** Bedrest, scrotal support, heat to the area, antibiotics if bacterial infection present.

Hydrocele is an accumulation of fluid in the scrotal tissues. **Tx:** Bedrest, scrotal support, surgery if condition persistent.

Hypogonadism is inadequate male hormones, resulting in delay of puberty if due to pituitary deficiency. **Tx:** Testosterone has to be given for life but will not correct sterility. **Klinefelter's syndrome** is a developmental abnormality. The tubules in the testes fail and sterility results. There is a chromosome abnormality. **Tx:** Testosterone will produce male characteristics but will not affect sterility.

Hypospadias is a condition in which the urethra opens to the outside other than at the end of the penis. The opening may be on the shaft of the penis or in the perineum. A fibrous band on the inside causes the penis to curve. **Tx:** Surgery to release the band followed by reconstruction of the urethra. Results are good.

Impotency is the repeated failure to achieve and maintain an erection of the penis. This may be due to insufficient blood supply caused by arterial disease, malfunctioning of the nervous system due to injury or emotional problems, abnormal amounts of hormones, or certain medications. Antihypertensives, antidepressants, sedatives, tranquilizers, or alcohol may be the cause. When the causative drug is stopped, the impotency subsides. Surgeries such as ileostomies may cause impotency because a nerve may be cut unavoidably. Paraplegics and quadraplegics may suffer from impotency. **Tx:** Hormones if that is the cause, a switch to a medication that does not have the side effect, penile implant.

Infertility may have many causes. Extensive testing may be needed. Hormones may help if there is a proven deficiency. Surgery may be needed if there is an obstruction anywhere in the sperm pathway. Artificial insemination using the ejaculate from several times from the husband, if the sperm count is low, may be successful.

Female

Amenorrhea, absence of menses, may be due to ovarian dysfunction or pituitary deficiency. Extensive testing may be required to find the cause. **Tx:** Hormone replacement if that is the cause.

Benign tumors of the uterus and ovaries are fairly common. The most common uterine tumor is "fibroids," or leiomyoma, which causes uterine enlargement, pressure, and, sometimes vaginal bleeding. **Tx:** Watch and wait if the tumor is small with no symptoms; remove the uterus if the tumor is large and is causing problems. Tumors of ovary may be solid or cystic. **Tx:** Resection of the cyst or removal of the ovary.

Cancers may occur in any structure. Cancer of the vulva is treated by surgical removal. Vaginal cancer is treated with radiation or surgery or a combination. Surgery consists of removal of the uterus and the entire vaginal structure. Cancer of the cervix may be cauterized if small or treated by a conization excision of the area or a vaginal hysterectomy. Cancer of the uterus is treated by removal of the uterus, both tubes, and both ovaries. A radium implant may be used before surgery. Cancer of the ovary is treated by removal of the uterus and both tubes and both ovaries. Advanced cancer requires radiation and chemotherapy.

Cancer of the breast is the most common site of cancer in women. There is a familial tendency. Cancer in one breast increases the chances of having cancer in the other breast. Any lump should be investigated. Every woman should examine her breasts just after the menstrual period; postmenopausal women can do the examination any time but routinely once a month. Biopsy should be performed on suspicious lumps. Early diagnosis is important. **Tx:** Removal of lump, removal of breast, radiation, chemotherapy, corticosteroids. Metastasis to other areas may require removal of ovaries, removal of adrenals, and removal of the pituitary.

Cystocele results from childbirth. The vaginal wall is weakened, and the bladder protrudes into the vagina. **Tx:** Exercises to strengthen muscles, surgical correction.

Dysmenorrhea is painful menstruation. This may be due to infection, misplaced uterus, tumor, or strictures of the cervix. **Tx:** Determine cause and treat the cause.

Endometriosis is a condition in which patches of the endometrium make their way into the pelvic cavity and adhere to tissue. Each month the patch goes through the cycle of menstruation and causes pain. **Tx:** Combined therapy of estrogen and progesterone; androgen therapy; surgery to remove the lesions or complete removal of uterus, tubes, and ovaries.

Erythroblastosis fetalis is a disease of the newborn. A mother with Rh− blood who carries a child with Rh+ blood develops antibodies in her blood. The first child will not be affected. The next child with Rh+ blood will receive the antibodies in the mother's blood, which will destroy their red blood cells. If the child does not receive exchange transfusions shortly after birth, damage to the CNS results. Cerebral palsy is a common result. The Rh− mother who delivers an Rh+ child is given Rhogam before 72 hours have elapsed to prevent antibody formation. Careful screening is done before administration of the Rhogam as there are subdivisions of the Rh factor. Mothers with Rh− blood who have miscarriages or ectopic pregnancies need to be immunized, also.

Fibrocystic disease of the breast occurs mostly in the 30 to 50 age group. Painful lumps appear and increase rapidly in size. Cysts of fluid may be aspirated for cytology studies. Solid cysts are removed if troublesome. Symptoms subside after menopause.

Infertility requires extensive testing. Any functional or structural abnormality is treated. Hormones are of value in many cases.

Leukorrhea is a whitish discharge from the vagina. This may be due to an inflammation of the cervix, decreased production of estrogen, or an infection. Microscopic studies or cultures will identify any organism. **Tx:** Antibiotics, local estrogen creams, specifics for organisms.

Rectocele occurs as a result of childbirth. The vaginal wall is weakened and the rectum protrudes into the vagina. Constipation may result. **Tx:** Surgical repair.

Toxemia of pregnancy is an acute hypertensive condition. It is called preeclampsia if no convulsions are present, eclampsia when convulsions occur.

The BP is high (140/90 or greater), there is edema, and the urine contains protein. **Tx:** Beginning symptoms may respond to thiazides, a diet high in protein, folic acid and pyridoxine, and a weight gain restricted to two pounds a week. Full blown toxemia requires hospitalization with careful monitoring of BP, urine albumin, and electrolytes. The patient is on bedrest, sedatives are given, diuretics may be used, and salt is restricted. If symptoms increase, labor is induced by rupturing the membranes when the pregnancy is of 33 weeks duration. A cesarean section may be necessary.

Venereal Diseases

Venereal diseases are sexually transmitted diseases (STD). Syphilis and gonorrhea are the ones most commonly associated with the word venereal.

Gonorrhea is an infectious disease caused by the Neisseria gonococcus. In the female, the infection starts in the urethra, Bartholin's glands, and the cervix, then progresses to the tubes, ovaries, and pelvic peritoneum. Gonorrhea is a common cause of pelvic inflammatory disease (PID). In the male, the infection begins in the urethra and progresses to the prostate, vas deferens, and epididymis. There is a mucopurulent discharge from the female vagina and the male urethra. Diagnosis is made by cervical and urethral smears for culture. **Tx:** penicillin, tetracycline, and kanamycin for those allergic to penicillin.

Herpes simplex virus-2 (HSV-2) is becoming a rapidly increasing problem. This is also called genital herpes. Blisters form on the genitalia, sometimes on the buttocks and thighs. The blisters are painful and may disappear for a time. Recurrences have different time intervals for different persons. The unborn child is in danger if blisters are in the birth canal at the time of delivery. A cesarean section may be required. Cervical cancer is eight times more likely in women who have HSV-2. **Tx:** There is no cure. Acyclovir is helpful; cleanliness during outbreaks is important to prevent bacterial infection.

Trichomonas vaginitis is caused by the trichomonas vaginalis flagellate. A thick, frothy, greenish-yellow vaginal discharge causes pruritis. Microscopic examination of the vaginal discharge or culture of the discharge provides definite diagnosis. **Tx:** Flagyl, Vagisec, acidic douches. The sexual partner must also be treated.

Disease-Causing Organisms

- Candida albicans
- Chlamydia trachomatis
- Hemophilus vaginalis
- Herpes simplex virus-2 (HSV-2)
- Neisseria gonococcus
- Staphylococcus
- Streptococcus
- Treponema pallidum
- Trichomonas vaginalis

SURGERIES AND PROCEDURES

Male

Circumcision is the surgical removal of a part of the foreskin of the penis. This is usually performed the day after birth. Men who have been circumcised have fewer cancers of the penis than those who were not circumcised. The wives of men who have been circumcised have fewer cervical cancers, exactly why is not known. If circumcision is not performed shortly after birth, it may have to be done later due to inability to bring the foreskin back over the glans of the penis. Circumcision is a religious ceremony for some groups.

Epididymectomy is the removal of or resection of the epididymis.

Hydrocelectomy is the removal of subcutaneous tissue of the scrotum that is involved in the edema.

Orchiectomy is the removal of one or both testicles. Cancer of the testes or prostatic cancer may require orchiectomy.

Penectomy is partial removal of the penis due to cancer or injury.

Penile implant is a device surgically implanted in the penis with a reservoir implanted under the skin to inflate or deflate the device. This allows erection for intercourse but does not restore ability to ejaculate semen.

Vasectomy produces sterility by cutting or removing a part of the vas deferens. A new method is insertion of a plastic plug into the vas deferens to interrupt the pathway. With this method, the plugs may be removed to restore fertility. Microsurgery is sometimes successful for restoring fertility when the vas has been cut.

Female

Amniocentesis is removal of fluid from the amniotic sac to study for certain genetic defects or to determine the cause of a problem in the pregnancy.

Anterior and posterior repair (A & P) tightens the muscular wall of the anterior and posterior vagina to correct cystocele and rectocele. Patient will have a Foley catheter inserted in surgery and left in place several days. A betadine douche and an enema are ordered preoperatively. The vaginal packing will be removed by the doctor.

Breast biopsy (BB) is removal of a growth for cytology study. This is usually done in the ambulatory surgery unit. The patient arrives in the morning and is discharged when recovery from anesthesia is complete. A general or a local anesthesia may be used depending on depth of the growth. A penrose drain may be inserted into the wound to assure drainage of blood and fluid. A frozen section (FS) may be studied immediately to give the doctor and patient a quick answer as to the cause of the growth.

Cesarean section is the removal of the baby through an abdominal or suprapubic incision and surgical opening of the uterus. Pre-op orders usually include type and cross for two units of blood. Post-op orders for IV fluids, Foley cath care, and ambulation in 24 hours are the usual routine.

Colposcopy is an examination with a scope of the recesses of the vagina and cervix.

Conization of the cervix is the removal of a cone-shaped portion of the cervix. The portion contains a small area thought to be cancer from results of a pap smear. This is used if the patient is young and desires children. Surgery is performed vaginally.

Dilatation and curretage (D&C) consists of enlarging the cervical opening with a speculum and scraping the surface of the uterine cavity. Excessive bleeding is often due to an abnormally thick endometrium, and a D&C will eliminate the excess tissue. A D&C may be performed in incomplete abortions to remove placental tissue. This is usually an ambulatory surgery case.

Episiotomy is an incision at the vaginal entrance and the perineum to enlarge the birth canal to prevent tears during delivery. The incision is closed after delivery. Sitz baths help heal the area.

Hysterectomy is removal of the uterus. The vagina is closed at the cervical junction. This may be performed vaginally or by abdominal incision. Permit will specify which method will be used.

Laparoscopy is visualization of the abdominal-pelvic cavity through a scope that is inserted through the navel; it is usually performed for sterilization purposes. An electric cautery instrument is inserted through a small suprapubic incision, and the scope enables the surgeon to see the fallopian tubes. The cautery burns a small section of each tube so the passageway is interrupted and the ova cannot enter the uterus.

Mammoplasty is reconstructive surgery of the breasts. Bilateral augmentation mammoplasty (BAM) is to increase the breast size. Silicone implants are used. The silicone is enclosed in a plastic material; all sizes are available. Bilateral reduction mammoplasty (BRM) is removal of fatty tissue and breast tissue to make the breasts smaller.

Mastectomy is removal of a breast. This may be because of cancer or repeated infections that do not respond to treatment. Small cancers may be excised by partial mastectomy or lumpectomy. A simple mastectomy is removal of the breast tissue. A modified radical mastectomy involves removal of axillary nodes and some muscle under the breast. A radical mastectomy involves removal of breast tissue, axillary nodes, and pectoral muscles.

Oopherectomy is removal of the ovary. The permit will state which one or if bilateral.

Pap smear (Papanicolaou) is a cytology examination of the secretions of the cervix taken from behind the cervix with a special tool. This may be done on a unit. If the test is positive, a cervical biopsy is performed. Results are reported as stages. Stage I is normal, Stage II and III are suspicious and require repeat examination, Stage IV and V are positive for cancer and require biopsy follow-up.

Pelvic examination includes visual exam of vagina and cervix with aid of a vaginal speculum and palpation of pelvic area to determine if there is any enlargement of the organs. The patient is in the lithotomy position with feet in the stirrups of the exam table. Examination under anesthesia (EUA) may be done to prevent pain or to give better visual evaluation.

Radium implants are used for cancer. For endometrial cancer a tandem is inserted into the vagina in OR. After the patient returns to her room, a cesium load is inserted in the tubes of the tandem. The tandem is removed after 48 hours. For breast cancer, a plastic tube is inserted through the tumor in OR. Iridium is inserted into the tube after the patient returns to her room. The length of time before removal depends on the extent of the tumor.

Salpingectomy is the removal of a fallopian tube; it may be one or bilateral. Removal of uterus, tubes, and ovaries is a hysterectomy with bilateral salpingo-oopherectomy (BSO). One tube may be removed in cases of ectopic pregnancy, pregnancy in which the embryo lodges in the tube and starts to grow there instead of moving down into the uterus.

Tubal ligation for sterilization requires an abdominal incision. The tubes are tied with non-absorbable thread or the tubes are cut and the ends tied. This is a major operation, and recuperation is longer than for laparoscopy.

LABORATORY EXAMS

- Antibody identification
- Antibody screen
- Antibody titer
- CBC
- Coombs
- Cultures
    Breast discharge
    Urethral discharge
    Vaginal discharge
- Cytology studies
- D^u
- Estrogen, 24 hr urine
- FSH
- ICSH
- LH
- Pap smear
- Pregnancy (HCG), urine and blood
- Progesterone
- Prolactin
- Testosterone
- Tests for syphilis
    FTA
    Kolmer
    RPCF
    RPR
    STS
    TPI
    VDRL

RADIOLOGY, NUCLEAR MEDICINE EXAMS

Amniography visualizes the placenta. A contrast material is injected into the amniotic sac via an abdominal puncture after the same volume of fluid is removed. Placental placement is important in bleeding during the third trimester and in presentation problems.

Bone scans determine metastasis and help determine cancer treatment.

Chest and skeletal x-rays show calcification and abnormalities caused by cancer.

Hysterosalpingogram visualizes the uterine cavity and the fallopian tubes; it is useful if a pathway obstruction is suspected in infertility.

Isotope placentography utilizes IV radioactive material which is attracted to the placental tissue to determine the location of the placenta.

Mammograms are studies of the breast tissue in three different views, one from above looking downward. Women who have cystic disease of the breasts should have mammograms at regular intervals. Any abnormality in the tissue is visible.

Pelvic arteriography uses IV dye to visualize arteries of the pelvis. Displacement of the arteries helps assess ovarian and uterine cancers.

Pelvic pneumography visualizes the uterus, ovaries, tubes, and ligaments. Carbon dioxide is injected into the peritoneal cavity. This helps establish the cause of infertility.

Thermography of the breasts is an aid in diagnosing cancer. Infrared photography shows areas of warmth. Cancers or inflammations are warm and show a contrast to normal tissue.

Ultrasound of the uterus may be used for diagnosis of cancer or may be used during pregnancy to determine the age and size of fetus or any abnormalities of the fetus.

Xeroradiography is an x-ray with more realistic bas-relief pictures of the skin and tissue of the breasts than the mammogram.

MEDICATIONS

Antibiotics

- erythromycin—IV for acute PID up to 4 Gm/d. PO—250 mg q 6 hrs for 7 days following 3 days of IV doses.
- penicillin—IM—in large doses for syphilis and gonorrhea.
- tetracycline—PO—for gonorrhea and syphilis, dosage varies.
- ampicillin—PO—500 mg qid for 5 days for hemophilus vaginalis and chlamydia trachomatis vaginal infections.

Antineoplastics

- cyclophosphamide
- 5-FU   in combination c̄ Prednisone
- nitrogen mustard   for metastatic breast cancer
- methatrexate
- melphalan is an effective drug for ovarian cancer, and multiple myeloma
- cyclophosphamide for ovarian cancer
- actinomycin D
- chlorambucil   combined for testicular cancer.
- mithramycin for testicular cancer that does not respond to other drugs.

Contraceptives

Contraceptive drugs and devices are used to prevent pregnancy. They are sometimes also used to correct menstrual irregularities.

Oral—protection not assured until second cycle.
- Enovid-E and Ovullen—PO—first day of menstruation is day 1, medication begins on day 5, one tab/d for 20 d.
- Demulen, Demulen 28, Ovulen 21, Ovulen 28 are packaged in rows with days of week above the tablets. Instructions are in the package.
Topical
- Encare is inserted into the vagina ten minutes before intercourse; it is effective for one hour.
- Delfen and Emko are aerosol foams for vaginal insertions.
- Koromex is a jelly for vaginal insertion.
Devices
- Condoms are coverings for the male penis to prevent the semen from entering the vagina.
- Diaphragms are made of latex rubber with a spring coil around the edge to fit over the cervix like a cap. These are used with contraceptive jelly or cream.
- Intrauterine devices (IUD) are inserted into the uterine cavity by a doctor. CU-7 and Tatum-T are copper and are shaped as their name implies. These may be left in place for as long as 36 months before replacement. Cramping, bleeding, and infection are fairly common side effects of copper.
- The Lippes Loop is made of polyethylene and is shaped like an S; it may be left in place for 2 years.
- Saf-T-Coil is a plastic double coil; it may be left in place for 2 years.

Hormones (dosages are individualized)

- Clomid (synthetic hormone-like) for infertility in women.
- diethylstilbestrol, PO and vaginal suppository, for vaginitis due to decreased hormone.
- estrogen in postmenopausal women with metastatic breast cancer.
- methosarb and calusterone (testosterone) for breast cancer with painful bone metastasis.
- methyltestosterone in small doses for dysmenorrhea.
- Pergonal for infertility in female. Dosage calculated from results of 24 hour urinary estrogen level.
- Pitocin, IV to induce labor.
- prednisone for ovarian polycystic disease to stimulate ovulation.
- Premarin vaginal cream for vaginitis due to decreased hormones.
- testosterone for testicular hypofunction of male.
- thyroid hormone for excessive uterine bleeding if tests show hyposecretion of thyroid.

Specifics for Vaginitis

- Flagyl—PO—250 mg tid for 7 days. Males are treated at same time to prevent re-infection. Used for trichomonas. Patients should be cautioned not to take alcohol during course of treatment.
- nystatin vaginal suppository daily for 2 weeks for Candida albicans.
- Tricofuron vaginal suppository twice daily for 1 week then daily till organism eradicted, used for trichomonas.
- Sultrin vaginal cream, one application daily for one week for Hemophilus and Chlamydia organisms.

Specific for HSV-2

- Contraceptive vaginal creams provide analgesic effect during blistering and ulceration.
- Acyclovir (zovirax) reduces time for recovery from an outbreak but is not a cure. Topical applications, IV for severe cases.

EXAMPLE OF PHYSICIAN'S ORDERS

Dx: Abdomonal pain,? Ectopic tubal pregnancy.

1. STAT ultrasound of pelvic cavity
2. NPO
3. CBC, ESR, UA ASAP
4. T&X for 2 units for use in OR
5. 5% D/W IV, use #18 angiocath
6. VS q 15 min
7. Notify me immediately if bleeding occurs
8. Abdominal and perineal prep on return from x-ray
9. Demerol 50 mg ⎫
   Atropine 0.4 mg ⎭   Im on call to OR
10. Permit for laparotomy with possible left salpingectomy

Post-op orders:

1. NPO
2. 5% D/W @ 125 cc/hr
3. I & O
4. VS q 15 min for 2 hrs, q 30 min for 2 hrs, q h for 6 hours, then routine if stable
5. H & H @ 10 PM tonite. Call results to me.
6. Demerol 75 mg q. 3–4 hrs prn for pain
7. Compazine 10 mg IM q 6 hrs prn for N/V
8. Electrolytes in AM
9. Connect Foley to continuous drainage.

REVIEW QUESTIONS

1. Problems of the reproductive system often involve the _____ system.
2. A pregnancy test is based on the _____ _____ hormone.
3. The main structures of the female reproductive system are the _____, _____, _____, _____ and _____.
4. List three diseases and disorders of the female reproductive system.

   _____

   _____

5. The main structures of the male reproductive system are the _____, _____, _____, _____, _____, _____, _____, and _____.
6. List three diseases and disorders of the male reproductive system.

   _____

   _____

7. Define the following:
   Gravida _____
   Neonatal _____
   Embryo _____
   Menarche _____
   Postpartum _____
   Infertility _____
8. State the meaning of the following abbreviations:
   BB c̄ FS _____
   BSO _____
   BAM _____
   A & P repair _____
9. List four radiology examinations of the reproductive system.

   _____

   _____

10. List six laboratory examinations relating to the reproductive system.

    _____

    _____

    _____

11. Classify the following medications:
    methotrexate _____
    tetracycline _____
    Ovulen-21 _____
    Clomid _____
    Pitocin _____
    Flagyl _____
    testosterone _____

12. A pregnant woman in her forties is worried that her child might be born with Down's syndrome. What examination would determine if this were true? _____

13. List three surgeries of the male reproductive system.

_____

_____

Chapter 19 | Conclusion

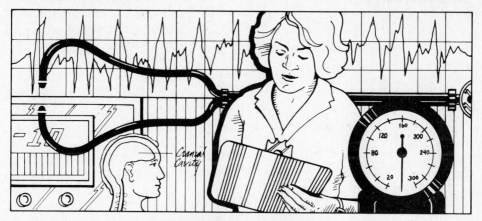

OBJECTIVES

Upon completion of this chapter, you will be able to:

1. Explain why a unit secretary must have a good working relationship with all the departments in the hospital.
2. Explain why it is important for the unit secretary to know the patients, the activities of the unit, and the assignment of each unit personnel.
3. Understand the exchange of information that is so important to the overall efficiency of the unit.
4. Explain why the knowledge of the unit secretary regarding information of patients and unit activities helps save time.
5. Discuss the different kinds of Physician's Orders for each of the nursing units.

You can now see that every department in the hospital has a part in the treatment of the patients. Departments depend on you to give them correct information, and you depend on them to report test results and other pertinent information to you. A good working relationship with all is an absolute must if the unit is to function efficiently and harmoniously.

So much depends on the unit secretary. The head nurse expects you to be her extra hand. To fulfill this expectation, you must keep in mind all that is happening on the unit. Each time a patient leaves the unit, you need to know where the patient is going and why. Many units have the secretaries listen to the shift report so that information concerning patients is obtained at the beginning of the shift. You also need to know what nurse has which patients. It is helpful to make a list and tape it to your desk area each day so that you don't have to keep looking at the assignment sheet.

Problems outside the work area should be left outside. If you start off the day in a bad mood, it soon permeates the entire unit and everyone with whom you come in contact. A smile accomplishes so much and costs so little. There are times when you may have to be forceful in expressing your opinions but that can be done in a nice manner.

There is a constant exchange of information between you and the personnel on the unit. The better you know your job, the easier that exchange becomes. You have probably thought that some of the information in this book would never be used. You will be surprised at the amount of information you will remember and how much it will help you communicate with the others on the unit. To be a part of the unit, you must speak the language.

Many times you will be the only person readily available when a doctor arrives on the unit. He/she may ask questions about a patient. If you are aware of what is going on, you will be able to answer the question and save valuable time. The same is true for the nurses on the unit; you can relate what the doctor has said and save them time.

Let's take a look at the units and review the kinds of orders for different patients. You need to know all the types because you may be hired as a float and be on a different unit each day.

The oncology floor is very quiet. Patients are quite ill and many are dying, but unit personnel maintain a cheerful atmosphere. Patients are allowed up as tolerated, and families may be around all day. Some rooms will be blocked for radiation. Patients in those rooms will have radioactive material inserted in the body. Everyone on the floor will have a tag to be worn when the room is entered. The tag tells the amount of radiation exposure the personnel on the unit have so that no one will be overexposed. Orders are mainly for blood tests, IVs, chemotherapy, and radiation therapy.

Eye cases are mostly surgical. Orders relate to eye drops, eye patches, and eye shields, and to assisting patients with activities and instructing them in home care when it is time for discharge.

Ear, nose, and throat patients may be medical or surgical. The medical cases probably have an infection so orders will pertain to antibiotics, gargles, ear drops. Surgery may be minor, with orders for humidity and removal of packing, or it may be major such as a radical neck with laryngectomy. Speech therapy is required for that type patient as well as tube feeding until the area heals. The patient also needs writing tools in order to communicate.

Genito-urinary (GU) patients may have catheters. Orders for irrigation of catheters and strict I & O, urine cultures, IVP x-rays, and straining urine are common.

Gynecology (GYN) patients are usually surgical. Orders for douches before surgery, vaginal instillations after surgery, packing removal, and sitz baths are common.

Orthopedic patients are almost always surgical. Orders deal with positioning, traction, casts, dressings, splints, equipment such as bedside commodes, crutches, walkers, special mattresses, PT and OT orders. X-ray examinations are pre- and postoperative.

Medical patients may have a problem involving any of the body systems. Orders will vary greatly. The majority will have to do with lab tests and x-ray exams. Medication orders may change daily. Some patients will go to dialysis. Chronic illness may require a long hospitalization; the patient becomes depressed, which adds to the problems already existing. All the special tests of the endocrine system will be seen on the medical unit. PT and OT help long-term patients.

The general surgery unit will have as much variety as the medical unit. Thoracic surgery patients may have chest tubes. G.I. tract surgeries will have nasogastric tubes and suction. Drains of all kinds will be seen. Orders will pertain to IVs, frequently changing diets, simple or complicated dressings, wound irrigations, measurement of drainage from the different types of drains, when to ambulate, and RT treatments to make sure the lungs function properly after an anesthetic.

CCU orders will mostly be drugs for arrhythmias, monitoring, special cardiology lab tests, and daily blood tests.

ICU will have medical and surgical patients so orders will change rapidly. IV orders will be complicated at times. Things happen so fast that many of the orders are already carried out before the doctor writes them. X-rays will be portable most of the time. Respirator orders change with the blood test results.

Pediatrics takes care of medical surgical cases. The same tests are used as for adults. Medication doses will be different. A nurse usually accompanies the child to x-ray or other departments for tests. Formulas for the infants are provided by dietary just as regular meals are; a supply is kept on the unit and restocked as needed. Mothers are allowed to stay most of the time. The unit will probably have a playroom with toys so the children will be able to play instead of being confined to their rooms.

The neurology unit will have orders for the different beds. PT and OT, as well as the speech therapist, work with most of the patients. CT scans are the most common examination. Monitoring of neuro signs is important.

Maternity orders are very routine unless the mother-to-be is having problems. There is a fast turnover in this department, so you will do lots of admissions and discharges. The same is true of the nursery.

All units, no matter what kind of patients, will have orders for the routine lab tests, diet orders, activity orders, IV fluids, narcotics, hypnotics, analgesics, tranquilizers, and sedatives so you will find many similarities even though diagnoses differ.

Now you are ready for the clinical experience where you can put this all together and see why accuracy is the first priority. You are entering a field that is changing rapidly. There are many exciting developments in the future.

REVIEW QUESTIONS

1. Explain why a unit secretary must have a good working relationship with all the hospital departments.

_____

_____

2. Explain how knowing the patients and being aware of unit activities can save time.

_____

_____

3. Which unit will use tags to record the radiation exposure of the unit personnel? _____

4. List three types of patients who may need the speech therapist.

   a. _____

   b. _____

   c. _____

5. Name one distinguishing factor regarding Physician's Orders for each of the following units.

   Neuro _____

   Ortho _____

   Medical _____

   Surgical _____

   Eye unit _____

   CCU _____

BIBLIOGRAPHY

Anthony CP, Kolthoff NJ: Textbook of Anatomy and Physiology. The C. V. Mosby Co., St. Louis, Missouri, 1975

Baker CE (pub): Physicians' Desk Reference. Medical Economics Co., Oradell, New Jersey, 1981

Boldeker EC, Dauber JH (ed): Manual of Medical Therapeutics, 21st ed. Little, Brown and Co., Boston, Massachusetts, 1974

Brady's Programmed Orientation to Medical Terminology. Robert J. Brady Co., Bowie, Maryland, 1970

Brunner LS, Suddarth DS: Textbook of Medical Surgical Nursing, 4th ed. J. B. Lippincott Co., Philadelphia, Pennsylvania, 1980

Bunn HF: Nonenzymatic glycosylation of protein: Relevance to diabetes. The American Journal of Medicine, Vol 70, pp 325–29, February 1981

Crossland J: Lewis's Pharmacology, 5th ed. Churchill Livingstone, New York, 1980

Cumming G, Semple SJ: Disorders of Respiratory System, 2nd ed. Blackwell Scientific Publications, Oxford, England, 1980

Gerald MC, O'Bannon FV: Pharmacology and Therapeutics. Prentice-Hall, Inc., Englewood Cliffs, New Jersey, 1981

Glover DW, Glover MM: Respiratory therapy: Basics for nursing and allied health professions. The C. V. Mosby Co., St. Louis, Missouri, 1978

Grollman S: The Human Body, Its Structure and Physiology. Macmillan Publishing Co., Inc., New York, 1974

Holvey DN (ed): The Merck Manual of Diagnosis and Therapy. Merck, Sharp and Dome Research Laboratories, Rahway, New Jersey, 1972

Hospital Research and Educational Trust: Being a Ward Clerk. Robert J. Brady Co., Bowie, Maryland, 1967

Kacmarek RM, Dimas S, Mack CM: The Essentials of Respiratory Therapy. Year Book Medical Publishers, Chicago, Illinois, 1979

Kessel RG, Kardon RH: Tissues and Organs: A Text-atlas of Scanning Electron Microscopy. W. H. Freeman and Co., San Francisco, California, 1979

Kogan BA: Health: Man in a Changing Environment. Harcourt, Brace and World, Inc., New York, 1970

Krupp MA, Chatton MJ: Current Medical Diagnosis and Treatment. Lange Medical Publications, Los Altos, California, 1979

Merritt HH: A Textbook of Neurology. Lea and Febiger, Philadelphia, Pennsylvania, 1979

Rosse C, Clawson DK (ed): The Musculoskeletal System in Health and Disease. Harper and Row, Hagerstown, Maryland, 1980

Schmidt A, Williams D: The Hickman Catheter, Sending your patient home safely. The Amazing Hickman and Its Easy Home Care, *RN Magazine*, pp 57–61, February, 1982

Shackelford RT, Zindema GD: Surgery of the Alimentary Tract, 2nd ed. W. B. Saunders Co., Philadelphia, Pennsylvania, 1978

Sheard C: Treatment of Skin Diseases. Year Book Medical Publishers, Inc., Chicago, Illinois, 1978

Sheperd JT, Vanhoutte PM: The Human Cardiovascular System: Facts and Concepts. Raven Press, New York, 1979

St. Joseph Hospital: Laboratory Manual. Albuquerque, New Mexico

St. Joseph Hospital: Medical Records Abbreviation List. Albuquerque, New Mexico

Strand MM, Elmer LA: Clinical Laboratory Tests, A Manual for Nurses, 2nd ed. The C. V. Mosby Co., St. Louis, Missouri, 1980

Watson JE: Medical Surgical Nursing and Related Physiology, 2nd ed. W. B. Saunders Co., Philadelphia, Pennsylvania, 1979

Widmann FK: Clinical Interpretation of Laboratory Tests, 8th ed. F. A. Davis Co., Philadelphia, Pennsylvania, 1979

Wiener MB (ed): Clinical Pharmacology and Therapeutics in Nursing, McGraw-Hill, New York, 1979

Williams RH (ed): Textbook of Endocrinology. W. B. Saunders Co., Philadelphia, Pennsylvania, 1974

Willson MS: A Textbook for Ward Clerks and Unit Secretaries. The C. V. Mosby Co., St. Louis, Missouri, 1979

Young JA, Crocker D: Principles and Practice of Respiratory Therapy. Year Book Medical Publishers, Inc., Chicago, Illinois, 1976.

APPENDIX I
ANSWERS TO REVIEW QUESTIONS

CHAPTER 1

1. The general duties of a unit secretary include all secretarial duties of the unit, communications to and from the unit, and the supervision of student secretaries.
2. Transcription of Physician's Orders will require most of the time and will involve communication with all departments.
3. You will use the telephone to call departments for information, make appointments, call doctors' offices, call patients' families, answer pages, initiate pages, and handle incoming calls.
4. You would locate and hand to the doctor the charts of his/her patients.
5. Transcription of Physician's Orders includes taking some action for each order written and recording the orders on the kardex card.
6. Census records include admissions, discharges, transfers, and deaths. Some hospitals include service transfers and passes.
7. Duties relating directly to patients' charts are: charting vital signs, transcribing Physician's Orders, filing reports, adding forms to the chart, and checking for proper identification.
8. You would not order supplies daily.
9. You would leave the unit to transport patients, to deliver specimens to the lab, and to photocopy parts of the chart.
10. Job qualifications may be checked against the list in Chapter 1.
11. Characteristics that are helpful in obtaining a job as a unit secretary may be checked by referring to the list in Chapter 1.
12. c
13. b
14. c
15. a

CHAPTER 2

1. The nuclear medicine department uses radioactive material prior to scanning.
2. The head nurse of the unit is your immediate supervisor.

3. The home health care department teaches patients self-care.
4. Medications are supplied by the pharmacy.
5. Patients' bills are handled by the business office and the admitting office.
6. The admitting office is usually the first department contact for the patient.
7. The laboratory does blood examinations.
8. Routine x-rays are taken in the radiology department.
9. Examinations of the heart are done in the cardiology department.
10. The public information officer or public relations officer dispenses information to the news media.
11. Applications for jobs are submitted to the personnel office.
12. Materials management or purchasing orders equipment.
13. Meals are served by the dietary department.
14. The housekeeping department or CS supplies the isolation carts.
15. To locate a doctor in a hurry, ask the switchboard operator to page "Any doctor call (unit) STAT." Special types of emergencies are explained in future chapters.
16. The rehabilitation department treats patients by physical means.
17. A special tray for a spinal puncture examination would be obtained from the central supply department.
18. The board of trustees or governing board sets the policies for the hospital.
19. An assistant director of nursing will assist the head nurse.
20. The medical staff determines the treatment for patients.
21. You would call the security guard for any disturbance that cannot be controlled by the unit staff.
22. The staff development personnel would conduct the class.
23. The administrator is responsible for the overall operation and sees that policies and standards are met.
24. Departments are supervised by department directors who report to an assistant administrator.
25. All requisitions must be addressographed by you.
26. c
27. a
28. c
29. a
30. b

CHAPTER 3

1. Communication is the act of one person or persons giving a message to another person or persons.
2. Receiving a message involves writing down the name of the person or department sending the message, the name of the person to receive

the message, and the message itself. It also includes repeating the message for accuracy. Be sure to give the message to the person for whom it is intended. Record the time you received the message.

3. To give a message, identify yourself and where you are calling from, give the name of the person to receive the message, give the message in simple language, and make sure it is understood.
4. Listening is as important as speaking.
5. If you can't supply information, ask the caller to hold the line while you find someone who can help.
6. Addressograph machines are for identification purposes.
7. You can talk with a patient over the intercommunication system.
8. The tube system transports papers.
9. The dumbwaiter may be used for delivering food trays.
10. The kardex is a record of the treatment for a patient.
11. Yes, special beliefs and customs must be respected.
12. Assignment sheets tell which person is responsible for which patient.
13. A unit blackboard may be used for listing patients having tests, or it may be used for an assignment list.
14. A communication notebook aids in listing and completing messages.
15. You give correct information, show an interest in the patient's welfare, and be kind and considerate to put the patient at ease.
16. Communication skills which build good personal relationships are dependability, tact, respect, tolerance, and sincerity. See the list in the chapter for others.
17. Posture tells others if you are interested in your work, eye to eye contact denotes attention, and sudden movements may denote hostility.
18. b
19. a
20. a
21. c

CHAPTER 4

1. Standard forms are those used for all patients. Supplementary forms are used for specific reasons.
2. Legally, all Doctor's Orders must be signed by the doctor. All forms in the chart must have the patient identification. Surgical consents must contain correct spelling with no abbreviations. Mistakes may not be erased but are corrected by lining through with ink, signing the correction, and writing the correct statement.
3. Refer to the list in the chapter.
4. The Diabetic Record, Laboratory Flow Sheet, Consults and Consents are supplementary. Refer to the chapter for others.
5. The unit secretary maintains the chart.
6. The medical records department types the history and physical.

7. The face sheet or the patient identification sheet contains the patient's address, telephone number, and name of the hospitalization insurance company.
8. The anesthesia record will contain the time and amount of any medication that was given in the operating room.
9. The social service worker writes on the progress notes to let the doctor know the progress of plans.
10. A patient's chart contains all the treatment a patient receives while in the hospital; it is a complete record.
11. You will tell the friend that you cannot discuss patients. Whatever you learn about a person while they are a patient must remain with you alone. The information you learn from working with the patient's records stays within your head and does not come out of your lips. Patients' charts are legal documents and are confidential. Revealing anything about a patient to another person could be grounds for a lawsuit.
12. b
13. a
14. c
15. b

CHAPTER 5

1. PO by mouth, per os.
   subl sublingual, under the tongue.
   IT Inhalation Therapy (also called Respiratory Therapy)
   IVPB intravenous piggyback medication
   SC subcutaneous, under the skin
   H hypodermic, a mode for medication administration
   IM intramuscular, into a muscle
   IV intravenous, into a vein
   Stat immediately
   Na sodium
   Cl chloride
   K potassium
   q d every day
   qid four times a day
   tid three times a day
   bid twice a day
   HS hour of sleep, bedtime
   pc after meals
   ac before meals
   c̄ with
2. A sedative is a drug that calms a person.
   A hypnotic produces sleep.

A narcotic produces sleep and relieves pain.

An analgesic relieves pain.

An antinauseant relieves or controls nausea.

3. 5cc = 1 dr = 1 tsp

240cc = 8 oz = 1 glass

1000cc = 32 oz = 1 quart or 1 liter

15cc = 4 dr = 1 tbsp

gr ī = 65 or 60 mg

4., 5., 6., and 7. Check your answers with the listing in the chapter.

8. A placebo is an inactive substance given in place of a drug. It may be given because a patient requests drugs frequently or it may be used in a drug study.

9. Controlled drugs are those which must be accounted for by law.

10. Pharmacology is the study of drugs.

11. Drugs are prepared in tablets, capsules, ampules, vials, tinctures, inhalers, ointments, aqueous solutions, elixirs, extracts—for complete list, see section on Types of Drug Preparation.

12. Accuracy is extremely important in drug orders because of the harm that could be done to a patient if an inaccuracy occurs. Everyone is responsible for their own acts and errors may involve only one person or several persons. You are responsible for accuracy when transcribing orders and must check the PDR if you are not familiar with a drug dosage and mode of administration.

13. a

14. c

15. c

16. c

17. b

CHAPTER 6

1. A kardex is the holder for patient care cards and the cards which contain a complete record of that patient's treatment.

2. BR <u>bedrest</u>

BRP <u>bathroom privileges</u>

DSD <u>dry, sterile dressing</u>

TCDB <u>turn, cough, and deep breathe</u>

U/O <u>urinary output</u>

BLESS <u>bath, laxative, enema, shampoo, shower or shave</u> (whenever patient requests)

LR or RL <u>Lactated Ringer's, an IV solution</u>

D5W <u>dextrose 5% in water, an IV solution</u>

NS <u>normal saline, 0.9% sodium chloride solution</u>

3. Your first priority is to check all charts for STATS, ASAPs, and now orders and complete those first. If there are several to be done, deter-

mine which to do first by the condition of the patients involved and the type of order.

4. Accuracy is always the first priority.

5. A medication is discontinued by tearing the card halfway and placing the card in the chart for the RN to check and entering in the kardex by lining through the order and entering a dc date or erasing the order according to hospital policy.

6. Computers contribute to patient care by making information more immediate, easier to access, easier to update, and always available.

7. Computers relay orders to other departments, relay interim reports to the nursing stations, print out patient care sheets, print out medication plans for each shift, and print daily census reports.

8. Tigan 250 mg tid standing order
Demerol 50 mg IM q 3-4 hrs prn for pian standing PRN order
Sitz bath qid and prn combination (standing and standing prn) treatment order
Solu-Cortef 60 mg IVP q 6 h standing order
1000 cc D5LR to run 8 hrs then dc limited time order
Give 2 units packed red cells today one time order

9. Check your answer against the list in the chapter.

10. The secretary is responsible for keeping an up-to-date and neat kardex card.

11. Transcription of Physician's Orders means activating each order that is written by the proper procedure and entering the order on the kardex card unless it is an ASAP, stat or now order.

12. Medication cards contain the patient's room number, the patient's name, the doctor who wrote the order, the medication ordered, the dosage of the medication, the mode, the frequency, the times if not a prn or ASAP, stat, or now order, the date ordered, a stop date if applicable, and the initials of the nurse who checks and signs the orders.

13. Drugs usually requiring renewal dates are antibiotics, narcotics, and anticoagulants.

14. c

15. d

16. b

17. c

18. b

CHAPTER 7

1. The Census Sheet records admissions, discharges, and transfers. Some hospitals include service transfers and passes.

2. The graphic sheet is started when a new patient is admitted by transferring the vital signs from the Admission Form that is completed by a NA or RN.

3. Discharge charts are sent to the Medical Records Department.

4. The volunteer bringing a new admission to the unit also brings the Identification Sheet or Face Sheet, the addressograph card, the Identification bracelet and the Admission Kit.

5. Emergency admissions may come from ER or OR.

6. Admissions, discharges, transfers, deaths, and passes are entered on the Condition Report for the supervisors.

7. Autopsy permits are obtained by the doctor. The unit secretary may complete the clerical portion of the form.

8. Patients to be autopsied are taken to the morgue.

9. Admissions to a hospital are arranged by a doctor.

10. Incident reports may involve a patient, a visitor, or an employee.

11. Discharges in which the patient leaves without the consent of the doctor are called AMA (Against Medical Advice) discharges.

12. The five types of isolation are: Enteric isolation for diseases transmitted by feces or urine. Respiratory isolation for patients with diseases that are airborne. Strict isolation for severe systemic infections. Wound and skin isolation for infected wounds or skin infections. Reverse isolation for patients with low resistance so the patient is protected from outside infections.

13. Four safety precautions you may use in the hospital are to have spilled material cleaned quickly so no one slips and gets hurt, notify maintenance to fix broken machinery instead of attempting to fix it yourself, be sure you know how to correctly operate a machine before attempting to use it, wear clothing that will be comfortable but pose no hazard.

14. Your duties in case of fire would be to close the fire doors and all the doors to the rooms, clear the halls of patients and visitors, then return to the desk and handle incoming calls. Hospital policy will dictate whether or not you are responsible for a patient list for evacuation purposes.

15. Your duties when a patient is ordered in isolation would be to order the cart for the room to be placed by the doorway (hospital policy dictates whether this would be ordered from housekeeping or central supply), notify admitting and make arrangements for a private room if that is necessary, notify housekeeping of the type of isolation, notify dietary, inform all personnel involved with the patient, be sure the escort service knows of the isolation if patient is to be transported, and when the patient is discharged or moved from the room, notify housekeeping so the room may be disinfected.

16. b

17. b

18. c

19. a

CHAPTER 8

1. The planes of the body are based on the body being in the anatomical position.
2. The frontal or coronal plane is vertical and divides the body into front and back portions.
3. The transverse plane is horizontal and divides the body into upper and lower portions.
4. Posterior or dorsal refers to the back.
5. Anterior or ventral refers to the front.
6. Superior means above, higher.
7. The cavities of the body are the dorsal, which consists of the cranial and spinal cavities, and the ventral, which consists of the thoracic, abdominal, and pelvic cavities.
8. Protoplasm is the living matter inside a cell membrane.
9. pH is the degree of acidity or alkalinity of a substance.
10. DNA is the chemical basis of heredity.
11. A gene is the unit of heredity.
12. A tissue is a group of cells that perform a specific function. The four main types are connective, epithelial, muscular, and nervous tissue.
13. An organ is a group of tissues that perform a complex function.
14. A system is a group of organs that perform a highly complex function.
15. Cancers are malignant tumors that invade surrounding tissues, are harmful, and are resistant to treatment.
16. Cancer is treated by surgical removal, chemotherapy, radiation therapy or hormone therapy or a combination of two or more.
17. A cell is the basic unit of life.
18. A chromosome is the part of the nucleus of the cell that contains genes.

CHAPTER 9

1. The outer layer of the skin is the epidermis.
2. The layer under the epidermis is the dermis.
3. The dermis is connected to a subcutaneous layer.
4. Hair and nails are appendages of the skin.
5. Sebum is produced by the sebaceous glands.
6. Perspiration is produced by the sweat glands.
7. Port-wine stains are treated with laser therapy.
8. Acne is a common skin disorder of adolescents and young adults that causes blackheads and whiteheads due to plugged follicles. Pimples, abscesses, and cysts may form in some cases.
9. Burns are a threat to life because of the systemic effects.
10. Melanoma is the skin cancer that is the leading cause of death in skin diseases.

11. A bedsore is a decubitus.
12. Benzoyl peroxide is in antiacne preparations.
13. Pruritus is itching.
14. Corticosteroids decrease inflammation and itching.
15. The skin protects the body from bacteria and sunrays, stores food and water to prevent dehydration, aids in regulation of body temperature, and manufactures Vitamin D.
16. Sun screens help prevent skin cancer.
17. Photochemotherapy is the interaction of ultraviolet rays with drugs to exert a beneficial effect in treatment of skin disease.
18. STSG means split thickness skin graft; only the top of the epidermis is used.
19. FTSG means full thickness skin graft; it includes all the epidermis.
20. Astringents are used to give tone to the skin and to check secretions.

CHAPTER 10

1. The three types of muscle are voluntary, involuntary, and cardiac.
2. Muscles make movement possible, maintain posture, and produce heat.
3. The skeletal system gives shape to and supports the body, provides movement, protects internal organs, stores mineral salts, and produces blood cells.
4. Hernias, cleft lip or cleft palate, and muscular dystrophy are diseases and disorders of the muscular system.
5. The membrane that covers bone is the periosteum.
6. Intervertebral discs are pads of cartilage filled with nucleus pulposus. They are found between vertebrae and absorb shock.
7. Contraction shortening of a muscle
   Dystrophy progressive wasting and weakening of a muscle
   Hernia a rupture of a muscle
   Paralysis inability to move; muscles have lost their ability to produce voluntary movement
   ROM range of motion, the movement a joint can make
   Spasm a sudden, uncontrollable contraction of muscle
   Cartilage connective tissue called gristle
   Cavity a hollow space
   Fracture a break in a bone
   Traction force in two directions to regain the normal position of bones and muscles
8. Abnormal curvatures of the spine are kyphosis, which is a hunchback condition; lordosis, which is a swayback condition; and scoliosis, which is a side to side curvature.
9. Five common diseases and disorders of the musculoskeletal system are

fractures, arthritis, ruptured discs, bunions, and internal derangement of the knee. For others, refer to the list in the chapter.

10. Medications commonly used for arthritis are Ascriptin A/D, Motrin, Clinoril, and Nalfon. Check the list in the chapter for others or look in the PDR.

11. Gout medications include colchicine for acute attacks, Colbenemid, and Zyloprim.

12. Muscle relaxants include Lioresal, Parafon Forte, and Valium. Check the chapter for others and look in the PDR.

13. Electrotherapy devices are Orthofuse, TENS, and EPC.

CHAPTER 11

1. The circulatory system consists of the blood, blood vessels, the heart, the lymphatic system, the spleen, and the thymus.

2. The blood carries food, hormones, and oxygen to all parts of the body and removes the waste products from tissues and carries them to organs for elimination.

3. Arteries carry blood from the heart to the body.

4. The function of the heart is to pump blood to the body and to receive the returning blood.

5. The atria are the upper chambers of the heart; the ventricles are the lower chambers.

6. The aorta is the largest artery of the body.

7. The vena cava is the largest vein of the body.

8. The spleen stores blood for emergencies, destroys microorganisms, removes old blood cells, and returns the iron to the blood.

9. Arrhythmias are irregular heart rhythms.

10. You first determine how the caller is related. Immediate family members would be told that there has been a change in the condition of the patient and that they should come to the hospital. Other than immediate family would be told to contact a family member because you cannot give information regarding patients.

11. A portable chest x-ray would be needed to determine if the catheter placement is correct.

12. A heart attack is also called a myocardial infarction or a coronary occlusion.

13. CPR means cardiopulmonary resuscitation, restoration of the activity of the heart and lungs.

14. The lymphatic system carries fluid to the tissues, produces lymphocytes and monocytes, and filters harmful substances from the blood.

15.
Leukemia	blood
Hodgkin's disease	lymphatic system
Thrombophlebitis	blood and blood vessels
Aortic stenosis	heart
Anemia	blood

16. Heart catheterization examination of the right or left heart with use of a catheter and the fluoroscopy machine. Dye is used to visualize the coronary arteries, and samples of blood are taken from the chambers of the heart
    Coronary bypass a surgery in which a leg vein is used to bypass a blocked section of the coronary artery
    Embolectomy surgical removal of a blood clot
    EKG electrocardiogram, a recording of the electrical activity of the heart
    Echocardiogram examination of the heart by the use of sound waves whose echoes produce a picture

17. Inderal — antihypertensive and antiarrhythmic
    heparin — anticoagulant
    Nitrostat — vasodilator or nitrate or antianginal
    verapamil — antiarrhythmic, calcium blocker
    Lasix — diuretic
    Vasospan — peripheral vasodilator
    Lanoxin — digitalis preparation

18. ACT, PT, and PTT are coagulation tests.

19. LDH, SGOT, CPK, and SGPT are all cardiac enzyme studies.

20. No, you would not. A Dr. Heart call is for emergencies or for persons not suffering a terminal illness. It would not be beneficial to the patient to be revived only to be claimed by death a few hours later. This patient's chart would probably be tagged DNR.

CHAPTER 12

1. Oxygen and carbon dioxide are exchanged during respiration.
2. Tomograms visualize all the sinuses.
3. The pharynx serves as a passageway for both the respiratory and the digestive systems.
4. Adenoids and tonsils are lymphatic tissue.
5. Cilia are hair-like projections that move in waves to move secretions upward.
6. Suctioning removes secretions when the patient is unable to cough.
7. A ventilator is a mechanical breathing device.
8. The nose, pharynx, larynx, trachea, bronchi, and lungs compose the respiratory system.
9. The respiratory system carries oxygen to all the cells of the body and disposes of carbon dioxide.
10. The most common diseases and disorders of the respiratory system are sinusitis, asthma, bronchitis, influenza, and tonsilitis. Review those listed in the chapter.
11. Benadryl — antihistamine
    Sudafed — decongestant and bronchodilator
    Aminophyllin — bronchodilator

erythromycin	antibiotic
Mucomyst	mucolytic
Prednisone	steroid
INH	specific for TB
amphotericin-B	antifungal

12. A lobectomy is the removal of a lobe of an organ; it refers here to a lobe of a lung.
13. A bronchogram is often performed with a bronchoscopy.
14. Thoracotomy means cutting into the chest.
15. Laryngectomy is removal of the larynx.
16. A tracheotomy is an opening into the trachea that is temporary; a tracheostomy is a permanent opening with a stoma.
17. Laboratory tests frequently performed in relation to the respiratory system are ABGs, sputum cultures with sensitivity testing, skin tests for TB or fungus, electrolytes (many of the bronchodilators decrease the potassium levels), cytology studies of sputum, bronchial washings, or pleural fluid.
18. You notify the nurse in charge of that patient so she may stop the O_2. The nurse will tell you the exact time she discontinued the O_2, and you notify the lab of the exact time the specimen is to be drawn. Complete a requisition or enter in the computer. Be sure the lab collects the specimen and notify the nurse after the specimen is drawn so that the O_2 may be started again.
19. Radiology and nuclear medicine examinations of the respiratory system include bronchograms, CT scans with perfusion studies, tomograms of sinuses or lungs, AP and Lat of the chest, arteriograms and venograms plus others listed in the chapter. Be sure that you follow through on diet restrictions when an examination dictates restrictions.
20. The RT department performs oxygen therapy, chest percussion, complete pulmonary function testing, and spirometry tests, provides humidifiers and vaporizers, administers IPPB Nebs and USN therapy, and supplies ventilators and oversees their use.

CHAPTER 13

1. The digestive system coverts food into nutrients for all the cells of the body.
2. The digestive system consists of the mouth, pharynx, esophagus, stomach, small intestines, and large intestines.
3. The large intestines are commonly called the colon.
4. The S-shaped portion of the colon is the sigmoid.
5. The liver and the pancreas are accessory organs or glands of the digestive system.
6. The divisions of the small intestines are the duodenum, the jejunum and the ileum.

7. g. (flatus)   gas in the G.I. tract
   d. (emesis)   to vomit
   j. (peristalsis)   wave-like movement
   a. (calculus)   stone
   h. (stoma)   surgically created mouth
   c. (hepar)   Greek word for liver
   i. (varices)   dilated veins
   b. (mastication)   chewing
   e. (defecation)   bowel movement
   f. (dysphagia)   difficulty in swallowing
8. Esophageal varices twisted, dilated veins in the lining of the esophagus
   Gingivitis inflammation of the gums
   Hepatitis inflammation of the liver
   Crohn's disease persistent inflammation which usually occurs in the small intestines
   Gastroenteritis inflammation of the stomach and intestines
   Peritonitis inflammation of the lining of the abdominal cavity
   Cirrhosis a chronic liver disease in which fibrous tissue or scarring causes impaired function
   Cholelithiasis presence of stone formation in the gallbladder
9. Mylanta   antacid
   Kefzol   antibiotic
   Parapectolin   antidiarrheal
   Antepar   anthelminthic
   Ilopan   antiflatulent
   Donnatal   antispasmodic
   Peri-Colace   laxative (stool softener)
   Tigan   antinauseant
   Tagamet   specific for peptic ulcers
10. G.B. series   radiology
    2 hr urine amylase laboratory
    Occult blood, stool laboratory
    Australian antigen laboratory
    Papida scan   nuclear medicine
    IVC   radiology
    Ba swallow   radiology
    CEA   laboratory
    BSP   laboratory
    U.G.I. series   radiology

CHAPTER 14

1. The urinary system filters wastes and helps regulate the composition of the blood.
2. The structures of the urinary system are the kidneys, ureters, bladder, urethra, and urinary meatus.

3. IVP is an x-ray that visualizes the kidneys, ureters, and bladder.
4. Dialysis is a process to remove wastes from the blood when the kidneys are unable to function properly.
5. The types of dialysis are peritoneal, hemodialysis, and CAPD.
6. Anuria absence of urine
   Pyuria pus in the urine
   Retention inability to empty the bladder
   Suppression failure of natural production of urine
   Uremia impaired renal function with retention of wastes in the blood
   Calculi stones
   Wilm's tumor an adenosarcoma that occurs in the fetus
   Cystoscopy an examination of the bladder with a scope while the patient is under anesthesia
   Bright's disease inflammation of the glomeruli
   Ileal conduit surgery to construct a pouch from the ileum and connect the ureters to the pouch and attach the open end of the pouch to the abdominal wall for a stoma
7. BPH benign prostatic hypertrophy
   TUR transurethral prostatectomy, a surgical procedure
   SPP suprapubic prostatectomy, a surgical procedure
8. Urised/analgesic and antibacterial
   Gantrisin/antibiotic
   Cystospaz/antispasmodic
   Imuran/immunosuppressive
   Septra/antibiotic
   Check the list in the chapter and the PDR.
9. Cystitis, pyelonephritis, uremia, acute renal failure, polycystic disease. Refer to the list in the chapter.
10. BUN, creatinine clearance, urinalysis, urine culture, acid phosphatase, PSP, and any others in the chapter.
11. Foley, French, Mushroom, and Urosan plus others in the chapter.
12. Nephrectomy, cystoscopy, ileostomy, kidney transplant. Check the list in the chapter.
13. CT scan, IVP, KUB, and cystogram. Refer to the list in the chapter.

CHAPTER 15

1. A hormone is a substance secreted by an endocrine gland and carried by the bloodstream to other organs, which they stimulate.
2. The endocrine glands are the pituitary, pineal, thyroid, parathyroids, adrenals, pancreas, thymus, testes in the male, and the ovaries in the female.
3. Diabetes insipidus   pituitary
   Graves' disease   thyroid
   Cushing's syndrome   adrenals

Diabetes mellitus	pancreas
Tetany	parathyroids

4. Tomograms of sella tursica — radiology
24 hr urine for 17-OHCS — laboratory
Cortisol test — laboratory
Echoscan of thyroid — radiology
Ketodiastix — nursing
5. propylthiouracil — antithyroid
Insulin — hypoglycemic agent or antidiabetic
Pitressin — pituitary hormone
Decadron — corticosteroid
Diabinese — oral hypoglycemic agent, antidiabetic
Cytomel — thyroid hormone replacement
Os-Cal — vitamin plus calcium

6. Thyroidectomy, adrenalectomy and hypophysectomy. Refer to the list in the chapter.
7. Tetany is a threat after a thyroidectomy.
8. A major concern in the special tests is that the lab tests are performed at the time specified.
9. A 2 hr PP requires a lab requisition and an entry in the kardex so that the RN will know to notify you as soon as the patient completes breakfast; you can then notify the lab as to the exact time to draw the blood specimen. Check to make sure the specimen is drawn at the correct time.
10. The insulin order would be handled as a now order because insulin is given before breakfast whenever possible. On new diabetics and ones who are being regulated, the doctor will order the insulin after receiving the FBS results for that day.
11. An order for BS today would be checked as a Random BS on the lab req.
12. Orders for sliding scale insulin involve a urine test before the insulin is given or a blood glucose level.

CHAPTER 16

1. The nervous system is composed of the brain, spinal cord, and nerves.
2. The function of the nervous system is to coordinate body activities by sending and receiving messages from all parts of the body.
3. The inability to speak or speak comprehensively or to understand speech is aphasia.
4. Glia is the supporting tissue of the CNS.
5. Kinetic refers to motion.
6. Inflammation of a nerve is neuritis.
7. Convulsion is a sudden attack of involuntary movement.

8. Epilepsy, headaches, narcolepsy, paraplegia, and meningitis are some diseases and disorders of the nervous system. Refer to the list in the chapter.

9. Evoked response tests — EEG
Carotid angiography — radiology
Craniotomy — surgery
CSF exams — laboratory
Myelogram — radiology
PET — radiology

10. Dilantin — anticonvulsant
amphoteric-β — antifungal
mannitol — diuretic for control of cerebral edema
Sansert — specific for migraine headache, adrenergic blocker
Mestinon — specific for myasthenia gravis, cholinergic
Ritalin — cerebral stimulant for narcolepsy
Larodopa — specific for Parkinson's syndrome

11. An electromyogram is performed by a neurologist to determine if the nerve in a muscle is active.

12. EEG is an electroencephalogram, a recording of the electrical activity of the brain.

13. The structural unit of the nervous system is the neuron.

14. The membranes that cover the brain and the spinal cord are the meninges.

15. A refex arc is the nerve pathway traveled by a stimulus and the response.

16. Decadron may be ordered in decreasing dosages with the order written for several days.

17. A spinal puncture or spinal tap requires a tray from central supply.

18. A Stryker frame, a circulo-electric bed, a Roto Rest Treatment Table or kinetic bed, and Craig bed are used on the neurology unit.

CHAPTER 17

1. The sclera provides protection for the eye.
2. The vascular layer of the eyeball is composed of the choroid, the ciliary body, and the iris.
3. The choroid layer gives color to the eye.
4. The retina contains receptors for light called rods and cones.
5. The cornea is the very center of the front of the sclera.
6. The blind spot is the optic disk.
7. The anterior cavity fluid is the aqueous humor.
8. The posterior cavity fluid is the vitreous humor.
9. Tears are produced by the lacrimal glands.
10. A cataract is a clouding of the lens so that light cannot pass through it to reach the retina.

11. Increased pressure in the eyeball is usually due to glaucoma.
12. The laser is used in photocoagulation to reattach the retina.
13. Three disorders of vision are diplopia, hyperopia, and myopia. Refer to the chapter for others.
14. Three surgeries of the eye are iridectomy, cataract removal, and blepharoplasty. Refer to the chapter for others.
15. The ossicles of the ear are the malleus or hammer, the incus or anvil, and the stapes or stirrup.
16. Miotics produce contractions of the iris and reduce pressure in glaucoma. Mydriatics cause the smooth muscle of the iris to relax. Cycloplegics cause the ciliary muscle to relax or to be paralyzed.
17. Auralgan Otic Sol'n is an analgesic for the ears. Orlex Otic Sol'n is an ear antibiotic. Antivert is an antivertigo drug that acts on the labyrinth of the ear to stop or reduce dizziness, vertigo, and nausea.
18. The three divisions of the ear are the external ear, the middle ear, and the inner ear.
19. The structures of the labyrinth are the vestibule, the semi-circular canals, and the cochlea.
20. Otitis media infection of the middle ear
    Meniere's syndrome dysfunction of the labyrinth with attacks of vertigo, nausea, headache, and incoordination
    Mastoiditis an infection in the mastoid bone
21. Three tests for ear function are the caloric test, audiogram, and testing with a tuning fork.
22. Three surgeries of the ear are myringotomy, stapedectomy, and tympanoplasty. Refer to the chapter for others.

CHAPTER 18

1. Problems of the reproductive system often involve the endocrine system.
2. A pregnancy test is based on the presence of increased HCG, human chorionic gonadotropin.
3. The main structures of the female reproductive system are the vulva, vagina, uterus, fallopian tubes, and ovaries.
4. Fibrocystic disease of the breast, endometriosis, and infertility are some diseases and disorders of the female. Refer to the chapter for others.
5. The main structures of the male reproductive system are the scrotum, penis, testes, prostate gland, vas deferens, Cowper's glands, and the seminal vesicles.
6. Epididymitis, hydrocele, and Klinefelter's syndrome are some of the diseases and disorders of the male reproductive system. Refer to the chapter for others.

7. Gravida <u>pregnant woman</u>
   Neonatal <u>the first four weeks after birth</u>
   Embryo <u>a fertilized egg up to eight weeks after conception</u>
   Menarche <u>beginning of the menstrual cycle for the first time</u>
   Postpartum <u>after a delivery of a child</u>
   Infertility <u>inability to conceive and give birth to a living child</u>

8. BB c̄ FS <u>a breast biopsy with a frozen section sent to the pathology lab for immediate evaluation</u>
   BSO <u>a bilateral salpingo-oopherectomy</u>
   BAM <u>surgical enlargement of a breast, bilateral augmentation mammoplasty</u>
   A & P repair <u>an anterior and posterior repair of the vaginal wall to correct a cystocele and a rectocele</u>

9. Mammograms, ultrasound of the uterus, amniography, and placentography are some radiology examinations of the female reproductive system. Refer to the chapter for others.

10. Pap smear, testosterone, estrogen, FSH, VDRL, and cultures of vaginal discharge are some of the lab exams relating to the reproductive system. Refer to the chapter for others.

11. methotrexate   <u>antineoplastic</u>
    tetracycline   <u>antibiotic</u>
    Ovulen-21   <u>contraceptive</u>
    Clomid   <u>hormone for infertility</u>
    Pitocin   <u>hormone used to induce labor</u>
    Flagyl   <u>specific for trichomonas</u>
    testosterone   <u>male hormone</u>

12. Amniocentesis examinations help identify congenital abnormalities.

13. Circumcision, orchiectomy, and vasectomy are some surgeries of the male reproductive system. Refer to the chapter for others.

CHAPTER 19

1. The unit secretary must have a good working relationship with all the hospital departments because the departments depend on the secretary for information and the secretary depends on the departments for accurate reporting of tests. All this aids in the efficient and smooth functioning of the unit.

2. The more the unit secretary knows about the patients and the unit activities the more she/he can help the doctors and the unit personnel when questions are asked.

3. The oncology unit uses tags to record the amount of radiation each person on the unit is exposed to for a period of time.

4. The speech therapist may work with stroke patients, brain-injured patients, and patients who have had laryngectomy surgery.

5. Neuro uses special beds
   Ortho will have orders for traction
   Medical will have lots of medication orders
   Surgical will have orders for dressings and drains
   Eye will have orders for eye drops, patches and shields
   CCU will have orders for monitoring of the heart

APPENDIX II
LABORATORY TESTS

ABBREVIATIONS

dl—deciliter, one-tenth of a liter
hpf—high power field
IU—International Unit
μ—micron, .001 cm
μm—micrometer, same as a micron
mμ—millimicron, one-thousandth of a micron
$\mu\mu$—micromicron, one-millionth of a micron
μg or mcg—microgram, one-millionth of a gram
ng—namogram, one-billionth of a gram
pg—picogram, one-trillionth of a gram

For ease in reporting, many lab results will have $\times 10^6$ or $\times 10$ to some power. This means that 10^6 is one million times the number given—$30 \times 10^6 = 30,000,000$ or 30 million. The easiest way to remember is that the number above the 10 means that many zeros are added. Portions of weights and measures are expressed decimally—$10^{-1} = 0.1$ or one-tenth, $10^{-6} = 0.000001$ or one millionth part. The number above the ten means that many numbers following the decimal point.

Tests are listed alphabetically with abbreviations first, since the doctors will order the test by abbreviation, then the full name of the test, patient preparation, normal values, explanation if needed, increased in what diseases, decreased in what diseases, and the section of the lab that performs the test. Values vary according to the method used. The values listed are the most commonly used.

ABG—arterial blood gases. Blood from an artery is drawn into a heparinized syringe, the needle is blocked, and the syringe placed in ice and taken to the lab immediately. If you are working in the special units, ICU, SAC, or CCU, you will be responsible for taking the ABGs to the lab. All ABGs are done in the Chemistry Lab.

- **PO_2**—partial pressure of oxygen—is dependent on the PO_2 of the inspired atmosphere, so it differs in different localities—normally given as 80 to 90 mm Hg. Your instructor can give you the reading for your area. This measures the amount of oxygen at the capillary membrane of the alveoli. It provides critical information in many pulmonary and cardiovascular diseases.

- **PCO_2**—partial pressure of carbon dioxide—34 to 46 mm Hg—increased in respiratory acidosis, unchanged or increased in metabolic alkalosis, decreased in metabolic acidosis and respiratory alkalosis.

- **pH**—7.35 to 7.45—increases in metabolic and respiratory alkalosis, decreases in metabolic and respiratory acidosis.
- **CO_2**—carbon dioxide—is controlled by the lungs and the respiratory center in the medulla—23 to 27 mEq/l—increased in respiratory acidosis and metabolic alkalosis, decreased in respiratory alkalosis and metabolic acidosis.
- **O_2 saturation**—90 to 98%—measures the availability of oxygen to the tissues.
- **HCO_3**—bicarbonate—21 to 26 mEq/l—an alkaline substance and a base that buffers the effects of CO_2 in the blood, controlled by the kidneys—increased in metabolic alkalosis and respiratory acidosis, decreased in metabolic acidosis and respiratory alkalosis.

ABO group—determines the type of blood. Blood bank.

ACT—activated clotting time—80 to 135 seconds—used in the control of heparin dosage. It is performed at bedside and results are available in a few minutes. Hematology.

Acetone—negative. The presence of acetone indicates diabetic ketoacidosis or severe starvation. Chemistry.

Acid hemolysin (Hamm test)—negative. If red blood cells are destroyed, it is an indication of a red cell defect that causes paroxysmal nocturnal hemoglobinuria (PNH). The first urine of the morning is dark due to the presence of hemoglobin. Hematology.

Acid phosphatase—0.0 to 2.0 IU/1—increased in prostatic carcinoma with bone metastases and in Paget's disease. Chemistry.

ACTH—adrenocorticotropic hormone—patient should have nothing by mouth except water for 8 hrs prior to the test—10 to 70 pg/ml—increased in Addison's disease, in stress, and after bilateral adrenalectomy—decreased in cancer of the adrenals and in parahypopituitarism. Chemistry.

Adenovirus—throat swab, rectal swab, stool, CSF, secretions of conjunctiva. Its presence shows one of a group of viruses that cause infections; virus isolation is needed to identify the type. A convalescent specimen is collected one week to two months after the acute specimen. Virology.

AFB culture—acid fast bacillus—sputum, urine, gastric washings. First morning specimens are needed for sputum and urine. A lab appointment is made for gastric washings, and the patient is on hold for breakfast. The test is done to determine if the Mycobacterium species is present; the most common one is tuberculosis. Microbiology.

AFB smear—also called gram stain—sputum, stool, throat swabs, CSF, wound exudate—shows the organism responsible for the disease so treatment may be started immediately without waiting for the culture results. Microbiology.

A/G ratio—albumin/globulin ratio—1.1 to 1.8—fractionation of serum proteins into the two main components—decreased in starvation, severe liver disease, bone marrow disease, nephrosis, and disease of the lymph nodes—increased in hypoglobulinemia. Chemistry.

Albumin—3.2 to 5.6 g/dl—decreased in nephrotic syndrome, hepatic cirrhosis, major infections, surgical and accidental trauma, malnutrition, eclampsia, and GI malabsorption. Chemistry.

Albumin (urine)—24 hr urine—50 to 100 mg/24 hrs—measures quantitative protein—increased in inflammatory or degenerative processes in the kidney structure. Chemistry.

Alcohol—toxic 80mg/dl—lethal over 400 mg/dl—helpful in differentiation of intoxication and coma from other causes. Toxicology. It may be reported as %—0.10% for threshold of legal intoxication, 0.20 to 0.25% for severe intoxication, 0.35 to 0.50% for life-threatening coma.

Aldolase—patient should be resting—1 to 6 mU/ml—increased in skeletal muscle disease, carcinomas, some leukemias, hepatitis and myocardial infarction. Chemistry.

Aldosterone—patient should be fasting—supine position is 2 to 9 ng/100ml or Mean 6 with the upright 2 to 5 times the supine—increased in adrenal cortical tumors, sodium restriction, diuretic therapy, and secondary aldosteronism—decreased in primary adrenal insufficiency. Chemistry.

Aldosterone, urine—24 hr urine—2 to 26 μg/24 hrs—increased in adrenal cortical tumors and secondary aldosteronism. Chemistry.

Alk. phos.—alkaline phosphatase—13 to 74 IU/1 for adults and 50 to 180 IU/1 for ages 1 to 15—increased in rickets, Paget's disease, osteogenic sarcoma, hyperparathyroidism, obstructive jaundice, biliary cirrhosis, infectious mononucleosis, viral hepatitis, and neoplasms of the liver. Chemistry, liver function.

Alpha-1-Antitrypsin—180 to 244 mg/dl—increased in pancreatitis, diabetes, renal, liver, and cardiac disease. An hereditary deficiency predisposes people to chronic lung disease and emphysema. Chemistry.

Amino acids—blood or 5cc random urine—if abnormal, written interpretation—screens for congenital metabolic disorders. Chemistry.

Ammonia—NH4—no food or drink for 8 to 12 hrs prior—18 to 80 mcg/dl—increased in hepatic coma, sometimes in severe heart failure, uremia, and erythroblastosis fetalis. Chemistry.

Amniotic fluid—measures the amount of bilirubin in the fluid. The results tell if the fetus is affected by hemolytic disease. Chromosome studies determine if the fetus has certain hereditary diseases. Chemistry.

Amoeba—sputum, gastric contents, stool—to detect parasitic infestations—presence and identification of the parasite gives a guide for treatment. Microbiology, bacteriology.

Amylase—60 to 160 U/dll—elevated in acute pancreatitis and falls abruptly 2 to 3 days after onset. An elevation for longer than 5 days suggests continuing necrosis or pseudocyst formation. It is also increased in mumps, perforated peptic ulcer, liver and gallbladder disease, peritonitis, intestinal obstruction, and ruptured ectopic pregnancy. Chemistry.

Amylase, urine—2 hr urine specimen—0 to 300 U/hr—increased in same diseases as serum increased values. Chemistry.

ANA—antinuclear antibody—negative—presence indicates an inflammatory process of the connective tissue, especially systemic lupus erythematosis. A complete **ANA profile** aids in differentiating the specific connective tissue disease. There are more than 20 nuclear antigens that give rise to antibodies. Microbiology.

Anaerobic cultures—specimen collected in specific manner to avoid exposure to oxygen. Special procedures most commonly used to obtain a specimen are transtracheal aspiration (needle is inserted through the skin into the trachea and sputum is removed by suction with a syringe), sinus tap drainage, culdoscopy aspirations, suprapubic bladder aspirations, surgical removal of tissue or abscess aspiration. There is a preliminary report in 48 to 96 hours, but some organisms may take a week to properly identify. Microbiology.

Antibiotic testing—blood levels are determined to see if there is enough antibiotic in the bloodstream to kill the organism causing a disease. Chemistry.

Antibody identification—to determine a specific antibody—useful in obtaining compatible blood for transfusion. Blood bank.

Antibody screen—to determine if patient has previously been sensitized to any blood group antigen. Blood bank.

Antibody titer—determines quantity of antibody. Blood bank.

Anti-smooth muscle antibody—negative—presence indicates liver disease. Chemistry.

Anti-thyroid antibodies—less than 1:32—increased in hypothyroidism called Hashimoto's disease and lymphadenoid goiter. Chemistry.

Antitrypsin level—0.59 to 1.07 mg T.I./ml (T.I. = trypsin inhibited) Congenital deficiency is associated with emphysema at an early age and neonatal hepatitis. Chemistry.

Ascorbic acid—0.2 to 2.0 mg/100 ml—determines level of vitamin C in the blood—deficiency causes tissue degeneration and anemia—increased amounts interfere with anticoagulant therapy and may cause renal calculi. Chemistry.

ASO—antistreptolysin 0 titer—50 todd units or less. Streptolysin is an enzyme produced by group A streptococci. Presence of elevated titer is indicative of strep infection in rheumatic fever and acute glomerulonephritis. Microbiology, bacteriology.

AuA (AA, HAA, HBAg, Australian antigen)—negative—presence is associated with type B hepatitis. Microbiology, serology slip.

A-V gases simultaneous—same studies as ABGs on arterial and venous blood at same time—the difference in the two is a good indication of left ventricular performance. Values vary so no normal is given; your instructor may give you the values used in your area. Chemistry.

Barbiturates—blood, urine, gastric content—therapeutic, toxic, and lethal levels depend on specific barbituate—purpose is to monitor dose and assess toxicity of an overdose. Chemistry.

Bence Jones protein—urine—negative—presence may indicate multiple myeloma. Hematology.

Bilirubin—total 0.1 to 1.0 mg/dl—direct 0 to 0.2 mg/dl. Direct bilirubin is increased in obstructive jaundice and hepatitis jaundice; indirect is increased in hemolytic, neonatal and hepatitis jaundice; total is increased in all types of jaundice. Chemistry.

Bilirubin, urine—present in liver disease and bile obstruction. Chemistry.

Blood crossmatch—the process of determining compatibility of blood for a transfusion. Procedure takes about 1 to 1½ hrs. Blood needed for surgery should be requested the day before. Blood bank.

Bone marrow aspirate—a small sample of marrow for studies in most anemias, leukemias, and multiple myelomas. Hematology with an interpretation by pathologist.

Bone marrow biopsy—a small sample of bone and marrow is collected by the

pathologist in cases of suspected metastatic malignancies, lymphomas, mye-
lofibrosis. Pathology—requires permit.

BSP—bromsulphalein. The patient is NPO for at least 4 hrs prior; the weight
of the patient is to be recorded on the requisition—A dye is injected into an
arm vein, and 45 minutes later a sample of blood is taken from the other arm.
0 to 5% retention is normal. Elevations indicate liver disease. Chemistry.

Buccal smear—taken from inside the cheek—smear for sex chromatin. Cytology.

BUN—blood urea nitrogen—9 to 19 mg/dl—increased in renal failure or in
heart failure with poor renal circulation, intestinal obstruction, GI hemorrhage, dehydration, shock, fever, cancer. Chemistry.

UN (urine)—24 hr urine—12 to 20 gm/24 hrs—increased in fevers and
other diseases that speed up tissue catabolism. Chemistry.

Ca—calcium—9 to 11 mg/dl—increased in hyperparathyroidism, bone disease,
excessive vitamin D—decreased in renal acidosis, rickets, nephritis. Chemistry.

Calcium (urine)—24 hr urine—50 to 150 mg/24 hrs—aids in the diagnosis of
parathyroid dysfunction—increased in osteoporosis. Chemistry.

Calcitonin—less than 0.40 ng/ml—aids in detection of medullary carcinoma of
the thyroid which produces excess calcitonin. Chemistry.

Cardiac enzymes—includes LDH, CPK, and the isoenzymes—see those listings.
Chemistry.

Carotene—50 to 300 mcg/dl—increased in hyperlipemia and hypocholestero-
lemia of diabetes—decreased in cases of lipid malabsorption and if patient
on low fat diet. Aids in diagnosis of cystic fibrosis of pancreas. Chemistry.

Catecholamines—24 hr or random urine—0 to 120 µg/24 hrs and 0 to 18 µg/
100ml for random—increased in pheochromocytoma of adrenal medulla.
Chemistry.

CBC—complete blood count—includes all tests listed below. All are done by
Hematology.

- **HGB**—hemoglobin—Females 12.4 to 16.4 gms/dl—Males 13.8 to 18.4 gms/
  dl—decreased in anemia and bleeding and in patients receiving drugs
  that repress marrow—increased in polycythemia vera, renal cysts, dehydration, CHF.
- **HCT**—hematocrit—Female 36 to 48%—Male 41 to 54%—same increases
  and decreases as hemoglobin.
- **RBC**—red blood cells—Female 4,500,000/cu mm—Male 5,500,000/cu mm—
  decreased in anemia and hemorrhage.
- **MCH**—mean corpuscular hemoglobin—27 to 31 pg—indicates how much
  Hgb each red cell has—increased in folate and Vitamin B_{12} deficiency—
  decreased in iron deficiency.
- **MCHC**—mean corpuscular hemoglobin concentration—32 to 36%—
  decreased in anemia.
- **MCV**—mean corpuscular volume—82 to 98 cu microns—aids in determining type of anemia.
- **WBC**—white blood cells—5,000 to 10,000/cu mm—increased in process of
  inflammation and in leukemia—decreased in malaria, viral pneumonia,
  viral hepatitis and toxic injury.

- **Diff**—differential cell count—100 WBCs are counted and then each type is given in percentage.
  Myelocytes—0%—presence indicates acute leukemia.
  Juvenile neutrophils—3 to 5%
  Segmented neutrophils—54 to 62%
  Lymphocytes—25 to 33%—increased in viral infections, CLL, and lymphomas.
  Monocytes—3 to 7%
  Eosinophils—1 to 3%—increased in allergic reactions and in parasitic infestations.
  Basophils—0 to 0.75%—increased in CML.
- **Platelet count**—150,000 to 350,000/cu mm—decreased in bleeding disorders and conditions producing bone marrow failure.
- **Reticulocyte**—0.5 to 1.5%—indicates function of bone marrow. If a patient has anemia, the bone marrow should produce an increased number of new erythrocytes.
- **Morphology** is the study of the shape and form. Shapes of RBCs and WBCs are indicative of specific diseases. Abnormal shapes are reported.

CEA—carcinoembryonic antigen—0 to 2.5 ng/ml for non-smokers—0 to 5.0 ng/ml for smokers—carcinoma of the GI tract causes CEA to be released into the connective tissue and then into the blood and lymph—used to monitor cancer patients who are receiving therapy—an increase after a drop to below 2.5 ng/ml suggests tumor recurrence, metastases, or resistance to therapy. Chemistry.

Cholesterol—120 to 270 mg/dl under 40 yrs—150 to 330 mg/dl over 40 yrs—elevated in nephritis, viral hepatitis, thyroid disease, and often in arteriosclerotic diseases. Chemistry.

Cholinesterase (Pseudo or Acyl choline)—3 to 8 units—increased in nephrosis, obese diabetes, and anxiety states—decreased in liver disease, pulmonary embolism, MI, muscular dystrophy, acute infections, anemias, malnutrition, and insecticide poisoning. Chemistry.

Cl—chloride—100 to 106 mEq/l—increased in severe dehydration, complete renal shut-down—decreased in vomiting, diarrhea, diuresis, edema, CHF, certain abnormal states of the CNS. Chemistry.

CO_2—carbon dioxide—see ABG. Venous blood—25 to 29 mEq/l.

Coccidioidin skin test—negative if less than 5 mm of induration—positive if 5 mm or greater of induration—intradermal skin test to aid in diagnosis of the fungus infection of coccidiomycosis. Immunology.

Coccidiomycosis (Valley fever, Desert fever)—acute and convalescent specimens are required—titers of 1:16 and 1:32 suggest infection—titers greater than 1:32 indicate active disease. Immunology.

Cold agglutinins—less than 1:32 titer—increased in atypical viral pneumonia and autoimmune hemolytic anemias. Immunology, Microbiology.

Coombs (direct and indirect)—positive direct is seen in hemolytic disease of newborn, autoimmune hemolytic anemia, and in hemolytic transfusion reactions. Indirect Coombs is useful in detection of IgG antibodies or determining antibodies in patients with autoimmune hemolytic anemia. Blood bank.

Cord blood—includes ABO group, Rh typing, and direct Coombs—a positive direct Coombs indicates incompatibility between the mother and infant. Blood bank.

Cortisol—15 to 25 mcg/dl at 8:00 AM—5 to 15 mcg/dl at 4:00 PM—increased values in severe hypertension, virilism, stress, infectious diseases, burns, Cushing's disease, pancreatitis, and eclampsia—decreased in adrenal insufficiency of Addison's disease and in panhypopituitarism. Chemistry.

CPK—creatine phosphokinase—0 to 78 IU/1—increased in MI, acute or chronic damage to skeletal muscle. Chemistry.

CPK isoenzyme—CPK has three isoenzymes; CPK-MB or CPK_2 is the myocardial one. CPK reaches maximum level 24 hrs after MI and falls to normal in two to three days; CPK-MB drops more rapidly. CPK-MB does not rise after pulmonary embolism, in CHF, or in angina pectoris with no necrosis; therefore, it aids in diagnosis. Chemistry.

Creatinine—0.5 to 1.5 mg/dl—increased in acute or chronic kidney disease. Chemistry.

Creatinine clearance—24 hr urine with serum creatinine collected (fasting) after the 24 hrs—70 to 130 mg cl/min—requisition must state height and weight of patient. Cr. clearance values closely parallel the percentage of functioning renal nephrons. Urine creatinine values are 16 to 22 mg/kg/24 hrs for female and 21 to 26 mg/kg/24 hrs for male. Chemistry.

CRP—C reactive protein—negative—presence indicates acute tissue injury—used to monitor acute inflammatory conditions such as rheumatic fever and rheumatoid arthritis. Microbiology.

Cryoglobulins—negative—presence of these abnormal proteins is suggestive of an autoimmune disease, multiple myeloma, or lymphosarcoma. Chemistry.

CSF—cerebrospinal fluid—specimens must go to lab immediately.
- **Appearance**—clear—cloudiness indicates presence of cells or bacteria. Appearance, color, cell count by Hematology.
- **Color**—colorless—yellow indicates subarachnoid hemorrhage; red indicates blood.
- **Cell count**—few RBC, less than five lymphocytes—bacterial and viral infections increase white cells; increased red cells may be due to hemorrhage or trauma during the spinal tap.
- **Total protein**—15 to 40 mg/dl—increased in infections, old hemorrhage, and multiple sclerosis. Chemistry.
- **Glucose**—45 to 85 mg/dl—decreased in bacterial and fungal infections, parasitic invasion of meninges, and TB of meninges.
- **Chloride**—118 to 132 mEq/l—decreased in tuberculous meningitis, other types of meningitis. Glucose and Cl in Chemistry.
- **Colloidal gold**—no reduction—presence of reaction may indicate neurological syphilis, multiple sclerosis, and meningitis.
- **Serology** (VDRL)—non-reactive—reactive indicates neurosyphilis. Involvement of the CNS occurs in about 25% of patients with syphilis. Immunology or Microbiology for VDRL and colloidal gold.

Cytology is the evaluation of cells to determine if malignant disease is present and to evaluate benign conditions. Sources:
- **Breast aspirations**—fluid or material from a cyst

- **Breast smears**—secretions from four quadrants of the breast
- **Bronchial washings**—collected during bronchoscopy
- **CSF**—collected during spinal tap
- **Fluids from body cavities**—collected during aspirations or centesis—include pleural, pericardial, peritoneal, and joint fluid.
- **Gastric**—esophageal washings—collected during endoscopy.
- **Sputum**—first morning specimen preferred.
- **Urine**—mid-morning specimen one hour after drinking several glasses of water—clean catch method, cath specimen for females.

Cytomegalic virus—negative—acute and convalescent specimens required. Presence indicates active infection, usually in infants up to 4 months of age. It is one of the Herpes family and is transmitted via the placenta to the infant. Immunology.

Cu—copper—70 to 155 mcg/dl—increased in cirrhosis of the liver, MI, carcinoma of the prostate when treated with estrogens—decreased in Wilson's disease of the liver. Chemistry.

Cu—copper—urine 0 to 30 mcg/24 hr—increased in Wilson's disease. Chemistry.

Cultures determine if an organism is growing in the specimen.

Diagnex blue test (tubeless gastric)—free gastric HCl should be present—packet of chemicals and instructions obtained from lab—two hour urine collected per instructions—absence of HCl suggests cancer of stomach, gastric polyps, pernicious anemia—decreased HCl is found in gastric ulcers. Chemistry.

Diff cell count—differential—see CBC.

Digitoxin—therapeutic range 20 to 39.0 ng/ml—used to monitor therapy. Blood drawn 6 to 8 hours after last dose of digitoxin. Chemistry.

Digoxin—therapeutic range from 0.5 to 1.5 ng/ml—used to monitor therapy. Blood drawn 6 to 8 hours after last dose. Chemistry.

Dilantin—therapeutic range from 1 to 2 mg/dl—toxic level is 4 mg/dl and produces respiratory depression—used to monitor therapy. Chemistry.

D^u—used in determining Rhogam candidacy of certain Rh negative mothers—positive D^u considered Rh − as recipients and Rh + as donors. Blood bank.

Electrolytes—includes Na, K, Cl, CO_2—Cl was discussed earlier.
- **Na**—sodium—136 to 145 mEq/l—decreased in cardiac failure, renal insufficiency, cirrhosis, and water intoxication and in conditions that increase ADH secretion.
- **K**—potassium—3.8 to 5.3 mEq/l—decreased in conditions that cause vomiting, diarrhea, and diuresis and in hyperaldosteronism.
- **Cl**—chloride—see Cl.
- **CO_2**—carbon dioxide content—25 to 29 mEq/l—this is venous blood, the CO_2 discussed before was arterial—increased in respiratory acidosis and metabolic alkalosis—decreased in metabolic acidosis, nephritis, eclampsia, and diarrhea.

Electrolytes are important in evaluating cardiovascular, renal, and pulmonary function. They are used to monitor post-op patients' fluid and acid-base balance. Chemistry.

Electrophoresis (serum)—fractionation of proteins by electricity. Chemistry.

- **Albumin**—3.5 to 5.5 gm/100ml—increased in fluid imbalance—decreased in liver disease, starvation, malabsorption, thyro-toxicosis, and nephrotic syndrome.
  Globulins:
- **Alpha-1**—0.2 to 0.4 gm/100ml—increased in inflammatory, degenerative, and malignant diseases—decreased in congenital antitrypsin deficiency associated with juvenile pulmonary emphysema.
- **Alpha-2**—0.5 to 0.9 gm 100ml—increased in acute inflammatory processes, nephrotic syndrome, trauma, burns, neoplastic diseases, polyarthritis—decreased in hemolytic anemia.
- **Beta-globulin**—0.6 to 1.1 gm/100ml—increased in liver and lipid disorders—decreased levels are not significant.
- **Gamma globulin**—0.7 to 1.7 gm/100ml—increased in chronic infections, chronic liver disease, myeloma, and malignant lymphoma—decreased in chronic lymphocytic leukemia and nephrotic syndrome.

Eosinophile (nasal or sputum smear)—less than 20%—increase indicates allergic reaction, used to distinguish between an infection and an allergy. Hematology.

Eosinophile count—see under differential of CBC.

ESR—erythrocyte sedimentation rate—sed rate—0 to 20 mm/hr for female—0 to 12 mm/hr for male—increased in inflammatory diseases and diseases that cause degeneration of the tissue—used to assess the progress and activity of certain chronic diseases such as rheumatoid arthritis. Hematology.

Estriol, urine—24 hr urine—value depends on week of gestation—should increase with each week of pregnancy—decrease occurs with fetal distress, placental insufficiency—increases may occur in erythroblastosis fetalis. Chemistry.

Estrogens (urine)—24 hr urine—4 to 60 mcg/24 hr for female—4 to 25 mcg/24 hr for male—increased in some tumors of ovary and adrenal cortex—decreased in deficiency or absence of ovarian hormones. Chemistry.

Ethanol—same as alcohol.

Factor VIII or Factor IX—cryoprecipitate—Factor VIII = 50 to 150%—Factor IX = 50 to 150%—values of trace to 25% occur in hemophilia. Blood bank.

Fat (qualitative, feces)—both neutral fat and fatty acids are reported as within normal range or increased or decreased—neutral fats increase in pancreatic insufficiency—fatty acids increase in intestinal malabsorption. Microbiology.

Fat (quantitative, feces)—72 hour collection—less than 15g—increased in malabsorption. Microbiology.

Fe—iron—75 to 175 mcg/dl—increased in hemolytic anemia—decreased in hemorrhage or slow, chronic bleeding, excessive menstrual flow, or inadequate iron intake. Chemistry.

Febrile agglutinins—includes typhoid fever, paratyphoid fever, salmonellosis, tularemia, and brucellosis—titers should be negative—acute and convalescent samples are required. Immunology.

Fi test (FDP latex test, Fibrin split products)—less than 100 mcg/ml—increased in venous and arterial thrombosis, pulmonary embolus—aids in diagnosis of disseminated intravascular coagulation (DIC) which occurs in shock, hyperthermia, extensive tissue damage, snake bites, obstetric complications, and acute intravascular breakdown of RBCs. Hematology.

Fibrinogen—200 to 400 mg/dl—increased in trauma, infections, neoplasms, and hemorrhage—decreased in DIC and post-cardiac bypass, congenital disorders such as afibrinogenemia and hypofibrinogenemia. Hematology.

Fluorescent antibody test—rapid method of testing for Group A streptococci by a routine throat culture and for Bordetella pertussis (whooping cough) by a nasopharyngeal swab—usually takes 24 hrs for culture reports but this method gives results in 8 hrs. Microbiology.

Folic acid (folate)—7 to 16 ng/ml—decreased in inadequate nutrition, interference of intestinal absorption, pregnancy, malignancy, chronic hemolytic anemia, and disturbances of folate metabolism. Chemistry.

Fragility (osmotic)—tests the reaction of red cells to NaCl solution—the resistance to hypotonic solutions is reduced in hereditary spherocytosis and some acquired hemolytic anemias. Hematology.

Free fatty acids—0.45 to 0.95 mEq/l—increased in all forms of functional hepatic disease, deficient glucose utilization, increased tissue insulin activity. Chemistry.

FSH—follicle stimulating hormone—6 to 30 mIU/ml for adult female—30 to 200 mIU/ml for postmenopausal female—increased in primary gonadal failure—decreased in hypothalmic or pituitary failure. Chemistry.

FSH (urine)—24 hr urine—less than 6 MUU (mouse uterine units)/24 hrs for children before puberty—6 to 50 MUU/24 hrs for adults and greater than 50 MUU/24 hrs for postmenopausal female—increased in primary failure of gonads due to non-producing ovaries, seminiferous tubular failure, and Klinefelter's syndrome—decreased in tumors of adrenals, ovaries or testis, anorexia nervosa, administration of estrogen. Chemistry.

FTA—fluorescent treponemal antibodies—negative—presence indicates syphilis—performed on spinal fluid as well as blood. Immunology or Microbiology.

Fungus culture (India ink prep, KOH prep)—includes smear—performed on sputum, tissue, bone marrow, skin scrapings, nail, hair—large numbers may indicate disease. Yeasts and actinomyces are normal in some areas of the body. Microbiology.

Gastric analysis—patient should be fasting for 12 hrs prior—lab may do by appointment or RN may do on unit according to individual hospital policies—0 to 30 mEq/l of free HCl and 5 to 40 mEq/l of total acid—if histalog is given, the free HCl is 30 to 125 mEq/l one hour after histalog and the total acid is 50 to 130 mEq/l one hour after histalog. Increased in duodenal ulcer and Zollinger-Ellison syndrome—decreased or absent in pernicious anemia, gastric cancer, rheumatoid arthritis, aplastic and hypochromic anemia. Chemistry.

Gastrin—0 to 300 pg/ml—NPO except for water 8 hrs prior—increased in Zollinger-Ellison syndrome, pernicious anemia, gastric ulcer, gastric cancer, and GI obstruction. In some cases of Z-E syndrome the increase may be slight but will increase after administration of calcium or secretin. Chemistry.

GGT—gamma glutamyl transferase—5 to 35 IU/l—increased in hepatobiliary and pancreatic disease, moderate increase in CHF and kidney disease. Chemistry.

Glucose (blood sugar)—65 to 110 mg/dl—FBS (fasting blood sugar) requires NPO except water for 8 hrs prior. 2 hr PC is drawn exactly 2 hours after diet or solution of 100 grams of glucose; you must notify lab of the exact time for blood to be drawn. Random BS may be drawn at any time of the day. Blood sugar is increased in diabetes mellitus, hyperthyroidism, hyperfunction of adrenal cortex, hyperpituitarism and decreased in hepatic disease, adrenal cortical insufficiency, anterior pituitary insufficiency, hypothyroidism and excessive insulin. Chemistry.

Glucose (urine)—24 hr urine—0.0 to 0.25 gm/24 hrs—increase usually indicates diabetes mellitus. Chemistry.

Glycosylated hemoglobin—Hb A_{1c}—0.4 to 4%—increases 3 to 4 times in red cells of diabetic patients. Reflects an average of blood sugar concentration over prior 2 to 3 months. Hematology.

Gram stain—smear—a rapid test to determine infection, type of organism as well as presence and type of inflammatory cells. Results can be obtained in about 30 minutes. Microbiology.

Growth hormone—may be called GH or HGH (human growth hormone)—0 to 10 ng/ml for adults—0 to 20 ng/ml for children—increased in acromegaly—decreased in dwarfism of children and in hypopituitarism in adults. Chemistry.

Growth hormone series—blood drawn for baseline, then L-Dopa is administered and blood drawn at 30, 60, and 90 minutes—normal persons will show increase after L-Dopa. Chemistry.

GTT—glucose tolerance test—NPO after midnight except for water—doctor specifies how many hours (1 to 6)—FBS and urine specimens collected, patient given 100 grams of glucose in a solution, blood and urine specimens collected at one-half hour and then hourly for specified time. If patient vomits, the doctor is notified to see if the test is to be continued or not. Normal values are 65 to 110 mg/dl for fasting, 110 to 160 mg/dl for ½ hr, 90 to 150 mg/dl for 1 hr, 65 to 110 mg/dl for 2 to 6 hrs. Diabetes mellitus produces a higher rise which stays higher longer. Hypoglycemia produces a fall to below 50 mg/dl after the high reading at the one-half hour interval. Chemistry.

GTT IV—glucose is given intravenously—same procedure otherwise—same values except the ½ hr may rise to 200 mg/dl— aids in identifying or eliminating intestinal malabsorption as a factor. Chemistry.

Guaiac—occult blood—random stool specimen—positive test indicates bleeding in GI tract—aids in diagnosis of tumors and ulcers. Microbiology.

HAA—see AuA, Australian antigen.

Hamm test—see acid hemolysin.

Haptoglobin—alpha-2-globulin, which is the primary plasma carrier of free hemoglobin—reported as normal, decreased, increased, or absent—increased in inflammatory disease and during steroid therapy—decreased or absent in liver disease. Absence may be congenital. Chemistry. (Some labs use 40 to 170 mg/dl as normal.)

HCG—human chorionic gonadotropin—5 to 30 IU/1—increased in pregnancy, hydatidiform mole, and choriocarcinoma. Immunology.

HCG (urine)—first voided morning specimen—positive if pregnancy has occurred. Microbiology or Immunology.

Hct—see CBC components.

Hemosiderin (urine)—early morning specimen preferred—negative—presence indicates destruction of red blood cells intravascularly. Hematology.

Herpes simplex—negative—positive titer indicates recent infection. Acute and convalescent specimens required. Virology.

Heterophile screen—monospot—negative—positive indicates an infectious mononucleosis. Immunology or microbiology.

Histamine—4 to 7 mcg%—increased in gastric carcinoid tumors. Chemistry.

Histology studies—any tissue studied for abnormality or disease.

Histoplasmin skin test—positive reaction indicates exposure to or infection by Histoplasma, a parasitic fungus that causes respiratory disease. Immunology or Microbiology.

5-HIAA—5-Hydroxyindole acetic acid—urine serotonin—24 hr urine—0 to 16 mg/24 hrs—increased in carcinoid tumors—decreased in renal insufficiency. Chemistry.

Hollander test—NPO after midnight except for water—a FBS and a 15 minute gastric content collection is made, then insulin is given IV—30 minute BS and 15 minute gastric content collections are made for 3 hours. The test is used to determine the completeness of vagotomy. There is an acid response if vagotomy incomplete. Chemistry.

IBC—iron binding capacity—250 to 410 mcg/dl—increased in iron deficiency—decreased in nephrosis. Chemistry.

ICSH—interstitial cell stimulating hormone—same as LH in males.

Immunoglobulins—proteins that act as antibodies and are designated as: **IgA**—50 to 200 mg/dl; **IgD**—no assigned value as the biological functions are not clearly defined; **IgE**—problems are rare so no value is given; **IgG**—600 to 1200 mg/dl—the only immunoglobulin capable of crossing the placenta and entering fetal circulation; **IgM**—50 to 175 mg/dl. Immunoglobulins help protect against infection. Congenital deficiencies cause the individual to have little or no resistance to disease. In nephrotic syndrome, ulcerative colitis, diseases of lymph vessels or intestinal tract, the immunoglobulins are decreased. Chemistry or Immunology.

Insulin—less than 20 µU/ml—increased in insulin producing tumors—Type I diabetes has very low or absent insulin levels. Chemistry.

K—potassium—see electrolytes.

Ketones (urine)—presence indicates uncontrolled diabetes, may occur in severe vomiting and diarrhea. Chemistry.

Kleihauer test—determines presence of fetal cells in mother's system—useful in determining amount of Rhogam to give to mother if fetal-maternal hemorrhage has occurred. Blood bank.

Kolmer—serological test for syphilis. Microbiology.

17-OHCS—17-hydroxycorticosteroids—24 hr urine—2 to 8 mg/24 hrs for female—3 to 12 mg/24 hrs for male—increased in Cushing's disease—decreased in adrenal virilism, adrenal cancer. Chemistry.

17-KGS—17-Ketogenic steroids—24 hr urine—5 to 23 mg/24 hrs for female—3 to 15 mg/24 hr for male—increased in hyperfunction of adrenal cortex and gonads; their hypofunction causes a decrease. Chemistry.

17-KS—17-Ketosteroids—24 hr urine—6 to 15 mg/d for adult female—9 to 22 mg/d for adult male—varies with age—increased in testicular tumors, Cushing's disease, adrenal tumors—decreased in Addison's disease, panhypopituitarism, hypogonadism, severe debilitating illness. Chemistry.

Lactic acid—lactate—6 to 16 mg/dl—increased in circulatory insufficiency, uncontrolled diabetes mellitus, severe liver disease, renal failure, lymphomas, and leukemia. Chemistry.

Lactose tolerance—NPO after midnight—FBS is drawn and patient is given 50 gms of lactose in solution. Blood is drawn every 30 minutes for 2 hours. Glucose levels should rise more than 20 mg/dl after lactose administration. Decreased rise indicates lactose deficiency, and the individual cannot tolerate lactose or milk sugar. Chemistry.

LDH—lactic acid dehydrogenase—125 to 270 IU/1—increased in MI, hepatic and renal damage, leukemia, malignancies, skeletal muscle injury, breakdown of RBCs. CSF LDH is increased in acute meningitis, leukemia, CVA, subarachnoid hemorrhage, and malignancies of brain and spinal cord. Chemistry.

LDH Isoenzymes—there are five components: **Fraction 1** is 20 to 30% of total, **Fraction 2** is 22 to 45% of total, **Fraction 3** is 15 to 30% of total, **Fraction 4** is 5 to 15% of total, and **Fraction 5** is 0 to 15% of total. Fractions 1 and 2 are increased in MI, renal infarction, and RBC destruction; Fractions 4 and 5 are increased in liver disease. Chemistry.

Lead—blood, less than 60 mcg/dl—urine, less than 100 mcg/dl in 24 hr specimen—increased levels indicate lead poisoning which is usually due to exposure to lead in industry. Chemistry.

LE Prep—test for lupus erythematosis—negative—positive in about 60 to 70% of individuals with SLE. Other autoimmune diseases may show a positive test. Hematology.

LH—luteinizing hormone—less than 25 mIU/ml for females—greater than 25 for post-menopausal females—less than 11 mIU/ml for males—increased in primary gonadal failure—decreased in hypothalamic or pituitary failure. Chemistry.

Li—lithium—therapeutic range 0.5 to 1.0 mEq/l—toxic above 2.0 mEq/l—used to monitor therapy in treatment of manic-depressive psychosis with manic episodes. Chemistry.

Lipase—0 to 1.0 U/ml—increased in pancreatitis, cancer of the pancreas, chronic biliary tract disease. Chemistry.

Lipids (total)—NPO after midnight—450 to 1000 mg/dl—increased in starvation, pregnancy, poorly controlled diabetes mellitus. Some cases of increased levels may be due to familial tendency. Chemistry.

Lipid profile—includes cholesterol, phospholipids, and triglycerides. See individual tests.

Lipoprotein electrophoresis—NPO after midnight—requires written interpretation by pathologist—aids in diagnosis of several deficiency diseases, genetic disorders, atherosclerosis, and coronary artery disease. Chemistry.

L/S ratio—lecithin: sphingomyelin ratio—amniotic fluid—2:1 indicates fetal lung maturity; enough surfactant is present to prevent hyaline membrane disease. Chemistry.

Liver profile—includes bilirubin, alkaline phosphatase, total protein, A/G ratio, SGOT, GGT, and prothrombin time. See individual tests.

Lymphogranuloma venereum—acute and convalescent specimens are required—used to verify infection by microorganism of Chlamydia family, a venereal disease. Immunology or Microbiology.

Malaria smear—negative—presence indicates invasion by plasmodium. Smear identifies the species (there are four), so that the accurate drug will be given. Hematology.

Melanin—fresh random urine—negative—presence indicates a melanoma. Chemistry.

Metanephrines (urine)—24 hr urine—0.3 to 0.9 mg/24 hrs—increased in pheochromocytoma, a tumor of the adrenal medulla. Chemistry.

Mg (magnesium)—1.5 to 2.5 mEq/l—increased in renal retention, dehydration, diabetic coma, depression of cardiac conduction, and neuromuscular activity—decreased in tetany, hepatic cirrhosis, pancreatitis, hyperparathyroidism, hypercalcemia, and severe diarrhea. Chemistry.

Mg (urine)—24 hr urine—2.5 to 5.0 mEq/L—uremia produces a high serum level and a low urinary level. Chemistry.

Monospot—see Heterophile.

Mucin test—good mucin—joint fluid coagulation activity—an infected joint would show poor mucin; rheumatoid joints show fair mucin. Chemistry.

Mumps skin test—positive test at onset of mumps-like disease indicates a past mumps infection to signify diagnosis is other than mumps. Immunology or Microbiology.

Na—sodium—see electrolytes.

Neonatal bilirubin—microbilirubin—increased in jaundice of the newborn—prime index for exchange transfusion in erythroblastosis fetalis. Chemistry.

O_2—oxygen—see PO_2 and O_2 saturation under ABG.

Occult blood (feces)—see Guaiac.

Osmolality—275 to 295 mOsm/kg—increased in hyperglycemia, uremia, alcoholic intoxication, diabetes insipidus—decreased in excess fluid intake and dysfunction of ADH secretion. Aids in fluid and electrolyte therapy for burns, shock. Chemistry.

Osmolality (urine)—300 to 1000 mOsm/kg—the urine to plasma ratio is decreased in renal disease, sickle cell anemia, diabetes insipidus. Chemistry.

O and P—ova and parasites—feces, sputum, and gastric contents—negative—presence indicates invasion of parasites—type will be reported. Microbiology.

Oxalate—24 hr urine—0 to 40 mg/24 hrs—increased in hereditary hyperoxaluria, inflammatory bowel disease, liver disease, massive doses of Vitamin C. Chemistry.

P—phosphorus—NPO after midnight—2.5 to 4.5 mg/dl—children 4.0 to 7.0 mg/dl—increased in hypoparathyroidism, renal failure—decreased in rickets, osteomalacia, renal acidosis. Chemistry.

Parathyroid hormone—NPO after midnight except for water—about 100 to 400 pg/ml—increased in hyperparathyroidism due to hyperplasia or tumor, chronic renal failure, malabsorption, Vitamin D deficiency—decreased in hypoparathyroidism from surgical trauma or unknown cause and in hypercalcemia from malignancy and sarcoidosis. Chemistry.

PBI—protein bound iodine—4.0 to 8.0 mcg/dl—increased in hyperthyroidism—decreased in hyperthyroidism, nephrosis, and malnutrition. Chemistry.

PCO_2—see ABG. Venous blood—38 to 53 mm Hg.

pH—see ABG. Venous blood—7.34 to 7.39.

pH (urine)—see Urinalysis.

Phenylalinine—0 to 3 mg/dl—deficiency results in CNS degeneration, phenyl-ketonuria (PKU). Some states require this test for all newborns so that treatment can be started if PKU exists; the test is usually performed at one or two weeks of age. Microbiology.

Phospholipids—NPO after midnight except for water—125 to 300 mg/dl—abnormal levels indicate liver dysfunction—increased in bile obstruction and biliary cirrhosis—decreased in some cases of atherosclerosis. Chemistry.

Pinworm prep—transparent tape is applied to perianal region on arising and then tape is pressed on glass slide—microscopic exam will determine if ova of pinworm is present. Microbiology.

Platelet count—see CBC.

Porphobilinogen (urine, qualitative)—random urine—negative—presence indicates porphyria, an inherited defect—May be present in lead poisoning and hepatitis. Chemistry.

Porphobilinogen (urine, quantitative)—24 hr urine—0 to 2 mg/24 hrs—increased in hereditary prophyria. Chemistry.

Porphyrins (urine, quantitative)—24 hr urine—corproporphyrin 50 to 250 mcg/24 hrs—uroporphyrin 10 to 30 mcg/24 hrs—both increased in congenital erythropoietic porphyria, acquired hepatic porphyrias. Coproporphyrins are increased in a condition called porphyrinuria which is caused by high fever, hemolytic or pernicious anemia, malignancies of the blood, acute pancreatitis, cirrhosis, and lead or arsenic poisoning. Chemistry.

PPD skin test—purified protein derivative of old tuberculin—Mantoux test—intracutaneous injection of solution of the mycobacterium tuberculosis organism. First strength is used if active TB suspected, intermediate dose used if doctor does not specify, second strength used if patient screened with first or intermediate strength. Induration read in 48 and 72 hours, negative is less than 5 mm; positive is 10 mm or more and indicates sensitivity but not necessarily active disease. If individual has had previous severe response to the test with no active disease, the test should not be given. Immunology or Microbiology.

Pregnancy test—first voided urine specimen in AM—slide test reports results in ½ hr—positive HCG levels of 2 to 5 IU/ml indicate pregnancy. Negative tests may be repeated using the 2 hr tube test method which detects a minimum of 0.5 IU/ml. Immunology or Microbiology.

Pregnanetriol (urine)—24 hr urine—0.2 to 4.0 mg/24 hrs for adults—less than 0.5 mg/24 hrs for children—increased in congenital adrenal cortical hyperplasia or adrenogenital syndrome. Chemistry.

Progesterone—male is less than 25 ng/100ml—female values vary according to time of menstrual cycle or pregnancy with greater than 100ng/100ml in follicular phase, greater than 400ng/100ml in leuteal phase, and greater than 800 ng/100ml during pregnancy. Decreased levels during pregnancy signal placental dysfunction. Increased levels found in adrenogenital syndrome. Chemistry.

Prolactin—2 to 30 ng/ml—increased in tumors of hypothalamus, some pituitary tumors, amenorrhea. Chemistry.

Protein (total)—6.0 to 8.2 gm/dl—decreased in malnutrition, bleeding, chronic illness—increased in dehydration due to diarrhea, vomiting, shock, burns. See A/G ratio and Albumin. Chemistry.

Protein (urine)—24 hr urine—10 to 150 mg/24 hr—increased in glomerulo-nephritis, cardiac disease, toxemia of pregnancy, liver disease, diseases with high fever. Chemistry.

Protein electrophoresis—see electrophoresis (serum).

Proteus OX-19—negative, 1:40 or less—suspicious, 1:80—evidence of Rickettsial infection, 1:160 or more. Rickettsia cause typhus and Rocky Mountain spotted fever. Immunology or Microbiology.

Proteus OXK—same as Proteus OX-19, a Rickettsial species.

Proteus OX2—same as Proteus OX-19, a Rickettsial species.

PSP—phenolsulfonphthalein—dye injected IV after patient voids and urine collected at 15 min, 30 min, 1 hr, and 2 hrs following injection—excretion of dye: 25 to 35% in 15 min, 40 to 60% total in 1 hr, 60 to 75% total in 2 hrs—increased in hypoalbuminemia—decreased in cardiac failure and diseases of the blood vessels of the kidneys. Chemistry.

PT—pro time—prothrombin time—10.6 to 13.0 seconds according to control—patient's seconds should be within one second of control—used to monitor coumadin and dicumarol therapy and detect deficiencies in coagulation factors of the blood. Hematology.

PTT—partial thromboplastin time—used to monitor heparin and ordered for one hour before heparin dose—detects deficiencies of the coagulation factors—activated normal 27 to 43 seconds. Hematology.

RA latex—rheumatoid arthritis latex—rheumatoid factor—positive denotes presence of macroglobulins which exist in chronic inflammatory diseases. Immunology or Microbiology.

RAST—radioallergosorbent test—blood sample for evaluation of allergies—mainly for food allergies. Chemistry.

RBC—red blood cell count—see CBC.

Renal calculi—analysis of stones from urinary tract—aids in diagnosis and treatment of patients with stone formation. Chemistry and Histology.

Renin—75 to 275 ng/dl—increased in ischemic kidney disease. Chemistry.

Reticulocyte count—see CBC.

RPCF—Reiter protein complement fixation test for syphilis. Microbiology.

RPR—rapid plasma reagin test for syphilis. Microbiology.

Rh—abbreviation for the rhesus monkey in which the Rh factor was first identified. Persons having the Rh factor in their red blood cells are Rh positive (Rh+); persons without the Rh factor in their red blood cells are Rh negative (Rh−). About 85% of the population is Rh+, and the other 15% is Rh−. There are several subdivisions of the factor which are of importance in determining if an Rh− pregnant woman will produce a child with erythroblastosis fetalis. Blood bank.

Rhogam—blood samples drawn within 24 hrs after abortion or delivery, cord blood also needed. This test assures that there is no incompatibility between the mother's cells and the immunoglobulin given to Rh− mothers bearing Rh+ children if the mother develops antibodies. Blood bank.

Routine cultures—determine presence of bacteria. Microbiology.

Rubella titer—German measles—titer of 1:20 or more indicates past infection and immunity. Immunology or Microbiology.

Salmonella—see febrile agglutinins.

Schilling test (Vitamin B$_{12}$ test)—NPO after midnight except for water—90 to 630 pg/ml for females—170 to 760 pg/ml for males—increased in acute and chronic leukemia, cirrhosis, infectious hepatitis, polycythemia—decreased in pernicious anemia, malabsorption syndrome, nutritional vitamin deficiency. Chemistry.

Schilling test (urine)—NPO after midnight except for water—patient voids at 8:00 AM and is given ^{57}CO-labeled Vitamin B$_{12}$. Two hours later, 1000 mcg Vitamin B$_{12}$ is given IM and then the patient may eat. 24 hr urine collected from time first medication is given. The test aids in diagnosis of pernicious anemia and malabsorption syndrome. Chemistry.

Semen exam—semen produced by masturbation and taken to lab ASAP. Used to determine fertility and to investigate completeness of vasectomy. Microbiology.

Sensitivity testing—performed in conjunction with cultures to determine which antibiotic the organism is sensitive to so that the proper drug will be used. Usually a culture and sensitivity test are done together (C & S). Microbiology.

Serotonin—50 to 200 ng/ml—increased in carcinoid tumors. Chemistry.

SGOT—serum glutamic oxalic transaminase—6 to 22 IU/l—increased in MI, liver disease, viral hepatitis, obstructive jaundice, and metastatic cancer of the liver. Chemistry.

SGPT—serum glutamic pyruvic transaminase—5 to 35 IU/l—increased in liver damage—decreased in Vitamin B$_6$ deficiency and in patients on dialysis. Chemistry.

Sickle cell prep—negative—presence indicates abnormal hemoglobin in red cells which causes a sickling effect when exposed to low oxygen tension. Sickle cell anemia occurs if the amount of abnormal hemoglobin is large. Hematology.

SMA—a profile of 20 commonly ordered tests—NPO after midnight except for water—includes FBS, BUN, creatinine, uric acid, Na, K, Cl, CO$_2$, total proteins, albumin, globulin, A/G ratio, iron, cholesterol, triglycerides, calcium, phosphorus, alk. phosphatase, SGOT, LDH, total, direct and indirect bilirubin. Chemistry.

Sodium—see electrolytes.

Sulkowitch (urine)—24 hr urine preferred—1+ to 2+—increased in hyperparathyroidism, diseases causing bone softening, hyperthyroidism, osteoporosis, excessive vitamin D—decreased in hypoparathyroidism, malabsorption, vitamin D deficiency. Chemistry.

Sweat chlorides—less than 40 mEq/l—increased in cystic fibrosis. Chemistry.

T$_3$—triiodothyronine—25 to 35%—increased in hyperthyroidism, metastatic cancers, severe liver disease, nephrosis, elevated before T$_4$ in Graves' disease—decreased in hypothyroidism. Chemistry.

T$_4$—thyroxine—5.4 to 13 mcg/dl—increased in hyperthyroidism, early hepatitis, acute thyroiditis, and by many drugs—decreased by many drugs and in cretinism, myxedema, hypothyroidism, chronic thyroiditis. Chemistry.

T$_4$ index (free T$_4$)—free thyroxine—1.0 to 2.3 ng/dl—increased in hyperthyroidism—decreased in hypothyroidism. Chemistry.

TBG—thyroxine binding globulin—2.1 to 5.2 mg/dl—increased in acute liver disease, congenital defects in the globulin, estrogen therapy, pregnancy—decreased in protein deficiency, chronic liver disease and TBG deficiency due to congenital defect. Chemistry.

Testosterone—25 to 100 ng/dl for female—300 to 800 ng/dl for male—increased in females having hirsutism and virilization syndrome—decreased in males in delayed puberty, hypogonadism—useful in differentiation of certain testicular tumors. Chemistry.

Toxicology—screening for toxic levels of drugs—if a particular drug is suspected, it is stated on the requisition. Results are reported in 3 to 4 hours if an emergency. Chemistry.

TPI—Treponema pallidum immobilization—non-reactive—positive test is diagnostic for syphilis. Microbiology.

Trichomonas—negative—presence indicates disease caused by the trichomonas vaginalis, producing vaginitis and chronic disease of genitourinary tract. Microbiology.

Triglycerides—30 to 135 mg/dl—triglycerides are neutral fats which are the body's major store of chemical energy—useful in determining type of hyperlipoproteinemia, managing diabetes, nephrosis, biliary obstruction, and in endocrine disturbances that cause metabolic derangement. Chemistry.

TSH—thyroid stimulating hormone—0 to 10 μIU/ml—aids in differentiating between primary hypothyroidism and secondary hypothyroidism—levels are high in primary type. Chemistry.

Type and screen—blood group is determined and screened for atypical antibodies—used preoperatively if certainty of transfusion has not been established. Blood bank.

Urea clearance—NPO after midnight except for water—24 hr urine with blood sample during that period—40 to 68 ml cl/min—used to measure renal function if urine excretion is 2 ml/min or more. Chemistry.

Urea nitrogen—see BUN.

Uric acid—1.5 to 6.0 mg/dl for females—2.5 to 7.0 mg/dl for males—increased in multiple myeloma, leukemia and polycythemia vera, gout—decreased in acute liver atrophy. Chemistry.

Urinalysis—UA, RUA—screening test for metabolic diseases, urinary tract infections, or renal disease. The test is performed in Hematology. It includes:
- **Color**—straw to amber. Products changing the color are drugs, hemoglobin, myoglobin, bile pigments, prophyrins, melanin.
- **Appearance**—clear. Bacteria or cells change appearance.
- **Specific gravity**—1.008 to 1.030—increased in chronic renal disease or excessive fluid intake—decreased in dehydration.
- **pH**—4.5 to 8.0—normal urine is acid to neutral—alkaline urine may be due to infections, metabolic disorders, diet, certain drugs.
- **Protein** (qualitative)—present in kidney disease.
- **Glucose** (qualitative)—present in diabetes mellitus.
- **Ketones**—present in starvation, diabetes mellitus, Cushing's syndrome, acromegaly, stress and high fever.
- **Blood**—present in inflammation of urinary tract.
- **Bile**—bilirubin—present in liver disease and in biliary obstruction.

- **Microscopic exam includes:**
  - **WBC/hpf**—more than 10 indicates infection.
  - **RBC/hpf**—presence indicates trauma or infection.
  - **Casts/hpf**—a rare hyaline cast is normal—others indicate renal dysfunction.
  - **Bacteria**—present in infection.
  - **Epithelial cells**—squamous type are normal, renal type are an indication of renal disease.
  - **Crystals**—normally found.

Urinary creatine—24 hr urine—0 to 150 mg/24 hrs for female—0 to 250 mg/24 hrs for male—increased in diseases that cause muscular destruction such as myositis, muscular dystrophy, hyperthyroidism, and muscular atrophy. Chemistry.

Urobilinogen (qualitative)—trace—increased in hepatitis—decreased in obstructive jaundice. Chemistry.

VDRL—STS—Venereal Disease Research Laboratory—serological standard test for syphilis—nonreactive—reactive result is diagnostic for primary and secondary syphilis, reverts to negative after successful treatment. Tertiary syphilis, the late stage which involves the heart, lungs and CNS, may show a negative serum but the CSF VDRL will be positive. Microbiology.

Vitamin A—Retinol—65 to 275 IU/dl—essential for vision, bone growth, maintenance of cell membrane, and spermatogenesis. Low levels are from inadequate diet or malabsorption. Chemistry.

Vitamin B$_{12}$—300 to 1000 pg/ml—increased in acute viral hepatitis, cirrhosis—deficiency may be due to inadequate dietary intake of the vitamin, lack of intrinsic factor, or intestinal malabsorption. Deficiency causes pernicious anemia and some neurological disorders. Chemistry.

VMA—vanillymandelic acid—for 3 days prior, diet must eliminate coffee, tea, chocolate, vanilla, foods containing vanilla, cola beverages and bananas—24 hr urine—0.7 to 6.8 mg/24 hrs—increased in pheochromocytomas. Chemistry.

Weil-Felix—demonstrates antibodies for Proteus OX-19, OX2, and OXK—see those listings.

D-Xylose test—NPO after midnight except for water—patient voids and is given D-Xylose according to his/her weight; urine is collected for 5 hours. Patients with hepatic or kidney disease should also have blood samples; fasting, 30 min, 1 hr, and 2 hrs. Urine excretion should be greater than 4 gm/5 hrs—blood level of 30 to 40 mg/dl within 30 to 60 minutes and maintained for another hour. The test measures the absorption ability of the duodenum and adjacent jejunum. Chemistry.

Zinc—60 to 148 mcg% for serum—445 to 840 mcg/24 hrs for urine—24 hr urine—increased in porphyria, acute rheumatic fever, and zinc poisoning. Chemistry.

APPENDIX III
ABBREVIATIONS

The abbreviations listed are those commonly used. The laboratory test abbreviations and chemical symbols are the ones used most often, and they are listed here and also in Appendix II. You may want to know an abbreviation before reaching the part of the text dealing with that test. For that reason, the most commonly used diagnoses abbreviations are included. Your instructor will probably indicate which abbreviations you should learn first.

Abbreviation	*Meaning*
$\propto$	alpha
@	at
AA	auto accident
	Alcoholics Anonymous
a̅a̅	of each
Ab	antibody
ab	abortion
abd	abdomen
	abdominal
ABE	acute bacterial endocarditis
ABG	arterial blood gases
ABO	ABO blood groups
a.c.	before meals
acc	accommodation
ACF	anterior cervical fusion
ACT	activated clotting time
ACTH	adrenocorticotrophic hormone
AD	axis deviation
A.D.	right ear
ADA	American Diabetes Association
ADH	antidiuretic hormone
ADL	activities of daily living
ad lib	as desired
adm	administration
	admit
	admission
ADT	adult diphtheria toxoid
AF	atrial flutter
	auricular fibrillation
AFB	acid fast bacillus

A/G ratio	albumin-globulin ratio
AGA	appropriate gestational age
AK	above knee
AKA	above knee amputation
alb	albumin
alc	alcohol
alk	alkaline
alk phos	alkaline phosphatase
ALL	acute lymphatic leukemia
ALS	amyotrophic lateral sclerosis
AMA	against medical advice
	American Medical Association
amb	ambulate
	ambulatory
AML	acute myeloblastic leukemia
amp	ampule
	amputation
amt	amount
ANA	antinuclear antibody
Anes	anesthesia
ant	anterior
ant. ch.	anterior chamber
ante	before
AP	anteroposterior
	apical pulse
A&P	auscultation and percussion
	anterior & posterior
AP & Lat	anteroposterior and lateral
approx	approximately
aq	aqua, water
	aqueous
Ar	argon
AR	atrial regurgitation
ARDS	adult respiratory distress syndrome
ARF	acute rheumatic fever
AS	aortic stenosis
	arteriosclerosis
A.S.	left ear
ASA	aspirin (acetylsalicylic acid)
ASAP	as soon as possible
ASCVD	arteriosclerotic cardiovascular disease
ASD	atrial septal defect
ASHD	arteriosclerotic heart disease
ASO titer	anti-streptolysin O titer
AST	antibody screening test
ASU	ambulatory surgery unit
ATF	atrial fibrillation
Au A	Australian antigen

ATS	anxiety tension state
A.U.	aures unitas, both ears
	auris uterque, each ear
AV	arteriovenous
AV diff	arteriovenous difference
ARV	aortic valve replacement
A&W	alive and well
ax	axillary
B	Bacillus
β	beta
B/A	backache
Ba	barium
BaE	barium enema (also B.E.)
BB	breast biopsy
	both bones
BAM	bilateral augmentation mammoplasty
BC	birth control
	bone conduction
BCC	basal cell carcinoma
BCBS	Blue Cross-Blue Shield
BE	barium enema (also BaE)
BFD	before discharge
BFR	blood flow rate
BID or bid	twice a day
bil	bilateral
bili; bilirub	bilirubin
BK	below knee
BKA	below knee amputation
Bkft	breakfast
BLESS	bath, laxative, enema, shampoo, shower, shave
BM	bone marrow
	bowel movement
bndg	bandage
BOW	bag of waters (amniotic sac)
BP	blood pressure
BPH	benign prostatic hypertrophy
BR	bed rest
BRM	bilateral reduction mammoplasty
BRP	bathroom privileges
BS	blood sugar
	bowel sound
	breath sound
BSC	bedside commode
BSO	bilateral salpingo-oophorectomy
BSP	bromsulphalein
BUN	blood urea nitrogen
bx	biopsy

C	carbon
	centigrade
	cervical
	cup
c̄	with
CA	carcinoma, cancer
Ca	calcium
	carcinoma
	cancer
CAB	coronary artery bypass
CAC	cardiac arrest cart
C&A	clinitest and acetest
CAD	coronary artery disease
cal	calorie
calc	calculus, stone,
	calculated
cap(s)	capsule(s)
CARVAS	cardiovascular
cath	catheter
	catheterize
C & S	culture and sensitivity
cath lab	catheterization laboratory
CBC	complete blood count
CBP	cardiac bypass
CC	chief complaint
cc	cubic centimeter
CCMS	clean catch midstream (urine specimen)
CCU	Coronary Care Unit
CD	closed drainage
	common duct
CDC	Center for Disease Control (in Atlanta, Georgia)
CDE	common duct exploration
CDH	congenital dislocation hip
CEA	carcinoembryonic antibody
cerv	cervical
CHF	congestive heart failure
chg or Δ	change
CHO	carbohydrate
chol	cholesterol
chole, choly	cholecystitis
	cholecystectomy
circ	circulation
	circulatory
	circumcision
ck	check (ed)
CL	corpus luteum
	critical list
Cl	chloride

CLL	chronic lymphocytic leukemia
cm	centimeter
CML	chronic myeloblastic leukemia
CNS	central nervous system
Co	cobalt
CO	carbon monoxide
	cardiac output
	corneal opacity
CO_2	carbon dioxide
c/o	complains of
COLD	chronic obstructive lung disease
comp	compound
compl	complaint
	complication
conc	concentration
cont	continue
COPD	chronic obstructive pulmonary disease
CPB	cardiopulmonary bypass
CPK	creatinine phosphokinase
cppb	continuous positive pressure breathing
CPR	cardiopulmonary resuscitation
CPT	chest percussion therapy
Cr	creatinine
C-R	crown-rump (with reference to length of fetus)
C.R.A.	central retinal artery
CRP	C-reactive protein
creat	creatinine
crit	critical
Cs	cesium
CS	Cesarean section
	central supply
CSF	cerebrospinal fluid
CTD	connective tissue disease
Cu	copper
CVA	cardiovascular arrest
	cerebrovascular accident
CVC	central venous catheter
CVP	central venous pressure
cysto	cystoscopy
Cx	cervix
cxl	cancel
CXR	chest x-ray
D	disease
	divorced
d	day
	dram
DAA	dead after arrival

DAT	diet as tolerated
DB & C	deep breathe and cough
DBE	deep breathing exercises
D/C, DC, dc	discontinue
	disconnect
	discharge (from hospital)
	direct current
D&C	dilatation and curettage
DC&A	dilatation and curettage, abortion
DD	dependent drainage
DDS	doctor of dental surgery
del	delivery
diag	diagnosis
diff	differential
Dig	Digoxin
DIP	distal interphalangeal (joint)
disch	discharge
disp	dispense
DJD	degenerative joint disease
D/LR	dextrose with lactated Ringer's
DM	diabetes mellitus
DNA	do not announce
	deoxyribonucleic acid
DNR	do not resuscitate
	dorsal nerve root
D.O.	doctor of osteopathy
DOA	dead on arrival
DOE	dyspnea on exertion
DPT	diphtheria, pertussin, tetanus
DPW	Department of Public Welfare
DR	delivery room
	dressing room
dr	dram
drge	drainage
drsg	dressing
DS	dead air space
D/S	dextrose and saline
D.S.	discharge summary
	Down's syndrome
DSD	dry, sterile dressing
DSU	day surgery unit
DT	delirium tremens
DU	duodenal ulcer
DW	distilled water
D/W	dextrose in water
D5W	dextrose (5%) in water
Dx	diagnosis
dysp	dyspnea

EBL	estimated blood loss
ECF	extended care facility
ECG	electrocardiogram
	same as EKG
ED	emergency department
EDC	expected date of confinement
EEG	electroencephalogram
EENT	eyes, ears, nose, and throat
EKG	electrocardiograph
	same as ECG
elix	elixir
EMG	electromyogram
EMT	emergency medical technician
ENA	extractable nuclear antigen
enl	enlargement
EOM	extraocular movements
	extraocular muscles
EPC	electronic pain control
ER	emergency room
ES	electric stimulator
ESR	erythrocyte sedimentation rate
ESRD	end stage renal disease
et al	and others
etc	et cetera, and so forth
ETOH	ethanol, alcohol
EUA	examination under anesthesia
exc	excision
exp	explore
	expired
ext	extract
ext cat	extraction cataract
F	Fahrenheit
FB	fingerbreadth
	foreign body
FBS	fasting blood sugar
FDA	Food and Drug Administration
fdg	feeding
Fe	iron
$FeSO_4$	ferrous sulfate
FF	fat free
F.F. or f.f.	force fluids
FFP	fresh frozen plasma
FHT	fetal heart tone
FIO_2	fractional inspired oxygen
FLB	funny looking beat
fld	fluid
fl dr	fluid dram

fl ext	fluid extract
FLK	funny looking kid
fl oz	fluid ounce
FME	full mouth extraction
FMG	full mouth gingivectomy
Fr	French
frac	fracture
freq	frequent
FS	frozen section
FSH	follicle stimulating hormone
FSP	fibrin split products
FT	fingertip (dilation cervix)
FTT	failure to thrive
FTSG	full thickness skin graft
F5U	fluorouracil
FU	follow up
FUO	fever of undetermined origin
Fx	fracture
Ga	gallium
GA	gastric analysis
GB	gallbladder
GC	gonococcus
GE	gastroesophageal
GI	gastrointestinal
GLU	glucose
GM	grand mal
gm	gram
GNC	gram negative coccus
GPC	gram positive coccus
GPA	gravida, para, aborted
gr	grain
GRP	group
Grp A Strep	Group A Streptococcus
GSW	gunshot wound
GTT	glucose tolerance test
GU	genitourinary
GYN	gynecology
GNR	gram negative rod
GPR	gram positive rod
H or Ⓗ	hypodermic
H	hydrogen
h	hour
HA	headache
H&H	hematocrit and hemoglobin
H&P	history and physical

H BAg	hepatitis B antigen
Hb, Hgb	hemoglobin
HBP	high blood pressure
HCl	Hydrochloric acid
HCS	human chorionic somatotropin
Hct	hematocrit
HCVD	hypertensive cardiovascular disease
hd	hand
	hard
	head
HEP	heparin
Hg	mercury
Hgb, Hb	hemoglobin
5-HIAA	5 hydroxyindole acetic acid
HLR	heart-lung resuscitation
HNP	herniated nucleus pulposus
HOB	head of bed
H_2O	water
H_2O_2	hydrogen peroxide
/HPF	per high power field
HPL	human placental lactogen
HR	heart rate
hr	hour
hrt	heart
HS, hs	hour of sleep
HSG	hysterosalpingogram
HSV-2	herpes simplex virus-2
ht	height
Hx	history
Hyst	hysterectomy
I	iodine
IABP	intra-aortic balloon pump
I&D	incision and drainage
IBC	iron binding capacity
ICCE	intracapsular cataract extraction
ICU	Intensive Care Unit
ID	identification
IDK	internal derangement knee
IFA	indirect fluorescent antibody
Ig	immunoglobulin
IHD	ischemic heart disease
IM	internal medicine
	intramuscular
IMP	impaction wisdom teeth
	important
	impression
IMV	intermittent mandatory ventilation

ing	inguinal
INH	isoniazid
inj	inject
inorg	inorganic
in situ	in natural or normal position
INT	internal
I & O	intake and output
IPPB	intermittent positive pressure breathing
IR	immunoreactive
IRRG	irrigation
IS	incentive spirometer
isol	isolation
IT	inhalation therapy
ITP	idiopathic thrombocytopenic purpura
IU	intrauterine
IUCD	intrauterine contraceptive device
IUD	intrauterine death
	intrauterine device
IV	intravenous
IVC	intravenous cholangiogram
IVP	intravenous pyelogram
	intravenous push
IVPB	intravenous piggyback
IVU	intravenous urogram
jc	juice
JCAH	Joint Commission on Accreditation of Hospitals
JRA	juvenile rheumatoid arthritis
K	potassium
k	kilo (prefix for 1000)
kg	kilogram
KCL	potassium chloride
17-KGS	17-ketogenic steroids
KO	keep open, see also TKO, KVO
17-KS	17-ketosteroids
KUB	kidney, ureter, and bladder
KVO	keep vein open
L or l	left
	liter
LA	left atrium
Lab	laboratory
LAD	left anterior descending (coronary artery)
	left axis deviation
lam	laminectomy
LAO	left anterior angiogram

LAP	left atrial pressure
lap	laparotomy
lat	lateral
lat decub	lateral decubitus
lax	laxative
lb	pound
LBP	low back pain
LDH	lactate dehydrogenase
LE	left eye
	lupus erythematosus
Lf	limit fluids
LESS	laxative, enema, shower, shampoo
L & F	laminectomy and fusion
LHAD	left heart assist device
LIB	left in bottle
liq	liquid
LKS	liver, kidney, spleen
LLC	long leg cast
LLQ	left lower quadrant (of the abdomen)
L/M	liters per minute
LMP	last menstrual period
LOA	leave of absence
	left occipitoanterior
LOP	left occipitoposterior
LOT	left occipitotransverse
loz	lozenge
LP	lumbar puncture
LPN	licensed practical nurse
LR	lactated Ringer's
	labor room
L-S	lumbosacral
LSK	liver, spleen, kidneys
LTA	laryngotracheal aspirator
LUL	left upper lobe (lung)
LUQ	left upper quadrant (abdomen)
LV	left ventricle
LVH	left ventricular hypertrophy
L&W	living and well
lytes	electrolytes
M	male
	married
m	meter
	milli-
	minim
	murmur
μ	micron
	micro-

MAR	medicine administration record
max	maximum
mcg	microgram
MCH	mean corpuscular hemoglobin
	maternal and child health
MCHC	mean corpuscular hemoglobin concentration
MCL	midclavicular line
MCV	mean corpuscular volume
MD	doctor of medicine
med	medicine
mEq	milliequivalent
mEq/kg	milliequivalent per kilogram
Mg	magnesium
mgm, mg	milligram
MI	mitral insufficiency
	myocardial infarction
MIC	minimal inhibitory concentration
micro	microscopic
min	minim
	minute
ml	milliliter
ml/min	milliliter per minute
mm	millimeter
mod	moderate
MOM	milk of magnesia
MR	mitral regurgitation
MRX1	may repeat 1 time
MR if Nec	may repeat if necessary
MS	mitral stenosis
	morphine sulfate
	multiple sclerosis
	musculoskeletal
MT	membrane tympanum (ear drum)
M.T.E.	maximum therapeutic effort
MVA	motor vehicle accident
MVD	mitral valve disease
MVR	mitral valve replacement
mx	mixed
	mixture
	multiple
N	nausea
	nitrogen
Na	sodium
NA	nurse's aide
	nursing assistant
NAK	no allergies known
NB	newborn

NBN	newborn nursery
Nebs	nebulizer treatment
neg	negative
NG, N/G	nasogastric (tube)
NGU	non-gonorrheal urethritis
NH$_4$	ammonia
NIH	National Institute of Health
NKA	no known allergies
NM	neuromuscular
noc, noct	night
NP	neuropsychiatric
NPO	non per os
	nothing by mouth
NRBC	nucleated red blood cell
NS	neurosurgery, neurosurgeon
	normal saline
NSR	normal sinus rhythm
NSG	nursing
NSY	nursery
NTG	nitroglycerin
N&V	nausea and vomiting
O	oral
	objective
O$_2$	oxygen
OB	obstetrics
obst	obstruction
occ	occasional
OD	right eye
	overdose
od	every day, daily
17-OH	17-hydroxycorticosteroid
OHD	organic heart disease
oint	ointment
OOB	out of bed
ophth	ophthalmology
OR	operating room
	open reduction
ORIF	open reduction, internal fixation
Ortho	orthopedics
os	mouth
OS	left eye
Osmol	osmolarity, osmolality
OT	occupational therapy
OU	both eyes
oz	ounce
P	phosphorus
	pulse

	plan
p̄	after
PA	physician's assistant
	pulmonary artery
	pernicious anemia
	posterior anterior
P&A	percussion and auscultation
PAC	premature atrial contraction
PAP	pulmonary artery pressure
	Papanicolaou
PAT	paroxysmal atrial tachycardia
path	pathology
Pb	lead
pc	platelet concentrate
	after meals
PCN	penicillin
pCO₂	partial pressure of carbon dioxide
PCW	pulmonary capillary wedge
PDA	patent ductus arteriosus
P/D	postural drainage
PDR	Physicians' Desk Reference
PE	physical examination
	pulmonary embolus
Peds	pediatrics
PET	positron emission tomography
PEEP	positive end expiratory pressure
peri	perineum
PERLA	pupils equal, react to light and accommodation
PFT	pulmonary function test
Ph	phosphate
pH	denotes acidity and alkalinity
PH	past history
phos	phosphorus
PID	pelvic inflammatory disease
PIP	proximal interphalangeal joint
pit	pituitary
	pitocin
PJC	premature junctional contractions
PKU	phenylketonuria
PNC	premature nodal contraction
PND	postnasal drip
PO	phone order
	postoperative
PO, po	by mouth
PO₂	partial pressure of oxygen
POC	products of conception
pos	positive
POS	problem-oriented system

post	after
	posterior
post-op	postoperative
PPD	post partum day
	tuberculin skin test
PPF	protein plasma fraction
	partial plasma fraction
PR	public relations
pre-op	preoperative
prep	prepare
primip	primiparous
prn	when necessary
	as required
pro time	prothrombin time
PT	physical therapy
	prothrombin time
pt	patient
PTT	partial thromboplastin time
PTVP	permanent transvenous pacemaker
PVC	premature ventricular contraction
PW	puncture wound
Px	physical examination
	prognosis
PZI	protamine zinc insulin
q	each, every
qd	every day
qh	every hour
q2h	every two hours
q hs	every night at bedtime
QID, qid	four times a day
QNS	quantity not sufficient
qod	every other day
qoh	every other hour
qs	quantity sufficient
qt	quart
Quads	quadricep muscles
R	rectal
	respiration
	right
RA	rheumatoid arthritis
	right atrium
Ra	radium
RIA	radioimmunoassay
rad	radical
	right axis deviation

RBC	red blood cell
	red blood cell count
RAO	right anterior angiogram
RDS	respiratory distress syndrome
RDU	renal dialysis unit
re	regarding
reg	regular
REM	rapid eye movement
resp	respiration
Ret. Det.	retinal detachment
Revas	revascularization
Rh	Rhesus (blood factor)
RHD	rheumatic heart disease
RL	Ringer's lactate
RLL	right lower lobe (lung)
RLQ	right lower quadrant (abdomen)
RML	right middle lobe (lung)
Rn	radon
RN	registered nurse
RNA	ribonucleic acid
RO	routine order
R/O	rule out
ROA	right occipitoanterior
ROM	range of motion
	rupture of membranes
ROP	right occipitoposterior
ROS	review of systems
ROT	right occipitotransverse
RR	recovery room
RSR	right sinus rhythm
RTC	return to clinic
RT	respiratory therapy
RUL	right upper lobe (lung)
RUQ	right upper quadrant (abdomen)
RV	right ventricle
Rx	prescription
	therapy
	treatment
S	subjective
s	left
s̄	without
SA	surface area
	sinoatrial
S&A	sugar and acetone
SAC	short arm cast
	special acute care

Sat	saturate
SBE	subacute bacterial endocarditis
SC, sc	subcutaneous
SDH	subdural hematoma
SD plasma	single donor plasma
sec	second (time)
sed	sedative
seg	segmented
SGOT	serum glutamic oxalocetic acid transaminase
SGPT	serum glutamic pyruvic transaminase
SGA	small for gestational age
SL, sl	sublingual
sl	slight
SLE	systemic lupus erythematosus
SLWC	short leg walking cast
SM	simple mastectomy
	systolic murmur
SMA	sequential multiphasic analyzer
SMR	submucous resection
SNF	skilled nursing facility
SO	salpingo-oopherectomy
SOB	short of breath
sol, soln	solution
SOM	serous otitis media
SOS	if necessary
sp	spirits
SPA	salt poor albumin
SPP	suprapubic prostatectomy
spec	specific
	specimen
sp gr	specific gravity
SQ, sq	subcutaneous
SRD	side rails down
SRF	subretinal fluid
$\bar{s}\bar{s}$	one-half
SS	soapsuds
SSE	soapsuds enema
ST	supportive therapy
Staph	staphylococcus
STAT, stat	at once, immediately
Strep	Streptococcus
STS	serological test for syphilis
STSG	split thickness skin graft
subl, SL	sublingual
subq, SC, sc, SQ	subcutaneous
supp	suppository
surg	surgery
sx	symptoms

T	temperature
T$_3$	triiodothyronine
T$_4$	thyroxine
TAB	therapeutic abortion
T&A	tonsillectomy and adenoidectomy
tab	tablet
TAH	total abdominal hysterectomy
TB	tuberculosis
tb, tbsp	tablespoon
TBG	thyroxine binding globulin
TCDB	turn, cough, deep breathe
T-D&C	therapeutic dilatation and curettage
TENS	transcutaneous electrical nerve stimulator
temp	temperature
THRA	total hip replacement arthroplasty
TIA	transient ischemic attack
TIBC	total iron binding capacity
TID, tid	three times a day
TKO	to keep open
TKRA	total knee replacement arthroplasty
TL	team leader
	total lipids
	tubal ligation
TLC	tender loving care
TNTC	too numerous to count
Tol	tolerated
TO	telephone order
TP	total protein
TPC	total patient care
TPR	temperature, pulse, respiration
TPN	total parenteral nutrition
tr	tincture
	trace
trach	tracheotomy, tracheostomy
trans	transfer
TSH	thyroid stimulating hormone
tsp	teaspoon
TTVP	temporary transvenous pacemaker
TUR	transurethral resection
TURP	transurethral resection of prostate
TV	tidal volume
	total volume
TWE	tap water enema
Tx	treatment
	traction
T&X	type and crossmatch (blood)
U	unit

UA	urinalysis
UAD	usual adult dose
UDO	undertermined origin
UGI	upper gastrointestinal
ung	ointment
U/O	urine output
URI	upper respiratory infection
USN	ultrasonic nebulizer
UTI	urinary tract infection

V	vacuum
vag	vagina, vaginal
VAH	Veterans Administration Hospital
VCU	voiding cystourethrogram
vent	ventricle
VD	venereal disease
vd	void, voided
VDRL	Venereal Disease Research Laboratory
VF	ventricular fibrillation
	visual field
VH	vaginal hysterectomy
Vit	vitamin
VMA	vanillylmandelic acid
VN	vocational nurse
VO	verbal order
vol	volume
VS	vital signs
VSD	ventricular septal defect
VT	ventricular tachycardia
	tidal volume

W	water
	widow
	widower
WA	while awake
WBC	white blood cell
	white blood cell count
WC	wheelchair
	Workmen's Compensation
Wd	ward
	wound
w/d	well developed
wds	wounds
wk	week
w/n	well nourished
WNL	within normal limits
WP	wedge pressure

wt	weight
w/u	work-up
x̄	except
X	times
X-match	crossmatch (blood)
y/o	years old
Zn	zinc
ZnO_2	zinc oxide

SYMBOLS

ʒ	dram
ʒ̄	ounce
/	per
∅	none known
>	greater than
<	less than
□, ♂	male
o, ♀	female
↑	increase
↓	decrease
±	more or less
≯	not greater than
≮	not less than

Index